PRAISE FOR *PUSHED*

"Were there ever any doubts as to the personal being political, this former editor at *Ms.* and editor of the revised *Our Bodies, Ourselves* convincingly lays them to rest in a gripping exposé of American obstetrics. With extensive field research and thorough historical contextualization, Block reveals some disturbing statistics in this country's birth management and shows how medical views of birth are as subject to change as the whims of fashion. . . A provocative and hotly controversial analysis of a side of reproductive rights feminism seems to have forgot."

—*Kirkus Reviews*, starred review
(A "Best Books of 2007" Selection)

"Why are so many C-sections performed in the United States? How many, if any, birthing choices are dependent on liability issues or convenience? What are the possible consequences for low-risk mothers seeking a more natural birthing experience in their own home? Block asks all of these questions and answers with a stirring discussion of reproductive rights, informed consent, and the rights of the mother vs. the fetus."

—*Library Journal*

"This provocative, highly readable exposé raises questions of great consequence for anyone planning to have a baby in U.S., as well as those interested or involved in women's health care."

—PublishersWeekly.com

"Jennifer Block has provided us with a well-researched, comprehensive, and in-depth critique of American birthways, showing everything that doesn't work about the American approach to birth and the little that does. A must-read for anyone wishing to understand why practitioners and women know so little about the normal physiology of birth and thus accept so many unnecessary and harmful interventions as normal and appropriate. Engaging, compelling, and insightful, this book draws

Pushed

The Painful Truth about Childbirth and Modern Maternity Care

Jennifer Block

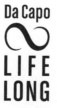

Da Capo

LIFE LONG

A Member of the Perseus Books Group

Many of the designations used by manufacturers and sellers to distinguish their products are claimed as trademarks. Where those designations appear in this book and Da Capo Press was aware of a trademark claim, those designations have been printed with initial capital letters.

Copyright 2007 © by Jennifer Block

Text design by Viewtistic, Inc.
Set in 11 point Adobe Caslon

Cataloging-in-Publication data for this book is available from the Library of Congress.

Da Capo Press
A Member of the Perseus Books Group
www.dacapopress.com

First Da Capo Press edition 2007
First Da Capo Press paperback edition 2008
HC: 978-0-7382-1073-5
PB: 978-0-7382-1166-4

Da Capo Press books are available at special discounts for bulk purchases in the United States by corporations, institutions, and other organizations. For more information, please contact the Special Markets Department at the Perseus Books Group, 2300 Chestnut Street, Suite 200, Philadelphia, PA 19103, or call (800) 255-1514, or e-mail special.markets@perseusbooks.com.

1 2 3 4 5 6 7 8 9

To my mother

Contents

Acknowledgments

This book would not have been born without the interest, passion, prodding, help, and influence of so many: Gloria Jacobs, Marcia Ann Gillespie, and the former editors of *Ms.* who mentored me; Geoffrey Cowley, who generously offered early thoughts and support; Laureen Connelly Rowland, who set me on the path to publishing; and Laura Conaway at the *Village Voice*, who taught me to "just tell the story," and who believed that *this* story was big enough to tell in a book.

In my travels from El Paso to Milwaukee to Richmond I've slept on many a guest bed, shared many a meal, and enjoyed many a conversation—I am grateful for them all. To the many women who revealed details intimate, humiliating, painful, and ecstatic; to the labor and delivery ward at St. Barnabas; to the midwives at Maternidad la Luz; to "Linda" and her clients for welcoming me and my notebook into their lives; to Cynthia for telling her story; and to all the providers, researchers, thinkers, and doers who answered questions large and small: thank you.

My agent Elizabeth Kaplan believed in this book from the start and imbued it with a sense of confidence and importance; my editor Marnie Cochran has been a limitless source of positivity and enthusiasm, and allowed me a wide berth in which to create. Lesley Rock Grisonich and the production staff were extraordinarily patient.

I owe thanks to the staff of the New York Academy of Medicine library; to Ashley Eldridge and Jaclyn Paris for their research assistance; to Laurel Maury, who generously read this manuscript page by page, with pencil in hand; to Virginia Vitzthum, for her constant support and sharp last-minute edits; and to Karen Rose, for her gusto and humor, and for calmly and expertly taking on the monumental task of fact-checking this book (though any mistakes are mine entirely).

I also must mention Janis Brody, Lisa Selin Davis, Trish Hickey, Jared Kelly, Pagan Kennedy, Phoebe Reilly, Tanya Stotsky, and Joanna Wheeler. Gabriel Willow patiently and lovingly made this work possible in so many ways. I also owe thanks to my family, in particular my aunt Audrey Block-Shnall, who gave me some ideas when she cut her own umbilical cord in 1992; my grandparents, all of whom I've been so blessed to know and love; my brother Adam and sister Steffany, for remembering to smile; my father Leonard Block; and my mother, Roberta Block, who wasn't sure I would make it out of the womb, but hasn't once doubted me since.

Preface to the Paperback Edition

The title of this book emerged long before the book itself. It seemed to encompass, in a monosyllable, everything I was learning about the typical American birth experience. Women were telling me (and still do) that they had entered their pregnancy wanting what was best for themselves and their babies. Most women would tell me they were just hoping for a *normal* birth—without much intervention, maybe without drugs if they could do it, and without surgery if at all possible. But women were also telling me they'd felt tremendous pressure from their medical providers to go against instinct and research—to induce labor, to schedule a cesarean, to lie back during labor when every cell in their body felt like moving. Women are supposed to *push* their babies out; instead, they felt they were being *pushed* around.

What I didn't realize in the beginning is that virtually everyone involved in maternity care is also on the receiving end of this pushing— the hospital, the doctor, the nurse, the midwife, the doula—all are caught in a system that discourages, to some degree, their providing optimal care. Obstetricians are pushed to intervene before it is necessary and with more

Introduction

On November 9, 1965, the United States Patent Office granted George Blonsky, a retired mining engineer, and his wife Charlotte, a former medical student, patent number 3,216,423 for their "Apparatus For Facilitating The Birth Of A Child by Centrifugal Force," or, simply, "The Blonsky." Specifications for the floor-to-ceiling contraption were precise: The Blonsky was to be constructed of heavy cast iron and aluminum, mounted on poured concrete, and surrounded by a circular "fence." The patient would be strapped horizontally along the radius of a circular platform and spun, like a merry-go-round, generating a force of up to seven G's (seven times the force of gravity). Perhaps best described as an amusement park ride based on a medieval torture device built like a NASA space-flight simulator, the machine was intended to create sufficient pull "to push aside the constricting vaginal walls, to overcome the friction of the uteral and vaginal surfaces and to counteract the atmospheric pressure opposing the emergence of the child," wrote the Blonskys. The baby, sucked out by a hyper-vacuum, would land in a basket built of a "strong, elastic material and supported under tension by tail ropes," lined with cotton padding. The physician, essentially reduced to ride operator, need employ an emergency brake only if the force of the ejected child failed to trigger an automatic shut-off mechanism.

Both inventors passed away, childless, before the turn of the millennium. Surviving cousin Gale Sturtevant and her husband Don, who were college students when the Blonsky was designed, attribute the apparatus to "Uncle George" and "Aunt Lotte's" fascination with a laboring elephant at the Bronx zoo: they spoke of the animal spinning around in a circle as it gave birth. In the elaborate eight-page patent application,[1] however, the couple mention nothing of the zoo, instead postulating that although "primitive" women have musculature suited to the task of childbirth, "civilized" women do not, and thus their machine would "assist the under-equipped woman by creating a gentle, evenly distributed, properly directed, precision-controlled force."

In 1965, civilized women weren't thought to be suited for much—not sport, industry, science, art, or home ownership. Having babies and raising them was firmly within their sphere, but statements about the modern woman's inability to give birth persisted in the medical literature and in the delivery room. There, women were typically strapped flat on their backs, wrists secured in leather straps and legs up in stirrups (pelvises tipped against gravity), and dosed with Demerol, or morphine and scopolamine, an amnesiac, to initiate "twilight sleep." While they were under, forceps (curved metal tongs), in combination with episiotomy (a cut to the vaginal opening), were frequently used to extract the infant. One can't blame the Blonskys for dreaming up a less invasive way.

The machine, never built, was of course clinically preposterous—astronauts experience only three G's upon liftoff and must wear special "G-suits" so as not to black out. In 1999, the Blonsky was rescued from patent lore and awarded an "Ig Nobel Prize" by the science humor magazine *Annals of Improbable Research (AIR)*. The Blonsky headlined the awards ceremony at Harvard University with a theatrical performance involving a spinning table, a doll, and an OB/GYN wearing a catcher's mitt. The "Igs" that year were specifically awarded for inventions that "cannot or should not be reproduced." The Ig category for the Blonsky was "Managed Health Care."

Normal, spontaneous childbirth is an automatic sequence, a series of internal and external movements, voluntary and involuntary, that a woman's body makes in order to have a baby. The pituitary gland releases the hormone oxytocin, which causes the smooth muscle lining of the uterus to contract rhythmically, and those contractions gradually accelerate and intensify. The lower portion of the uterus, the cervix (Latin for "neck") softens and opens into the vagina; the pelvic joints and ligaments become pliant; the amniotic sac—the membrane that surrounds the fetus and fluid—ruptures. The baby descends into the pelvis and through the dilated cervix, and, with the aid of muscular efforts, bodily movement, and the stretching of the pelvic anatomy, is expelled from womb to world.

This physiological sequence continues after the birth as well. The uterus contracts further; the remaining blood flows from the placenta to the fetus through the umbilical cord; the placenta detaches and is expelled. Still more contractions follow, which retract and repair the extensive network of uterine blood vessels left enlarged and exposed by the shorn placenta. The breasts, meanwhile, produce colostrum—highly concentrated breast milk—in the mammary glands. Both magnificently dynamic and somewhat predictable, the duration of each stage of the birth process, and even to some extent the order in which they occur, vary from woman to woman and birth to birth.

But very few women in the United States experience this physiological sequence. The strap-in, switch-on Blonsky method may seem comical today, but most American women give birth wired to a rig of machines.

Walk into any freshly occupied U.S. hospital "LDRP" room—it stands for labor, delivery, recovery, and postpartum—and you will find the expectant patient lying in a recumbent position on an obstetric bed. One of her arms is connected, by thin tubing that extends from a vein on the back of her hand, to a plastic IV bag suspended above her head; the other is probably wrapped at the bicep with a nylon and Velcro blood pressure cuff that automatically contracts every ten minutes or so. A finger might be ensconced in similar material, measuring her pulse and blood oxygen levels. An elastic band tethers her belly to an electronic fetal monitor, a machine that rhythmically prints out a paper trail of fetal heartbeats like an accountant's register and displays the reading on a flat-screen monitor mounted at the bedside. She's likely to have several other appendages as well: an epidural catheter extending into the space between her vertebrae and spinal cord, a Foley catheter threaded into her urinary tract, an intrauterine pressure catheter inserted through her cervix and into the uterus, and circulation stockings on her legs. At any one time, she might have five or more drugs pulsing through the IV line. Altogether, she may have up to 16 different tubes, drugs, or attachments.[2]

Each of these devices performs a separate function. Through the IV, doctors can deliver fluids, sleep aids, narcotics, antibiotics, blood anticoagulants, or acid-reflux drugs. They can also speed up and strengthen contractions with the drug Pitocin, a synthetic version of the hormone oxytocin. To make sure the artificial contractions don't come too fast or too hard, which could deprive the baby of oxygen, the electronic fetal monitor assesses the duration of each contraction and the fetal heart rate, and alerts staff if that rate is "nonreassuring." The intrauterine pressure catheter gauges the power of each contraction, determining whether the level of Pitocin is adequate. The continuous drip, into the epidural, of paralyzing agent combined with a narcotic blocks the pain caused by contractions and weakens sensation and motor control, which is why the urinary catheter is needed. The circulation stockings counter the effects of immobilization, which can lead to blood clots. The other devices record vital signs, ensure that fluid levels are adequate, and check that infection is not present. Recently approved by the FDA, another device (bringing the total to 17) may become a common feature of maternity care: two electrodes planted inside the vagina on either side of the cervical opening to continually measure dilation and alert staff when a woman is "complete," at 10 centimeters.

American women are aggressively monitored, screened, and tested throughout pregnancy and childbirth. Labor is often started artificially or accelerated with drugs and instruments: well over half of labors are chemically induced or augmented with synthetic oxytocin, and two-thirds of women have their water broken manually.[3] Just as few modern American labors begin on their own or progress on their own time, most do not conclude on their own, either. In 2005, 30.2% of U.S. women gave birth by cesarean section,[4] and of those giving birth vaginally, one-third had an episiotomy, a surgical incision to widen the vaginal opening.[5] About half of all C-sections are scheduled prior to the due date, avoiding the labor sequence altogether.[6]

Even though the United States has the most intense and widespread medical management of birth—99% of women give birth in a hospital—

we rank near the bottom among industrialized countries in maternal and infant mortality. In spite of our vigilance, preterm births are on the rise,[7] cerebral palsy—thought to be caused by fetal distress—rates have remained stagnant,[8] and in 2002, infant mortality rose for the first time since 1958.[9] According to the World Health Organization, we rank second to last among 33 industrialized countries in this regard[10] and 30th for maternal mortality.[11] Although we are superior in saving the lives of infants born severely premature, women are 70% more likely to die in childbirth in the United States than in Europe.[12] Black women are four times more likely to die than white women.[13]

In the countries with the best maternal and infant outcomes—the Netherlands, Sweden, and Denmark—women and babies benefit from lifelong universal healthcare, but that care is markedly different: obstetricians attend only high-risk pregnancies. The vast majority of laboring women get individual support from a midwife, are free to move about and birth in whatever position feels best, and are rarely induced, anesthetized, or cut. These countries have between a 14% and an 18% cesarean rate,[14] and in the Netherlands some 20% to 30% of births happen at home with virtually no medical intervention at all.[15] Their approach, opposite to that of the United States, is to support physiological birth, allowing labor to begin and progress in its own time, and intervening only when necessary.

Are U.S. women less capable of giving birth than their Scandinavian sisters? Is technology being overused at the expense of women and babies? As one leading obstetrician put it to the *New York Times* in 1989, when one-quarter of U.S. women were undergoing cesareans, "I can't believe that 25 out of 100 women cannot deliver a baby normally."[16] I've undertaken this investigation because I can't believe it either.

Karen Wacker is a postpartum nurse at Winthrop Hospital on Long Island, New York. She's been caring for women and babies for 23 years. Cesareans, she's noticed, have been steadily on the rise. One summer day in 2006, she scanned the 33-bed ward and counted 28 patients recovering from C-sections. "When moms have C-sections, they tie up our beds," Wacker told me. "When we're full, we send moms to the high-risk ward. When high-risk fills up, moms have to stay on the labor floor. Overflow happens all the time."

Winthrop reported a cesarean rate of 41% in 2004. In the New York metro area, several hospitals report rates of between 30% and 45%.[17] Rates vary around the country. The average in Broward County, Florida, is 39%;[18] in King County, Washington State, it is 30%,[19] and in Brattleboro, Vermont, it is 26%.[20] The vast range among comparable populations tells us that much of what dictates care is, in effect, local fashion, not medical necessity. Meanwhile, cesarean section has been the most common major surgery performed in the United States for 26 years running. (Hysterectomy—removal of the uterus—ranks a close second).[21]

Winthrop Hospital, it should be noted, was once at the vanguard of another trend, that of "natural childbirth." In the 1980s the hospital installed jacuzzis in every birthing suite and boasted the then-radical "rooming in" option, in which babies could stay with their mothers rather than in the nursery. Today the tubs are rarely used, and to "room in," women have to forgo visitors and pay out of pocket for a private room. The nurse manager says that the trend is toward more cesareans. "Physicians are moving away from vaginal birth."

I've talked to many birth practitioners who have said the same, that surgical birth is en vogue. "Cut 'em out, cut 'em out, cut 'em out," said one obstetrician. "You laugh, but that's what we're coming to." In Champaign, Illinois, which has a C-section rate 15 points lower than on Long Island, I met a nurse-midwife who predicts that in 20 years, all women will give birth by cesarean. He (yes, he) also wasn't laughing. In the summer of 2006, Dr. Kenneth Trofatter, a perinatologist in Greenville, South Carolina, told a local paper that the cesarean rate is "not going to get any better . . . I really do envision a time when all patients deliver by C-section."[22] Others have suggested in peer-reviewed journals that this might actually be advisable.[23]

The current media buzz is over a woman's "right to choose" an elective cesarean. At the same time, however, there are actually limits on a woman's right to choose a normal birth. The LDRP "attachments" are often mandatory in hospitals. Due dates are increasingly tantamount to deadlines. Women who've had a previous cesarean, for instance, are in many cases being denied vaginal birth altogether. In the hope of achieving a normal birth, women with means are paying as much as $2000 out of pocket for a private *doula* who will accompany them to the hospital for patient advocacy as much as labor support. A 2004 publication called

What Every Pregnant Woman Needs to Know About Cesarean Section points out, "As cesarean rates continue to rise, it may be much harder to reach a goal of avoiding a cesarean than [of] having one."[24]

The old debate over "natural childbirth" seems quaint at this point. I don't have much use for the term, which has become synonymous with vaginal birth. What's happened to normal birth—what *is* normal birth? Not simply nonsurgical birth. (Imagine the Blonsky in every hospital and pregnant women waiting in line as though for a ride at Six Flags!) Not simply unmedicated, either. It is natural, after all, to want to alleviate pain. The term I find most useful to describe normal birth is *physiological* birth: labor begins and progresses spontaneously, the woman is free to move about for the duration, and she pushes in advantageous, intuitive positions.

We know that if we take our otherwise healthy patient in LDRP, release her cuffs and bands, unplug the probes and sensors, and turn off the Pitocin and morphine, 9 times out of 10 her body will birth a baby with minimal interference or injury, especially if she has the one-on-one support of a skilled caregiver. We know this from the experience of other countries, but also from studies of American women who choose to birth with certified midwives in birthing centers or in their own homes. The most recent study, of 5000 low-risk women who had planned home births, found home to be just as safe as the hospital. Only 3.7% of these women underwent cesareans, 2.7% received Pitocin, and 2.1% got episiotomies. Low-risk women giving birth in hospitals have far higher rates of intervention and surgery, yet the same number of neonatal deaths.[25] Indeed, the World Health Organization concludes that "Midwives are the most appropriate primary health care provider to be assigned to the care of normal birth."[26] In 2006, the British health secretary announced plans to encourage all UK women to consider giving birth at home. "The Government is planning a 'strategic shift' in childbirth policy away from hospital delivery," reported the London *Independent*, to "challenge the assumption that births should take place in hospitals."[27]

Christiane Northrup, MD, obstetrician-gynecologist and author of the best-selling *Women's Bodies, Women's Wisdom*, surprised a New York audience when she said that she'd told her own daughters that they should not give birth in a hospital. "For well-nourished women," she said, "the safest place is home."[28]

For women who want to avoid the hospital, however, the alternatives can be hard to come by, unaffordable, and even illegal. Birthing centers are few and are buckling under malpractice insurance, and hospitals have disbanded nurse-midwifery practices across the country. Health insurers and Medicaid often refuse to cover midwives, and in many states, certified professional midwives can't be licensed and are legally prohibited from attending home births. Experienced midwives may even be subject to criminal investigation, prosecution, and jail. In some places, women who want a home birth must go underground to hire a midwife. And as they give birth, these mothers are accomplices to a felony. Since when is normal birth a crime?

In 1975, Suzanne Arms published *Immaculate Deception*. The book was a *New York Times* bestseller and Book of the Year. Her groundbreaking exposé reported how women in childbirth were routinely separated from their partners, physically restrained at the wrists and ankles, lowered into the stirruped lithotomy position, administered drugs without their consent, given episiotomies without their consent, discouraged from breastfeeding, and denied their babies following delivery.

At the time of that book's publication, most obstetric practices hadn't been studied rigorously, if at all. Today we know better, yet much of Arms's critique still stands. Leather restraints, and even stirrups, are delivery room relics, but I've heard women say things like "You're pretty much tied to bed," "You're pinned down," and "You won't be allowed to move around." I've heard from women who were given episiotomies without their consent, and sometimes despite their express refusal. And I've heard from women with previous cesarean scars who are being given no choice but a repeat cesarean.

Arms published *Immaculate Deception* when *Roe v. Wade* was still news; today we can evaluate maternity care in terms of reproductive rights. Do women have the right to give birth with whom, where, and in the manner in which they choose? And if so, is that right being upheld?

In Arms's day, women suffered physically—60% to 90% of women giving birth got episiotomies[29]—but the effects were also psychological and emotional, and they translated into social change. The fallout was the natural childbirth movement and significant changes in hospital protocol. Men were allowed in, babies were allowed to stay in rooms, lactation consultants materialized, and episiotomy rates declined. But in 1975, the cesarean rate was less than 15%,[30] the threshold at which the World Health Organization has documented that the risks of surgery begin to outweigh the benefits.[31] Today, we need to consider the consequences of 1.2 million cesarean sections each year. A woman is four times more likely to die having a cesarean section than a vaginal birth.[32] Some physician researchers fear we will soon see a rise in maternal mortality as a result.

Today, what's normal is being redefined: from vaginal birth to surgical birth; from "My water broke," to "Let's break your water;" from "It's time" to "It's time for the induction." As medical anthropologist Robbie Davis-Floyd writes, "in the early twenty-first century, we do not know what normal birth is."[33] Most practicing obstetricians have never witnessed an unplugged birth that wasn't an accident. Women are even beginning to deny normal birth to themselves: if "normal" means being induced, immobilized by wires and tubes, sped up with drugs, all the while knowing that there's a good chance of surgery, well, might as well just cut to the chase, so to speak. "Just give me a cesarean," some are saying. And who can blame them? They want to avoid what they think of as normal birth.

It turns out that the elephant the Blonksys saw chasing its tail at the Bronx zoo was not acting as elephants normally do in labor. In the herd, an elephant labors and gives birth surrounded by other females. They gather—in a circle—and maintain that sphere until the new calf is born. The elephant at the Bronx zoo was simply making do.

CHAPTER 1

Arranged Birth

HURRICANE CHARLEY WAS NOT SUPPOSED to hit Florida Hospital Heartland Medical Center. Tracy Lethbridge, a labor and delivery nurse there at the time, remembers asking her boss early on Friday, August 13, 2004, whether the hospital would call a "code orange" to bring in extra staff, discharge noncritical patients, and shoo all guests and visitors home. It wouldn't. Highlands County and its county seat Sebring, where the hospital is situated, had always been considered a safe haven, and meteorologists expected the storm to hug the West Coast and move north toward Tampa.

Charley made landfall at Port Charlotte, 80 miles to the southwest of Sebring that afternoon with winds of 150 miles per hour. Confounding predictions, the storm took a sudden northeast tack, heading toward Orlando, where tourists were lined up under hotel porticoes videotaping nature's distinctly Floridian performance. Lethbridge remembers the storm pounding 70–80-mph winds and rain on the hospital's windows and roof at about 6:00 p.m. She and her colleagues shuttled postpartum patients from their windowed birthing suites to a central storage area they'd cleared out, just in case. "There were two fresh deliveries," Lethbridge remembers. She was able to usher one new mother into the safe room; the other, still waiting to regain motor function after an epidural, stayed on a gurney in the hallway. A few miles to the south the town's radio tower fell. In Bartow, to the north, a 50-foot deep sinkhole swallowed a car whole. The winds brought down several power lines, knocking out electricity across three counties.[1]

Hunkering down that evening was a minor interference compared to the week that followed. The hospital's emergency generator kicked in, but, like the rest of the town, the facility lost main power until the following Friday. With only enough generator capacity to run essential functions, there was no air-conditioning and no lab capabilities. That meant that the 13-bed labor and delivery ward wasn't a very comfortable place to either labor or deliver, nor did it have the lab setup required to manage epidural anesthesia safely. Lethbridge and her colleagues had to treat their patients much differently.

"We canceled all labor inductions," recalls Lethbridge. Normally, two beds a day would have been reserved for inducing women into labor, an often lengthy process that begins with drugs that "ripen" and dilate the cervix (Cervidil or Cytotec) and contract the uterus (Pitocin). Normally, even women who arrived in early labor—when the cervix is minimally dilated and contractions are several minutes apart—would often be encouraged to stay and would be administered Pitocin to hasten contractions. Lethbridge observed that under normal circumstances, the vast majority of babies were delivered during the day. But without the impetus to free beds for scheduled inductions, and because it made no sense to admit women in early labor to sweat in the steamy ward, the L&D staff became more selective. "We admitted only women who were in active labor—regular contractions and progressive cervical dilation," says Lethbridge. "If they were not in active labor, we'd send them back home."

Working just a few days in this altered universe, the nurses began to notice some marked changes. "Women were delivering within hours of arriving, even first-time mothers, without any Pitocin," says Lethbridge. She recorded other anomalous phenomena—she was studying for her master's degree at the time and was so struck by Charley's unexpected impact that she planned to write her thesis on it. "We had no cases of fetal distress during labor and no respiratory distress of neonates following delivery," she wrote in an e-mail shortly after the hurricane. "We had an incredibly low cesarean rate. Amazingly, the babies were about evenly distributed between day and night shifts."

In 2004, Florida Hospital delivered 951 babies, 29.4% by cesarean section.[2] With two labor inductions per weekday—about 40 a month, or nearly 500 a year—induced labor would have accounted for about half of all births. Under Charley's spell, between September 13 and September 20, seventeen women gave birth: one was induced, two had scheduled repeat cesareans, and just one had a cesarean for "failure to progress." That works out to a cesarean rate of 17%; excluding the repeat cesareans, it was 6%.

Lethbridge's observation about nine-to-five births is backed by national data: in 2004, the most recent year for which data are available, an average of 11,235 infants were born per day. But they were much more likely to be born Monday through Friday. During the week, about 12,000 babies were born per day; on Saturdays and Sundays, the tally dropped to about 8,000. (The most popular day to be born was Tuesday, at 13,045.)[3] The Centers for Disease Control and Prevention (CDC) calls this a "weekend birth deficit."[4] At Florida Hospital during the week following Charley, however, "women were coming in at night and delivering," says Lethbridge. "What happened was, women were going into labor all on their own, having good labor courses, and delivering healthy babies. Even the women who were scheduled to be induced that week, three-quarters of them came in and delivered anyway. And basically, they did better than if they had been induced. We thought, wow, this is amazing!"

Hurricane Charley was not only unexpected, it was statistically improbable: only 22 hours before Charley touched down, Bonnie had struck northwestern Florida, making Friday, August 13, the first recorded instance in which two major storms struck the same state in the same day. In maternity terms, Charley was a surprise twin. And it was as if the eye of this strange, errant hurricane had settled over Florida Hospital for the next week, buffering it from the normal pushes and pulls of labor management; as if the swirling weather overhead had somehow turned back the clock to a less rushed, less regimented, less technologically driven era. Charley provided a window into normal, physiological birth.

At the time, Lethbridge had been a nurse for 8 years, in labor and delivery for 4 years. The following year, she quit. Several things were bothering her. Safety protocols seemed to have no bearing on actual practice; she saw too many women induced or wheeled to the operating room, she felt, because the floor needed a bed free or because the physician had to be somewhere; and she blamed the hospital's concern over the bottom line for supplying the ward with too few nurses, which hampered their ability to give quality care. "We were not delivering care the way we should have," says Lethbridge. "I guess what it comes down to is you wake up in the middle of the night—at 3 a.m., after you've fallen asleep at midnight so you can wake up at 5 o'clock to leave the house at 10 after 6 to get to work on time for the 7 o'clock shift. You wake up with your heart pounding because you can't remember if you told the incoming shift what kind of pain medication you gave somebody; you can't remember whether you charted a monitor reading properly. You spend a lot of money on Imodium A-D."

Lethbridge finally expressed her views to management—and was told she could look for new work if she wasn't happy. But it was the hurricane, she says, that stopped her from going back to L&D altogether. "I remember thinking at the time, this is the way birth is supposed to be," she tells me, "let your body do what it needs to do, allow your body to take its own time." At Florida Hospital, at least, this approach was incompatible with the clinical setting. "Once you hit the hospital, a time clock begins ticking. I have only so many beds available," Lethbridge explains. Physicians would routinely rupture waters artificially and order Pitocin to achieve a birth by day's end, she says. During the hurricane, they left those amniotic sacs intact and sent the women back home. "And I don't think any of the patients were at all unhappy about going into labor on their own," adds Lethbridge. "Nobody complained that by gosh they wanted Pitocin." Nor did anybody complain about being told to spend early labor at home. "In all honesty, you're probably better off at home," says Lethbridge. "You'll be more relaxed, you can eat, you can shower, you can walk around. If you stay in the hospital, you're going to be locked down in a bed."

When the nurses reviewed the records the week following Charley, they felt they had proof to back up their concerns. "We went to our nurse manager and said, 'Look! This primip [first-time mother] came in at 4 o'clock and gave birth at 8!' But she was just as powerless as we were."

Within the next year, four out of the five nurses on Lethbridge's team left Florida Hospital.

YOU'RE GOING TO MEET YOUR BABY TODAY!

A woman in her last month of pregnancy is experiencing random uterine contractions, and her cervix is fading throughout. It is a slow and erratic dance at first; labor is when the dance acquires a rhythm, then a crescendo, leading to a climax.

Hospitals are accustomed to ordering chaos—the lacerated, broken, gasping trauma patient is wheeled into the ER, where staff swiftly open the airway, stop the bleeding, and set the bone. They stabilize. Childbirth, on the other hand, is chaos that the body can resolve itself. If everything goes normally, order will come—a baby will be born, creation will trump destruction. The birth attendant can help support the maternal body's own resolution, or the birth attendant can manage and control the process with modern means. Support versus stabilize.

In the vast majority of U.S. hospitals today, birth is stabilized. And the ability to stabilize, to bring the chaos of labor under control, is a relatively recent development in human history made possible by synthetic oxytocin, brand name Pitocin. Not unlike the Blonsky, the machine that would do for the body what the body could do on its own, Pitocin is used to replicate or accelerate the body's own childbirth sequence. The synthetic hormone is controlled via a computerized drip, which can be programmed to release the drug in precise increments directly into the bloodstream via the IV. Contractions can be turned up or down by the nurse or doctor like the volume on a stereo.

According to the CDC, induction of labor has risen sharply over the past 15 years, from 9.5% in 1990 to 21.2% in 2004.[5] But "these numbers are believed to be underreported," cautions Joyce A. Martin of the National Center for Health Statistics, which compiles the data. Independent studies and expert opinion strongly suggest that a solid majority of women in the United States are receiving synthetic oxytocin sometime during childbirth to either induce labor or "augment" it. A 2006 study in the *New England Journal of Medicine* of 5500 low-risk, first-time mothers at large teaching hospitals reported that among the sample, 40% of the women were induced into labor and 70% reccived Pitocin at some point during labor.[6]

In 2002 and again in 2005, the patient advocacy and research organization Childbirth Connection hired the polling firm Harris Interactive to survey more than 3000 recently pregnant women across the country. The *Listening to Mothers* surveys, as they are called, found that the induction rate is more than twice what the CDC reports: providers tried to induce labor in four out of ten women surveyed. Among the women surveyed in 2005, 65% were given amniotomies, the procedure in which the provider manually breaks the water; half reported that their labors were sped up with synthetic oxytocin. The women surveyed were considered "low-risk," a mix of first-time mothers and women who had given birth before.[7]

Such reports suggest that Florida Hospital is not unlike most hospitals in the United States, that nearly half of labors today begin artificially with a combination of synthetic hormones and deliberate rupture of the amniotic sac, and that even women for whom labor begins spontaneously often get Pitocin to speed things up. In posh Livingston, New Jersey, physicians say that virtually all of their patients receive Pitocin to either induce or augment labor. "Once you're admitted, my feeling is that we should be advancing our cause," one physician there told me. In inner-city Chicago, a nurse reports that most of her patients are induced. A physician in Champaign, Illinois, reports a 31% induction rate and a 34% augmentation rate in 2005. In Keene, New Hampshire, a nurse estimates that half her patients are induced. In Highlands County, Florida, Tracy Lethbridge says induction is "the norm, not the exception." Atlanta obstetrician Michael Randell, MD claims he induces labor in 90% of his patients. "We live in a Palm Pilot society. Everything is planned," he told the Associated Press.[8] Induction is even a commodity: Adeza Biomedical, a California-based company, is seeking FDA approval for a diagnostic test that will *predict* a woman's induceability.

Are women, for whatever reason, not going into labor on their own and not progressing fast enough? Or is it our American tendency to favor speed, control, and technology that has led us to what Robbie Davis-Floyd calls this "technocratic" model of birth?[9]

- In 2002, Michelle McSweeney was induced before labor in New York City. The birth of her daughter began and ended not with her body's own execution of the childbirth sequence, but rather with a series of drugs, instruments, and machines. She was called in to OB triage on a Sunday afternoon for what she thought was an ultrasound check, when a nurse pulled back the curtain and told her, "You're going to meet your baby today!" The nurse had spoken to McSweeney's obstetrician, who prescribed an induction over the phone.

  McSweeney was admitted, and a resident inserted Cervidil, a prostaglandin suppository that looks like a flat tampon, into her vagina. Nurses started an IV in her arm and strapped an electronic fetal monitor around her belly. After a few hours McSweeney was given a sleep aid and told to rest. At 8 a.m. her doctor arrived, did a vaginal exam, and then inserted a crotchet-hook-like instrument through her cervix, puncturing the amniotic sac. She ordered an IV infusion of Pitocin. At that point McSweeney agreed to an epidural, a catheter inserted into a space between her vertebrae and spinal cord, which would deliver a continuous flow of anesthetic and narcotic, blocking pain sensation from the waist down. Following that, a nurse inserted an intrauterine pressure catheter and a urine catheter, because McSweeney would no longer be able to feel the urge to urinate or walk to the bathroom. An automatic blood pressure cuff was fitted around her bicep and a pulse oximeter around her finger. Eighteen hours later, the induction unsuccessful, McSweeney was wheeled into the operating room, and the obstetrician surgically removed her baby via cesarean section.

- Candice Hilton, in Jackson, Mississippi, was scheduled for an induction in October 2000. Upon her admission to the hospital, staff broke her water, started an IV, strapped her to a fetal monitor, and administered Pitocin. She coped with the pain for 3 hours and then asked for an epidural; soon after that, a nurse inserted a urinary catheter. Within a few hours Hilton was fully dilated and told to start pushing. Hilton pushed for 2 hours, lying flat on her back. As the baby's head emerged, a nurse threw her weight on Hilton's abdomen—this is known as applying fundal pressure—and the obstetrician cut an episiotomy.

- Renee Johnson, in Richmond, Virginia, got up to pee at about 3 a.m. on January 16, 2004. After a few trips to the bathroom she realized it was amniotic fluid—her water had broken—and she called her physician. "She said, 'Hurry up and come over to the hospital,'" says Johnson. There, Johnson was told she had dilated 2 centimeters. She was admitted, hooked up to a fetal monitor and a blood pressure cuff, and an IV was inserted into her arm. At 9 a.m. Johnson's doctor examined her: 4 centimeters. "She said, 'You know you're not dilating as quickly as I thought you would, so we're going to give you something to help,'" Johnson recalls. Two hours later, she was pushing her baby out.

Neither Johnson, Hilton, nor McSweeney was considered "high-risk" and all three women intended to go into labor naturally and give birth with minimal intervention. Why did their doctors not allow labor to start or progress on its own?

Gary Hankins, MD, professor and vice chair of obstetrics and gynecology at the University of Texas Medical Branch at Galveston and chair of the obstetric practice committee of the American College of Obstetricians and Gynecologists (ACOG), says nobody should be doing inductions without a good reason. "That's not good medicine." Although ACOG does condone inductions for "psychosocial" or "logistic" reasons,[10] Hankins says he personally never induces for convenience. "An induction absent a solid indication absolutely increases all risk to mom and baby," he says. Laura Riley, MD, medical director of labor and delivery at Massachusetts General Hospital and Hankins's predecessor as chair of the ACOG practice committee, which releases guidelines on such practices, agrees. "Ideally you wait for natural labor," she told me. "Just by the mere fact of induction, you've now intervened in a pregnancy that otherwise would have continued, and you've already increased the risk of a C-section."

Hospital staff did not tell McSweeney about any risks, but they gave her three ostensibly medical reasons for the intervention: she was 11 days past her due date, her baby was "measuring big," and her amniotic fluid looked low. The reason given to Hilton was that she was overdue. The reason for Johnson's Pitocin was that her water had broken, and the baby was at risk for infection.

These justifications are common, but all are controversial. Inducing labor for a baby that looks large, called "suspected macrosomia" in the literature, is supported neither by research nor by ACOG. "That's saying, 'Well, the baby is getting big, and if it keeps on getting this big, it's not going to fit,'" explains Jacques Moritz, MD, director of obstetrics and gynecology at Roosevelt Hospital in New York City. "Well, Guess what? We're not that smart." Ultrasound estimates can be off by more than a pound on either side; in fact, studies have shown that palpating the belly with the hands yields a more accurate estimate.[11] And counterintuitively, babies don't necessarily keep growing the longer they're left in the womb. Statistically, fetal size appears to level off after 40 weeks gestation.[12] "Macrosomia is not a reasonable indication for induction," says Riley.

There's also the question of how big is too big? "Macrosomia" is itself an uncertain diagnosis, defined as either larger than 4000 grams (8 lb 13 oz) or larger than 4500 grams (9 lb 14 oz), depending on which study you're looking at. In 2003, Harvard researchers mapped out 1999–2000 U.S. birth data, which included 6.7 million infants, and found that roughly 15% of term babies weighed 4000 grams or more.[13] Are 15% of babies abnormal? Furthermore, studies of large babies have shown that 90% of those weighing more than 4000 grams can be born vaginally when given the opportunity.[14] The chance that a baby will weigh more than 4500 grams is about 3%.[15]

The sense among physicians and women that babies are getting bigger isn't necessarily wrong. Harvard researcher Emily Oken, MD, who led the birth weight analysis, explains that statistically, the average birth weight is slightly skewed by the increase in truly macrosomic babies born to mothers who have insulin-dependant diabetes prior to conceiving—about 3% of childbearing women.[16] But babies in general are bigger than they were in the baby boom, because they are being born to mothers who are well fed and to more mothers who are considered obese. "The trend in the first half of the century was to limit growth," says Oken. Physicians had their patients on strict diets and weren't discouraging smoking. The historians Richard and Dorothy Wertz write that "between 1920 and about 1975, three generations of women starved themselves during pregnancy to keep their weight gain below the recommended twenty-pound limit, thereby producing untold thousands of low-birthweight infants and possibly causing some neonatal deaths."[17] By the 1970s and 80s, the trend reversed, and women were told to pack on pounds, perhaps too many, during pregnancy. "The concern became having babies that weren't too small," says Oken. Now, public health authorities are revisiting the caloric intake recommendations.

Doubt of the maternal pelvis's ability to allow the fetus passage has been a feature of obstetrics for centuries. In the 1800s physicians used the pelvimeter, an instrument that looked like a protractor and a compass combined, to predict whether a baby would fit. And well into the 1960s pregnant women were routinely X-rayed to screen for "cephalopelvic disproportion," or CPD, a rare condition in which the baby's head is too big to clear the pelvis. But research shows that even modern, sophisticated measurements tell us little about the pelvis's competence, because the pelvis expands during childbirth.

Ellen Hodnett is a professor of nursing at the University of Toronto, a special advisor to the World Health Organization Department of Reproductive Health and Research, and a member of the Cochrane Collaboration's Pregnancy and Childbirth review team, which conducts systematic reviews of the available literature on all maternity practices. Cochrane is considered the authority on evidence-based maternity care. "That one kills me," she says of the idea that babies can't fit. "The maternal pelvis is a very well-constructed and flexible body structure in late pregnancy."

Much of the worry over size turns out to be a series of "if-thens." It isn't that the baby is too big, per se, but that what's called a shoulder dystocia might occur—a rare complication where the head emerges but the shoulders get stuck, in which case it is too late to do a cesarean—and that the baby might suffer damage to the brachial plexus nerve, located between the neck and shoulder (even rarer), and that there might be permanent damage in the form of Erb's palsy, a paralysis of the arm (rarer still). But the argument that inducing labor will prevent a shoulder dystocia doesn't stand up to scrutiny: just because a baby is small doesn't mean the risk disappears—half of all shoulder dystocias occur in babies under 4000 grams.[18] Inducing labor increases the odds of an emergency cesarean section, along with its attendant risks, without improving fetal outcome.

Some physicians suggest skipping induction and moving straight to elective cesarean for big babies, an approach that is similarly problematic.

Amniotic fluid is also estimated by ultrasound, and the literature does not support it as a reason to induce. "An ultrasound is not exactly a Kodak picture of the baby," says Hodnett, although the results given to women often read like a page out of a field guide: weight, fetal head measurement, amniotic fluid levels, and length are expressed down to the second decimal point, giving the numbers an aura of certainty. Amniotic fluid shifts constantly, with more being produced all the time. "The predictive ability of amniotic fluid volume as an indicator of anything for an otherwise healthy pregnancy is extremely low," says Hodnett. "There's just not the evidence to support it."

The question of whether to induce a pregnancy that is "overdue" is less clear-cut, and requires a bit of a statistics lesson. A baby is considered "term," or mature, if it is born between 38 and 42 weeks gestation. The due date is estimated as 280 days—40 weeks—from the first day of the woman's last menstrual period and also by ultrasound. Forty weeks is the median of the normal range, explains Philip Hall, MD, professor and director of maternal-fetal medicine at St. Boniface General Hospital in Winnipeg, Manitoba. "People seem to have thought for a long time that 40 weeks is some magic number," he says. Rather, it is just a midpoint. In other words, if we were to distribute a large sample of normal pregnancies along a graph, we'd see a bell curve. Forty weeks would be the height of the curve, and an equal number of women would give birth before and after. "Two standard deviations is within the normal range," explains Hall, "and that's 13 days on either side." Thus, a due date would be expressed more accurately as a "due month."

It used to be that a pregnancy lasting beyond 42 weeks was considered "post-term." But today, inducing on or before 41 weeks is fairly standard across North America. "The biggest indication for induction is post-term pregnancy—41 weeks and beyond," says Hankins. This shift came after a large study found that a stillbirth is more likely to occur after 41 weeks.[19] But the absolute risk is extremely small, the difference between .5 stillbirths per 1000 at 40 weeks and 1 per 1000 after 41 weeks.[20] And Hall argues there's no evidence that time spent in the womb is to blame. "The babies who are stillborn at 41 weeks die for the same reasons as babies who are stillborn at 39 weeks," he says. Between 15%

and 20% of pregnancies reach the 41-week mark, so potentially removing that tiny risk requires subjecting a very large number of women and babies to the risks of artificial labor, the consequences of which have not yet been fully teased out (see page 134). Hall calls such a policy "nonsense." "Women should not be led to believe that 'another few days will kill my baby,'" he says.

To the contrary, the French obstetrician and author Michel Odent, also a critic of the induction "epidemic," as he calls it, argues that labor begins when the baby is ready to be born (see page 139). Odent likens gestation to apples ripening on a tree: "You wouldn't pick them all on the same day, would you?" (There are other metaphors: water molecules boiling, popcorn popping, leaves falling—nature provides a range of normal.) Requiring an induction for every woman by 42 weeks is "a little bit childish, a little bit irrational," says Odent. "If you induce all women over 41 weeks, this leads to a higher rate of cesarean section."

Another reason for inducing is to minimize the risk of infection. It's not uncommon for a woman's water to break hours before contractions begin. This is labeled PROM, short for either *prelabor* rupture of the membranes or the more judgmental *premature* rupture of membranes. There is a label because there is a concern: the membrane holding the amniotic sac and "mucus plug" that rests at the base of the cervix protects the fetus from exterior microbes. The worry is that if labor doesn't quickly progress following loss of that protective barrier, infection will set in. Since the 1960s the "24-hour rule" has held: birth must happen within 24 hours, one way or another. Accordingly, in order to beat the clock, artificial oxytocin is given to stimulate contractions.

Hodnett co-authored a study of 5000 women in 1996,[21] the largest to date, and found no increase in neonatal infection in PROMs that were watched for up to *4 days* after rupture. The vagina is a nearly airtight passageway, so loss of the plug and rupture alone don't significantly increase the risk of infection, she explains. Vaginal exams, however, *do*, and should be kept to a minimum following rupture. Hodnett's research protocol prohibited them. But that caution is not usually heeded, she tells me. Indeed, women typically experience several vaginal exams during labor to determine how many centimeters the cervix has dilated, sometimes by different practitioners.

Thus, administering Pitocin in an effort to shorten labor and thereby reduce the risk of infection may actually increase that risk because it occasions vaginal exams and the use of internal monitors, both of which provide pathways for microbes. The Israeli company Barnev's device, approved by the FDA in early 2007, electronically monitors dilation with ultrasound probes affixed to either side of the cervix in lieu of multiple vaginal exams. Of course, any internal instrument, including Barnev's, will still increase the risk of infection.

Most women, some 60%, will go into spontaneous labor within 24 hours of their water breaking, and 95% will begin labor within 72 hours. Nevertheless, hospital protocol is usually clear on the 24-hour rule. And in some hospitals and among some practitioners, the window is 12 hours or less. "We feel a sense of pressure to get things moving," Laura Riley in Boston told me. "My own practice is that I give people about 8 to 10 hours." What these time limits mean is that once a woman's water is broken—spontaneously or deliberately—she is on a deadline. Once McSweeney's doctor broke her water (a procedure to which McSweeney had not consented), she was told she had 24 hours to push the baby out or she'd need a cesarean. Had her OB not broken her water, she might have turned off the Pitocin and let nature take its course; instead, McSweeney was locked into position. "I sort of felt like a prisoner," she told me.

Most women go into labor within a safe amount of time following membrane rupture, and the vast majority of women go into labor before 42 weeks; in one study using ultrasound dating, only 3.5% had not given birth at 42 weeks.[22] That leaves a minority who would be outliers, who might indeed benefit from an induction or augmentation. Instead, a majority of women are sped up. Is so much use of synthetic oxyocin remotely justified? Hodnett says no. "It just defies logic that half of women get an artificial version of a hormone that the body normally produces during labor."

CONVENIENCE

Kathleen Rice Simpson, PhD, a professor of nursing at St. Louis University School of Nursing, says the increasing tendency to speed up or

jumpstart labor has nothing to do with the women's bodies. "It's convenience," she says. "Convenience. Convenience. Convenience." Simpson
has been a labor and delivery nurse for 30 years, has published dozens of
journal articles, has conducted several studies—her curriculum vitae is 33
pages long—and has authored safety manuals for the American Society
for Healthcare Risk Management, the American Hospital Association,
and the Association of Women's Health, Obstetric, and Neonatal Nurses,
or AWHONN (pronounced A-1). AWHONN's *Perinatal Nursing* and
other publications are endorsed by ACOG. Simpson says that labor
induction and augmentation are not only more prevalent than the CDC
reports but often violate safety standards. She is frequently called on to
evaluate a labor and delivery ward following a bad outcome or to review
a malpractice case. Mismanagement of Pitocin, she says, is the leading
cause of liability suits and damage awards.[23]

"It's convenience for the physician mainly, but convenience also for
patients," says Simpson. "And absent any data to tell them that it's not
OK, they say, 'Well, maybe I'll have my baby this day or that day.' I firmly
believe that mothers are not informed enough to know that this is not a
good idea, and that any woman who has the right information would not
want to have her baby induced." Inducing tends to create longer, more
difficult, more painful labors in general, and it ups a woman's chance of a
C-section by two to three times.[24] The midwife Gail Hart notes, "We
can make a woman have contractions, but we don't always succeed in
forcing her body to release the baby and give birth. If we start a labor with
chemicals, we may very well have to finish it with a surgeon's scalpel."[25]
Pitocin also summons contractions that are stronger and more frequent
than those produced by the body, which, if they are not monitored
properly, can lead to *hyperstimulation* of the uterus—contractions that
come too hard and too fast—which can cause fetal hypoxia, or oxygen
deprivation.[26]

"The number-one problem I see is that there is a push to get the
baby delivered earlier or faster, and so nurses are often pressured to continue increasing the oxytocin, despite there already being too many contractions," says Simpson. "Interview any nurse and they'll tell you the
number-one issue in clinical conflict in labor and birthing in the United
States right now is oxytocin. There is a continuing push–pull kind of
thing going on."

The push–pull she's referring to is the tension between nurses, who are providing the bulk of maternity care in hospitals on set work-shifts, and doctors, who are directing that care while managing their own practices. "There's a common misperception that when women give birth it's like *The Cosby Show*," says Tracy Lethbridge in Florida. "That the doctor meets you at the hospital and sits up with you all night." At teaching hospitals, residents manage labor along with the nurses, but at community hospitals (about 80% of hospitals in the United States), "the vast majority of nurses are managing labor entirely by talking to the doctor on the phone as needed," says Simpson. When the doctor arrives, it is often just to deliver the baby. "That's completely normal and common. And I don't think people understand that. They come to the desk and say, 'Well I'm here, my doctor is going to be meeting me.'"

This system creates two competing agendas, which are often played out on the Pitocin dial—and on women and babies. "The physician would like to have the baby delivered as soon as possible, and the nurse is much more willing to let labor go as it is going," says Simpson. "It's really frustrating. You want to do right by your patients." Simpson led a 2006 study of nurse–physician communication in labor and delivery. In it 54 nurses and 38 obstetricians were interviewed. "There were two distinctly different views on use of oxytocin. Nurses felt pressured by their physician colleagues to 'push the Pit,'" writes Simpson. "In contrast, most physicians were concerned with increasing the oxytocin rate to 'keep labor on track' and 'get her delivered.' They repeatedly used 'aggressive' to describe their preferred method of nurse administration of oxytocin." One physician said, "The main thing is to have a nurse who is not afraid of Pit, who can actively manage the labor and be aggressive in turning it up on a regular basis." Another remarked, "When I hear I've got a nurse who will go up on the Pit, I know it's going to be a good day."[27]

At St. John's Mercy Medical Center in St. Louis, Simpson frequently greets patients who arrive for an induction unaware of the reason. "I've been hearing this for a while," says Simpson. "When I admit a patient, I say, 'So, what brings you in today?' And they say, 'Well, my doctor told me I'd have a baby today.' I say, 'Oh, well, what's the indication?' 'Well, my doctors just told me.' They don't have any knowledge of the risks of induction." Jill Jernigan, a registered nurse and director of childbirth education at Florida Hospital, told me that the ward is now doing three inductions per day. "They bring them in for induction in the morning, rupture the membranes, put them on Pitocin all day, and then they section them at 5 or 6 in the evening if they haven't made progress."

Although McSweeney, Hilton, and Johnson were given medical reasons for the intervention, they all report being encouraged to induce early on for no particular reason. "It started at 39 weeks," says Hilton. "She said, 'When do you want to be induced?' I said, 'I don't.' She said, 'Well, I'll give you one more week and that's it.'" At her 40-week appointment, Hilton says her OB asked, "So are you ready to have a baby?" and offered to schedule her the following day.

"All I had to do was say the word and I could have been induced on my due date," says McSweeney. At age 35, McSweeney thought she could relax once she got pregnant. But as the days went by with no signs of labor, she had never heard her biological clock ticking so loud. Each day, allowing labor to begin on its own became an increasingly tense negotiation with her doctor. A week later, still no labor, and her OB "started coming down on me," says McSweeney. "OK, we really need to start talking about inducing," she remembers her saying. "How's Friday?"

Johnson's practice offered. "It was presented as an option, if I wanted to ensure that my doctor would be the one to deliver the baby. But I said no," she told me. "I just wanted the baby to come when he was ready."

In the fall of 2004, I put word out that I was looking to speak with patients or attendants who had any experience with labor induction. I got dozens of responses from women, doulas, and labor and delivery nurses across the country. Many of them spoke of the push–pull articulated by Simpson. Carey Johnson, who lives in Brooklyn, New York, was offered an induction again and again. "My OB really, really wanted to induce me during my second pregnancy," she wrote over e-mail.

> It was so weird! Literally the day after my due date, she offered to strip my membranes. I asked if there were any medical concerns that made her want to induce, and she said no. The next week, she offered to admit me right there for Pitocin. Again there were no medical concerns, and again I declined. She insisted I come in every day from then on, and at each visit she offered to induce. After I declined on the tenth day "late," she

made an appointment for induction in two days. I went into labor without induction or intervention that evening and had my baby 7 hours later. I still don't know what the hurry was! A "due date" is a midpoint in a curve, right?

"Stripping" or "sweeping" the membranes is a technique whereby the practitioner inserts a gloved finger into the vagina to jostle the mucus plug and lift the amniotic sac off the cervix, with the goal of stimulating prostaglandin production and labor. This is considered a method of induction, and carries with it a risk of infection, but many providers report using the technique routinely at the end of a woman's pregnancy. In New Jersey, a physician I spoke with has a reputation for effective stripping, and she says her partners make sure to rotate their patients to her at 39 weeks so she can work her magic. "We don't do many inductions," she boasts. Of course, if her patient's water breaks (another risk of stripping) and she's not in active labor, the physician will start Pitocin immediately.

One in ten women surveyed in 2005 said they were pressured to induce.[28] Ellen Hodnett is concerned about this phenomenon and is convinced that women are needlessly experiencing long, exhausting, invasive labors or surgery as a result. Her latest research endeavor is a large study of early labor care in hospitals spanning the United States. She says that moms-to-be, unfamiliar with true labor, very often come to the hospital long before it's necessary. In years past, she says, they would have been sent back home, but today that doesn't seem to be the case. Echoing what Tracy Lethbridge saw in Florida, Hodnett reports, "What we're hearing from the nurses is how they have to guard and almost protect these women from automatic admission into labor and delivery so that doctors can start an induction."

Simpson, too, is conducting a clinical trial on informing women of the risks of elective induction before they're admitted. "We are trying to see if we can intervene," she says.

ACTIVELY MANAGED

Oxytocin got its name in 1909, after Sir Henry H. Dale, a physiologist, discovered that the extract of the human postpituitary gland contracted the uterus of a pregnant cat. After the delivery of a litter of kittens in what was probably record time, he named the drug by marrying the Greek words for "fast" (*oxy*) and "birth" (*tocos*).

Following Dale's discovery, slaughterhouses began harvesting the postpituitary extract of cattle, called it Pituitrin, and marketed it to physicians. A popular saying of the day was "Throw away your forceps and use Pituitrin!" Pituitrin replaced derivatives of ergot, a toxic fungus endemic to rye crops (from which LSD was later synthesized) that had been observed to cause uterine contractions during outbreaks. Ergot was unpredictable—it might cause no contractions or dangerous ones. Pituitrin offered the practitioner a more reliable means to control labor, and it grew popular over the next decade.

Pituitrin, however, had its own problems: adverse reactions to the animal proteins, contractions that accelerated out of control, uterine ruptures and embolisms, maternal and fetal deaths. The term *Pituitrin shock* was coined, and use of the product waned. In 1928, scientists further purified the formulation, and the pharmaceutical company Parke Davis sold the substance under a new name, Pitocin. It remained animal-derived for the next two decades, and its effects were still somewhat unpredictable. It was injected intramuscularly, and in the event of a bad reaction, there was no recourse other than waiting for the come-down.

It wasn't until the 1950s that expediting childbirth began in earnest. Call it better birthing through chemistry. Vincent du Vigneaud, the chemist son of a Chicago machine inventor who had led the Cornell research team that synthesized penicillin, did the same with oxytocin in 1953. For this du Vigneaud was honored with the 1954 scientific award of the American Pharmaceutical Manufacturers Association, presented by the vice president of Hoffman-LaRoche, and in 1955, he won the Nobel Prize. By the 1960s, physicians were following protocol that called for the dilute solution, administered via IV, that is still used today. For the first time in obstetrics, physicians had a relatively safe, reliable means by which to control labor.

The CDC didn't begin tracking Pitocin use until 1989, but in some hospitals that kept records, mostly among private, wealthy patients, it became routine. In New York City, nearly 50% of patients in 1955–56 were receiving the drug to stimulate labor "electively."[29]

Also in the 1950s, a young obstetrician from New York, Emmanuel Friedman, began studying the average length of labor. What would soon become known throughout the Western world as the Friedman curve had some nuance—the doctor mapped several stages of active labor and the respective rates of progress for each on "partograms." But the research was interpreted in its simplest terms: dilation should occur at the rate of 1 centimeter per hour. After his findings were replicated elsewhere— whether Pitocin was speeding up the observed labors is not known—the curve gained widespread acceptance as the minimum speed on the child-birth highway: anyone moving more slowly should get a tow.

By the 1970s, routine use of Pitocin was codified in a method called active management of labo(u)r, the brainchild of Kieran O'Driscoll, MD, and fellow obstetricians at the National Maternity Hospital in Dublin, Ireland, one of the largest obstetric centers in the British Isles. Their reasoning was influenced by Friedman. That is, if normal birth was to occur within a certain timeframe, then making "prolonged labor" go faster would reduce complications and cesarean sections, which the doctors claimed were happening too frequently (the rate was 4%). Working with Friedman's centimeter-per-hour rate, O'Driscoll and his colleagues set time limits. Labor that lasted longer than 12 hours they called *dystocia*, a word that previously had been used only to describe mechanical failure of the baby to descend.

The Dublin trials, or Dublin protocol, as it is called, were first published in an influential 1969 article entitled "Prevention of Prolonged Labor."[30] In these trials, 200,000 women were studied over 25 years. The protocol, designed for first-time mothers, employed several elements: women had their waters manually broken upon admission to the hospital and were assigned a midwife "to monitor the labor and encourage the mother." If labor did not progress at 1 centimeter per hour, artificial oxytocin was administered by IV and was increased until five to seven contractions were occurring every 15 minutes.

One key aspect of active management was vigilant evaluation of women prior to admission in the hospital: the National Maternity Center in Dublin admitted only women in true, active labor. A woman dilated 2 centimeters without regular contractions was told to go for a walk and come back when she meant business. The physicians argued that "efficient uterine action is the key to normality," and they gave every patient "two firm assurances . . . that labor will not last longer than 12 hours and that she will never be left without a personal nurse by her side at all times."

Under the protocol, the cesarean rate gradually *increased* over the years (from 4% to 9%), 40% of women received artificial oxytocin, and the hospital saw a 12-fold increase in the number of women requesting epidural anesthesia, possibly an indication that artificial oxytocin causes more unbearable pain.[31]

In the 1980s, some U.S. physicians, themselves concerned with a cesarean rate that had tripled (from 5% to 15%) during a single decade, began testing active management as a means of bringing that rate down. Results were mixed. Nevertheless, active management soon migrated west and spread, shedding one significant trait along the way: one-on-one support of midwives. Subsequent research shows that practitioners had neglected to study the necessary element: it isn't amniotomy or oxytocin that lessens cesarean frequency but, rather, the constant presence and support of a caregiver.[32] In Dublin, 80% of laboring women are still attended solely by a midwife.[33] Most women in the United States do not get one-on-one care, let alone that of a midwife trained to support the normal birth process.

O'Driscoll's Dublin study set a standard that still prevails in U.S. hospitals today: childbirth is given a window of opportunity. It must progress at a minimum speed and occur within a maximum duration. The *Mothers* surveys found that the average length of labor in 2002 and 2005 was 10 hours, almost exactly matching the Friedman curve and active management protocol.

A key question, of course, is whether Friedman had originally captured the time parameters of normal birth. According to Kathleen Rice Simpson, Friedman probably wasn't seeing much Pitocin use, but what he was seeing was only part of the picture. He had no knowledge of how long the woman had been laboring at home prior to arriving at the hospital. Second, he was observing birth prior to the epidural. Careful to pass no judgment on it either way, Simpson says the epidural "changes the course of labor. Even the most conservative literature says it increases it by 40 to 90 minutes. And it's usually more." Thus, applying the Friedman curve to women today is like expecting a sailboat facing headwinds to keep pace with a high-speed ferry. With an 80% epidural rate[34] and a tendency to admit women before they are in active labor and immobilize them, we can't expect the "efficient uterine action" that Friedman observed.

O'Driscoll framed his method as preventing pathology, what he called "prolonged labor." Consequently, as labor has come to be more actively managed, the range of what is considered normal has narrowed. "The definition of the normal upper limit to labor has been reduced from 36 hours in the 1950s to 24 hours in the 1960s to 12 hours in 1972 when active management was introduced," writes Marsden Wagner, MD, a neonatologist and former director of Women's and Children's Health at the World Health Organization.[35] With fewer women considered normal, it follows that more would be considered pathologic. The number of women diagnosed with dystocia, now known as "failure to progress," more than tripled between 1970 and 1989, from 3.8% to 11.6%.[36] And dystocia has apparently risen since, now accounting for as much as one half of cesarean sections in first-time mothers.[37] Similarly, the number of cesareans attributed to "fetal distress" rose from 1.2% in 1980 to 6.3% in 1989.[38] A similar change occurred when Pituitrin entered the market in the 1910s: the diagnosis of "uterine inertia" increased along with the substance's popularity—set against an artificially expedited length of birth, the body's own speed was seen as sluggish.[39] But what really happened? Did birth become more pathologic, or did we at some point begin seeing the normal variation in labor as abnormal? As the sociologist Barbara Katz Rothman puts it, "Have our uteri somehow lost the knack this generation? Or have our doctors speeded up the clocks on us?"[40] Or is there a third possibility, that active management practices have inflicted complications of their own making?

THE RUSH

The philosophical underpinnings of active management predate Blonsky, Friedman, and the Dublin trials by decades. In 1920, the highly respected Chicago obstetrician Joseph DeLee, founder of the Chicago Lying In Hospital, spoke to an annual meeting of the American Gynecological Society, of which he was then president. In a now legendary speech on "The Prophylactic Forceps Operation,"[41] the persuasive orator laid out step by step his method for managing normal birth: administer morphine and scopolamine, then ether, then cut an episiotomy; extract the infant with forceps, sew up the incision, and give more morphine/scopolamine "to prolong the narcosis for many hours postpartum, and to abolish the memory of the labor as much as possible."

Among the justifications for this method, DeLee cited pain relief, preventing morbidity (injury and disease), and "supplementing and anticipating the efforts of Nature." Whereas in years prior, physicians generally looked on childbirth as a normal, physiological event to be directed by the woman's body, DeLee's presentation, which was subsequently published as the lead article in the inaugural issue of the *American Journal of Obstetrics and Gynecology*, called labor "pathogenic," meaning unhealthy, a procedure to be directed by the woman's physician. The speech breathed life into what we know as modern obstetrics. This was the philosophy of active management, before it was given that name, and it shaped maternity care in the twentieth century.

The years following DeLee's proposition were somewhat of an identity crisis for obstetricians. The Flexner report, released in 1910, revealed that 90% of practicing physicians had no college education and that most had substandard training.[42] Meanwhile, epidemiological data showed that midwives attending home births had fewer maternal deaths.[43] Physicians had to decide: was it the role of the attendant to remain hands-off as much as possible, or was it the attendant's role to intervene in normal birth and try to control it in order to *prevent* complications? Today, the former is called expectant management, the latter active management.

The physician Brooke Anspach would have fallen into the expectant camp: "[W]e should endeavor to surround the patient and the attending obstetrician with the most ideal conditions, so that *whenever labor begins* the patient will have adequate and skilled attention throughout, *no matter how long it lasts*," he said in 1923.[44] DeLee argued otherwise: "I claim that the powers of natural labor are dangerous and destructive in many instances to both mother and child, and that interference by a skilled *accoucheur* at the proper time can prevent a goodly portion of this danger and much of this destruction."[45] Anspach was aware that he was in a shrinking minority. "At present day, Nature no longer dominates the practice of obstetrics," he said. The physician "is not content even to await the onset of labor but takes steps to induce it at the time when he believes the process should occur. . . . [H]e completes the delivery at once by means of episiotomy and the aid of forceps. If the case promises to be difficult, he ignores the natural channel of expulsion and delivers the child through the abdominal incision."[46]

Even before DeLee, childbirth wasn't necessarily actively managed, but it was often physiologically hindered, a legacy that may have prompted the doctrine of preemption. During the 1800s, mobility during labor was gradually eliminated and the position in which women gave birth flipped from vertical to horizontal.[47] Whereas women had formerly played an active role in childbirth, sitting, standing, squatting, or kneeling to push out an infant under the care of midwives, who were the primary attendants of birth in North America and elsewhere up until the twentieth century, doctors typically had women lie down in bed—modesty required it, authority presumed it—and the interventions and anesthesia that followed kept them there.

The movement away from upright, physiological childbirth can literally be measured in inches, in the evolution of the low birth stool, of which there are depictions dating back to ancient Egypt, to the birth chair, which then morphed into the modern stirruped obstetric table.[48]

Women were further immobilized by the Victorian era: even their bone structure, musculature, and organ placement were altered by the active "waist training" of corsets, if not by disease, and their vitality and health were undermined by the cultural aversion to female activity. By the twentieth century, a popular movement for chemical relief from the pain of childbearing took hold—inspired by Queen Victoria in England and led in the United States by a female homeopath in Boston. Nevertheless, as some physicians of the day and historians have argued, the pain may have actually been made worse by women's generally debilitated state and the psychosocial conditions of the Victorian era.[49] Except for the blip of the natural childbirth movement of the 1970s, the demand for chemical relief has remained robust. Chloroform and ether begot morphine and scopolamine, or "twilight sleep"; twilight sleep begot the spinal; and the spinal begot today's continuous epidural.

When DeLee proposed managing childbirth, one of his motivations was to minimize injury and death. The removal of women's active participation in birth necessitated, to a degree, the use of forceps, episiotomy, manual pressure on the abdomen, and drugs to restart contractions stalled by the knockout analgesia, and the survival of mother and baby some-times depended on such heroic maneuvers. These birth aids had been developed to treat abnormal, critical cases. Forceps, for example, were invented by a barber surgeon in early seventeenth-century England who was sick of having to crush a term fetus and extract it in parts, which had for centuries been the only remedy for hopelessly obstructed labor. As anesthesia became routine, so did intervention. In effect, by the Victorian era, many births were *rendered* abnormal, requiring chemical and instrumental assistance. Without active physiological childbirth, the birth process needed active management.

The spinal was a one-shot dose of anesthetic injected into the spinal fluid that came into popular use when women abandoned twilight sleep. A physician, now in his fifties, whose father was also an obstetrician, recalled the spinal/forceps routine prior to the era of obstetric anesthesiologists and modern epidurals. "You'd have an IV of Demerol or whatever, and the OB would give the spinal. You had a nurse on either arm, you'd put on the forceps, you pulled a lot, she screamed a lot, and then the baby was out. . . . The patient was so out of it she didn't know why she was screaming, and she couldn't push anyway."

Today's epidural is a combination of anesthetic and narcotic—each anesthesiologist has his or her own signature formulation—administered continuously into the lumbar spine via a catheter and programmed drip similar to the Pitocin. It is a marked improvement over the anesthesia of old. Women are no longer unconscious or paralyzed from the waist down. And they are usually able to push. The "walking epidural," which involves an even lower dose of anesthetic, is a misnomer, however. Few women are physically capable of walking, and almost none are allowed to. The bedridden legacy of the Victorian era remains. *Listening to Mothers* found that once admitted to the hospital with regular contractions, three-quarters of women did not walk around. For delivery, more than half of respondents lay on their backs, pelvises tipped against gravity.

Forceps are nearly museum relics, but the second stage of labor—the pushing part—is still actively managed by what's called directed pushing, or "purple pushing." For decades, women who weren't completely numb have been told to hold their breath and *Push!* for ten full seconds, usually while a nurse counts out loud, a process that is repeated until the baby is out. In 1957, Constance L. Beynon, a British obstetrician, began doubting the ritual after observing a woman who birthed without incantation. It was accidental; she was attending a first-time mother for a colleague and tried to stall the delivery so he would arrive in time. "We ignored the patient's early straining efforts and when finally the head reached the pelvic floor, just allowed it to emerge slowly on minimal pushing, hoping every minute that her doctor would walk in," wrote Beynon. "The baby (8 pounds, 3 ounces) was born before the doctor arrived but with practically no effort on the part of the patient and an intact vagina and perineum. The peacefulness and obvious ease of the birth were most impressive."[50]

Further research revealed to Beynon that in women with physical disabilities or heart conditions, who were physically unable to push, "easy labor is remarkably common." Beynon then carried out a trial at Sussex Maternity Hospital with 100 first-time mothers and compared them to nearly 400 who were typically managed. For the study, the caregivers were not to suggest that the mother push; if they had to say the P-word, the case was recorded a failure. Of the 100 women, 83 delivered spontaneously within an hour and 98 within 2 hours, without any suggestion of what to do. Beynon wrote, "For many years now I have adopted the practice of allowing my patients to follow their own inclination in the second stage, forbidding all mention of pushing by those in attendance."[51]

Active management in the broad sense is not limited to labor and delivery but is also applied in what is known as the third stage, after the emergence of the baby. By the 1950s it was routine to clamp and cut the umbilical cord immediately, and the practice is still standard today. The baby is then typically placed in a tray under a heat lamp for measurements, footprints, and a battery of tests and prophylactics, and blood is drawn from the cord for testing. Left alone, the umbilical cord will continue pulsing for several seconds, allowing the remaining blood to flow from the placenta as the baby takes his or her first breath. There is no research evidence to suggest any benefit to immediate cord cutting, and some evidence suggests it causes harm by depriving the infant of nutrient- and oxygen-rich blood.[52] One obstetrician, writing in 1941, equated cutting the cord to submitting the baby to a "rather severe hemorrhage."[53] The cord left intact, on the other hand, mechanically ensures immediate skin-to-skin contact on the mother's warm belly—nature's heat lamp— and immediate mother–baby interaction, which is considered optimal.

depictions of birthing stools, women knew that upright positions allowed easier stretching of this part of the anatomy—the first midwifery texts, published in the early sixteenth century, never failed to mention it.[63]

Modern studies show that squatting, for instance, increases the diameter of the pelvic outlet and that upright positions, especially hands and knees, decrease the length of labor, shorten the pushing stage, increase the fetus's blood oxygenation, and protect the perineum.[64] Roberto Caldeyro-Barcia, a Uruguayan physician who studied birth positions in the 1950s, said, "Except for being hanged by the feet . . . the supine position is the worst conceivable position for labor and delivery."[65]

Cutting the perineum was first mentioned in the literature in the eighteenth century as a last-ditch effort to free a stuck child, "as if it were contained in a Purse." One hundred years later, it was proposed by doctors as a method to preempt and redirect a severe perineal tear away from the anus when the physician thought such tearing to be "inevitable."[66] At the end of the nineteenth century, there was a small but marginal cadre of physicians calling for "liberal" use of episiotomy, but the obstetric leadership of the time still saw birth as a physiological event, to be governed by "natural law: . . . normally every perineum will properly distend to allow the exit of the child, leaving all the tissues intact," wrote William Dewees, a Kansas obstetrician, in 1889. Indeed, in the late 1800s there was a lively debate on how best to *protect* the perineum.[67] This was "the highest object attainable," wrote Dewees, and to that end he recommended hot compresses, perineal massage "freely using inunctions of lard," and a side-lying position for delivery, with hands on the perineum providing counterpressure as the head emerges.[68] Others recommended massaging with warm olive oil. In 1915, a survey of obstetricians indicated that they cut the purse strings in only 5 of every 100 cases.[69]

But in 1918, a prominent obstetrician suggested, "Shall we cut and reconstruct the perineum for every primipara?"[70] These were the words of R. H. Pomeroy, who interpreted childbirth as violence; the fetus's head "a battering ram wherewith to shatter . . . a resisting outlet." His words were reinforced by the call of DeLee and others for complementary episiotomy with forceps, a tool that was already in wide use at the time, and the cut became more and more common. By the 1930s, episiotomy was prevalent in textbooks, and professional allegiance to "natural law" was crumbling. One physician wrote in 1930 that "the tissues of the modern women do not well withstand the tension and stretching incident to the average normal labor."[71] DeLee, after all, had called women "nervous inefficient products of modern civilization."[72] In a complete reversal of the previous generation's trust in the agility of the female form, an obstetrician at the University of Texas wrote in 1937 that episiotomy "is *unnecessary* in approximately 10 percent of primipara" (my emphasis).[73]

As in active management, the justifications of episiotomy were prevention of morbidity thought to be the result of "pathologic" labor—overstretching and prolapse of the pelvic floor, a muscular diaphragm that holds the pelvic organs in; loss of sexual function; and fetal distress. Perineal tears are classified by four degrees, with first-degree tears being superficial and healing on their own. Fourth-degree tears extend through the anal sphincter and require restorative surgery. Episiotomy creates a second-degree tear, requiring stitches inside the vagina as well as on the perineum. Proponents argued that a clean, straight cut was easier to sew up than a jagged tear, and that it was more prudent than risking the possibility of a severe tear.

Speed was another justification, enthusiastically articulated by the trailblazing founder of the American Medical Women's Association, Bertha Van Hoosen. In her autobiography, Van Hoosen looks back on episiotomy much as her homebound peers adulated the washing machine: "The most widespread innovation in modern obstetrics is the cutting of the muscles at the vaginal outlet," she wrote. She believed that a tear was not only more difficult and time-intensive to repair, but also more injurious. On the other hand, she did not appear to think of episiotomy as injury at all: "Older midwives and obstetricians made an art of the slow and careful delivery of the baby's head without inflicting any injury to the muscles of the perineum," she wrote, but now, "the obstetrician assumes the responsibility for the time when the baby shall come, and the depth to which the mother shall be laid open to hurry the birth."[74]

In less than 30 years—the same 30 years in which the rate of hospital births increased from 25% to 90%[75]—episiotomy was entrenched in routine obstetric practice. The tenth (1950) edition of *Williams Obstetrics* reported that aside from the cutting of the umbilical cord, episiotomy had become the most common operation in obstetrics.[76] Data from individual hospitals show that between 50% and 100% of women had the procedure in the 1950s and 1960s. In 1979, the first year that national data were available, 65.1% of women giving birth vaginally were cut.[77]

Routine episiotomy had never been studied, but it persisted in the United States even as forceps declined, well into the 1980s. It also became sacrosanct: the first physicians to question it had to do so anonymously. J. K. Russell, a British professor of obstetrics, later claimed penning an anonymous editorial in the *Lancet* in 1968, which called on his American colleagues, including the authors of *Williams Obstetrics*, to revisit the practice.[78] Five years later, another anonymous commentary appeared in the *British Medical Journal*. Later claimed by Robyn Pogmore, an Australian-trained physician living in England, it called episiotomy "deliberate mutilation of the maternal perineum."[79] The first critiques by U.S. physicians came a decade later and were published in marginal journals and books, such as *Contemporary OB/GYN* and *21st Century Obstetrics Now!*, after women's health activists had launched a consumer movement against the procedure and demanded scientific research on its claimed benefits. The first randomized controlled trials of episiotomy were not published until 1984.

The logic of episiotomy was that a second-degree tear would prevent a third- or fourth-degree tear, but studies conducted through the 1980s and 1990s found the opposite to be true. One study found that episiotomy makes such an injury *nine times* more likely.[80]

ACOG issued a practice bulletin against routine use of episiotomy in March 2006, following the publication of a systematic review in the *Journal of the American Medical Association* that found "no benefits from episiotomy. . . . Indeed, routine use is harmful."[81] Others saw cause for a moratorium much earlier. Michael House, a British obstetrician, reviewed the medical literature in 1981 and wrote: "[I]t would be expected that for a standard procedure that is performed hundreds of thousands of times every year that there would be solid evidence in the world literature comparing the results of delivery without episiotomy. . . . In fact, no such evidence exists."[82] In 1982, CDC researchers Stephen Thacker and David Banta published an exhaustive review of the literature dating to 1860, which concluded that no scientific evidence supported episiotomy. They called on obstetricians to end its routine use.[83]

In the mid-1980s several studies on episiotomy emerged, with many authors echoing Banta and Thacker's recommendation. In 1985, European and American regional offices of the WHO and the Pan American Health Organization held a conference on appropriate technology for birth. One of their recommendations: "The perineum should be protected wherever possible. Systematic use of episiotomy is not justified."[84] *Williams Obstetrics*, which had for decades echoed Pomeroy's battering ram metaphor, countered that "It can be said with certainty that, since the era of in-hospital deliveries with episiotomy, there has been an appreciable decrease in the number of women subsequently hospitalized for treatment of symptomatic cystocele, rectocele, uterine prolapse, and stress incontinence!"[85] It did not withdraw this claim until 1993, advising, "Episiotomy should not be performed routinely."[86]

Today there is broad consensus among researchers that routinely cutting the vagina causes undue harm. Rather than preventing complications, it seems to promote them: episiotomy has been associated with higher rates of third- and fourth-degree lacerations, infection, urinary and fecal incontinence, prolonged pain, and sexual problems. What the scientific community recommends be a rare, emergency procedure is still used in *one-third* of women giving birth vaginally, mostly first-time mothers.[87] The best-selling pregnancy guide *What to Expect When You're Expecting*, which that has sold more than 12 million copies, still calls episiotomy a "minor surgical procedure."[88]

Candice Hilton of Mississippi was cut without being told—she didn't feel it because the epidural had cut off sensation. "Ten minutes after the birth the doctor was still at my vagina, and I said, 'What are you doing?' She said, 'Well I'm sewing you up.' I said, 'Did I tear?' and she said, 'No, I cut you.'"

THE MACHINE

In 2000, the FDA conditionally approved a a device called OxiFirst®, which was designed to estimate a fetus's blood oxygen levels during birth. The device's purpose was essentially to boost the accuracy of another device, the electronic fetal monitor. The thinking was that confirming "non-reassuring" fetal heart tones might prevent unnecessary cesareans, and a preliminary study suggested it would. However, in November 2006, a large randomized, controlled trial funded by the National Institutes of Health found otherwise.[89] The absence of any benefit was so stark that it prompted researchers to cut the study short. They commented that the study represented a success in medical research: it had prevented a useless, invasive product from being incorporated into routine medical practice. "This genie has not yet escaped from the bottle," one obstetrician opined.[90]

Unfortunately, another genie already had. At about the same time that the doctrine of active management solidified Pitocin's share of the market in the 1970s, another product, the electronic fetal monitor, was making its way into the delivery room, creating a doctrine all its own. Like Pitocin, it promised practitioners an unprecedented tool with which to manage labor, to control its natural chaos.

Using Doppler ultrasound technology developed in the 1960s for the U.S. military, the electronic fetal monitor could pick up the fetus's heartbeat continuously, which at the time seemed to be a major improvement from a nurse or doctor listening frequently with a specially designed stethoscope, called a fetoscope. Presumably, the new machine would be more likely to detect heart rate problems and alert hospital staff to impending fetal demise in time for them to intervene. In 1969, a small company called Corometrics Medical Systems put the monitor on the market, and with it the promise of a perfect outcome.

Three physicians on Corometrics's own board of directors conducted the studies that would be used to sell the machine to hospitals across the country. The marketing blitz was a resounding success, and revenues soared from $467,000 in 1969 to $5 million in 1973, a nearly 1000% increase. Like other interventions that came to be routine, electronic fetal monitoring (EFM) was originally intended for use in managing abnormal, high-risk pregnancies: fetuses that were premature, underweight, or otherwise compromised. But investment literature from the early 1970s prophesied widespread, routine use: "We can see the time when the fetus will be monitored from several months after conception until birth by a series of electronic devices. . . . When this happens, the market for equipment and disposables will be in the billion dollar range." When American Home Products purchased Corometrics in 1974, it was worth $1.9 million. Company insiders, including prominent Yale and Harvard physicians who had originally "tested" the product, held more than half of the company's stock.[91]

Today most fetal monitoring is done externally, but the original models were applied internally. The monitor was a wand-like device with a sharp steel screw at the tip, which was inserted through the cervix and driven into the fetus's scalp. Corometrics experts claimed EFM would reduce the chance of infant death and mental retardation,[92] but by 1976, questions about its efficacy and safety were surfacing. The first randomized studies—those conducted by researchers without financial ties to the manufacturer—were under way and were showing increased rates of maternal infection and cesarean section among those monitored electronically, as well as increased fetal injury in the form of head wounds and infection.[93]

In 1976, Congress passed the Medical Devices Amendments, which required the U.S. Food and Drug Administration to approve any electronic medical device for safety and "effectiveness." By this time, however, almost every maternity ward in the country had purchased one or more electronic fetal monitors and was using them on the majority of labor and delivery patients. The EFM machine was grandfathered in. It would require no FDA review.[94]

Albert D. Haverkamp, MD, an obstetrician who spent 4 years researching EFM at a large Denver hospital, testified before a Senate Subcommittee on Health in 1978 that the machine had become ubiquitous in the absence of any randomized, controlled studies.[95] Haverkamp presented his own ongoing research. In two studies of high-risk women assigned to either EFM or frequent listening by a nurse with a fetoscope, use of EFM was found to impart no benefit, but it more than doubled or tripled the cesarean rate. "At a time when most thoughtful obstetrical authorities are urging universal electronic fetal monitoring, the study results appear unbelievable," he told the committee. "I really believe we are over-selling our technology." Haverkamp also reported that much larger studies showed that EFM had no impact on infant mortality. "Yet, many hospitals won't allow a patient to labor without a monitor and many doctors won't accept a patient who will not have a monitor because of their medical legal fears," he continued. "That's an awful lot of monitoring in normal term pregnancies to gain an unclear benefit."

EFM exploited those medical legal fears, heightening the influence of malpractice on a physician's practice and on a woman's birth experience. It may have even helped *create* the litigious climate among obstetric patients. The "strip," as the paper readout is called, has been admissible courtroom evidence since the 1980s, so in most hospitals, continuous electronic fetal monitoring is mandated. It is their paper trail.

The number of cesarean operations tripled between 1968 and 1976, the first year that the procedure made the list of the ten most frequently performed surgeries in America.[96] Thacker and Banta, the same team that would scrutinize episiotomy, prepared a 1978 government report that concluded EFM to have little benefit and to be a costly and dangerous procedure. Their estimate of annual expenditures related to EFM, including unnecessary cesarean surgery, was $411 million. "The diffusion of EFM into virtually every obstetrical setting represents a failure of public and private policies and officials," they wrote.[97] By 1983, the cesarean had become the second most common surgery in the United States.[98]

In 1985, the National Center for Health Services Research reviewed more than 600 studies on EFM and concluded that continuous EFM had yet to show improved fetal outcome, except in the case of very small babies.[99] The reports, the hearings, and the conferences were mounting evidence that the machines should have been scrapped long before; instead, hospitals upgraded. In the mid-1980s, Corometrics, which is now owned by General Electric, introduced a new feature: "central" monitoring. This allowed nurses to monitor multiple patients simultaneously from the nurses' station. The machine had initially transferred attention from the patient to the reading, and now central monitoring enabled the attendants to work even more remotely and expanded the standard patient-to-nurse ratio to 2:1, though nurses often report being assigned to three patients. In Dublin, O'Driscoll had envisioned one-on-one care as standard, but EFM made standard care less personal and yet more costly: a 1988 government report estimated the annual price tag for this technology at $1 billion.[100]

For the natural childbirth movement, the emergence of the monitor was unfortunate timing. Just as activists were urging women to get up and birth, hospitals reined them back down in bed and strapped them, both physically and psychologically, to a machine that falsely promised a safe birth. At the time, one of the main worries was a baby born with cerebral palsy following a traumatic birth. It turned out that just a fraction of cerebral palsy cases are attributable to delivery, and that EFM is no better at detecting fetal distress than the humble feto-scope, and, in fact, that the machine is more likely to be wrong. A study of more than 150,000 births in California found that EFM falsely pre-dicted cerebral palsy 99.8% of the time, making it "the only laboratory test in current use that, when abnormal, is wrong most of the time," as one obstetrician put it. Not surprisingly, there has been no reduction in cerebral palsy in three decades, nor a reduction in babies who die or end up in the neonatal intensive care unit (NICU).[101] And even though the device may give the impression of high-tech precision, physicians and nurses report heavily relying on their intuition to interpret the readings.[102]

The World Health Organization recommends intermittent moni-toring with either a fetoscope or a handheld Doppler ultrasound, a rechargeable cordless device that allows the laboring woman freedom of movement. The Doppler, they write, is "a clear example of appropriate technology."[103] ACOG considers continuous monitoring and inter-mittent monitoring to be of equal value, and is out of step with its UK, New Zealand, and Australian counterparts,[104] as well as with the U.S. Preventative Services Task Force, a part of the Department of Health and Human Services that is charged with evaluating research on screening and prevention. The task force recommends that "Electronic fetal moni-toring should not be performed routinely on all women in labor."[105] However, intermittent monitoring is effective only when the patient-to-nurse ratio is 1:1. For women to be monitored this way, the hospital would need more hands.

In spite of the evidence, women continue to be told they must wear a monitor, and therefore that they must stay in bed. In 2005, nearly all women giving birth in a U.S. hospital had the sensor bands strapped around their bellies—the *Mothers* survey counted 93%. Most respondents to the survey were in fact bound several times over: 83% had an IV line in their arm, 56% had a urine catheter, and 76% had epidural or spinal anesthesia. It is unclear which gets attached first, but the primary reason women gave for being prostrate was not that they were numb but that they "were connected to things."

Michelle McSweeney in New York City had originally wanted an unmedicated birth but gave in to an epidural because "I couldn't get up anyway," she recalls. "I've got these belts around my gigantic stomach, I've got a catheter, I've got a thing on my finger, I've got an IV in my arm. I felt like a science project."

THE WOODEN SPOON

Scottish epidemiologist Archie Cochrane died before the term *evidence-based medicine* made it into print. But his book *Effectiveness and Efficiency: Random Reflections on Health Services*, published in 1972 and translated into several languages, essentially argued for it. In less than 100 pages, Cochrane critiqued medicine for having embraced treatments in the stark absence of scientific study.

Cochrane harbored particular venom for obstetrics, awarding it a wooden spoon (as opposed to the silver spoon he bestowed on phtisiology, the study of tuberculosis). Iain Chalmers, a young obstetrician in Wales, took up Cochrane's challenge. Frustrated by the contradictory management practices he saw in labor wards, Chalmers left clinical obstetrics and began what would be a lifelong pursuit of research and practice evaluation. In 1976, he made waves by writing a very controversial chapter in an already controversial book suggesting that common maternity care practices not only might be ineffective but might also be causing harm. He called for trials "in which there is no intervention except continuous emotional support."[106]

Two years later, Chalmers was tapped by the British National Health Service to found and direct the National Perinatal Epidemiology Unit at Oxford University, where he and a team of researchers spent the following years compiling thousands of randomized controlled trials on obstetric practice and conducting systematic reviews of available data on every obstetric practice. With the help of a grant from the Rockefeller Foundation, Chalmers and his team finally published their results in 1989 in a two-volume, 1500-page tome, *Effective Care in Pregnancy and Childbirth*,[107] and a truncated paperback called *A Guide to Effective Care in Pregnancy and Childbirth*.[108] The research team surveyed some 300 common obstetric practices and classified them along a continuum from "beneficial" to "ineffective or harmful." For example, physical, emotional, and psychological support during labor and birth is deemed "beneficial;" freedom of movement during labor, "likely to be beneficial;" and active management of labor as having "unknown effectiveness." Routine intravenous fluid is called "unlikely to be beneficial," and separation of mother and baby, "likely to be ineffective or harmful." (See Appendix A for excerpt.)

With *Effective Care*, Chalmers and his group had done something unprecedented in medicine. Whereas systematic reviews had at that time been conducted on specific conditions such as breast cancer and heart disease, *Effective Care* was the first systematic evaluation of an entire specialty. For all its heft, however, the text was more of a testament to what was unknown than to what was known. "Most of what we were doing we didn't know one way or another if we were doing harm," Chalmers told me. Of hundreds of practices evaluated, nearly one-quarter fell in the limbo category, one-third were either unlikely to have any benefit or likely to do harm[109]—it was unclear from the available evidence whether much of what went on in maternity wards was effective or even safe.

To some, Chalmers's work was an insult, literally 1500 pages charging that obstetricians didn't know what they were doing. "We were called an obstetric Bader-Meinhof gang," recalls Chalmers, referring to the violent postwar Marxist group in Germany. But a World Health Organization survey of routine obstetrical interventions in 1983 backed the review: it had found only 10% of maternity care justified by scientific evidence.[110] To Archie Cochrane, who wrote a foreward to the unabridged version months before his death, *Effective Care* was a model for other areas of medicine to follow, "a new achievement," he wrote, "a real milestone in the history of randomized trials and in the evaluation of care." It so impressed him that he lifted the curse of the wooden spoon.

In 2000, *Effective Care* went electronic as the Cochrane Pregnancy and Childbirth Database, named after Chalmers's mentor. Today the database has expanded into the Cochrane Collaboration, which conducts systematic reviews of practice in more than 50 medical subspecialties, from wound care to depression. The approach devised by Chalmers and his colleagues to evaluate obstetric care thus paved the way for the movement, across many medical specialties, toward evidence-based medicine.

Friedman and O'Driscoll and those who had come before had painted birth as a predictable, linear process, a one-size-fits-all approach. Deviations were abnormal, dysfunctional. The goal of obstetrics was, as the New Jersey obstetrician succinctly put it, "to advance the cause."

Effective Care turned this fundamental assumption on its head and suggested that less is usually more, even for pregnancies that are deemed high-risk. Chalmers and his team wrote that instead of artificial oxytocin, "simple measures, such as allowing the woman freedom to move around, and to eat and drink as she pleases, may be at least as effective and certainly more pleasant for a sizeable proportion considered to be in need of augmentation of labour." In the updated *A Guide to Effective Care*, the authors could find no evidence "to justify forcing women to lie flat during the second stage of labour."[111]

The same year that *Effective Care* was published, in 1989, a report by the United States Public Health Service, commissioned by the NIH National Institute of Child Health and Human Development, said much the same about prenatal care. The report stated the findings of a panel, chaired by Mortimer G. Rosen, head of obstetrics and gynecology at Columbia Presbyterian Hospital in New York. For low-risk women, the panel recommended 7 or 8 prenatal visits rather than the usual 13. It also found no benefit to routine pelvic exams, urine screening in early pregnancy, pap tests, and frequent blood pressure readings. The headline in the *New York Times* read, "Less Prenatal Care Urged for Most Healthy Women."[112]

It was also in 1989 that a landmark study of birthing centers was published in the *New England Journal of Medicine*.[113] Nearly 12,000 low-risk women giving birth under the care of midwives at 84 centers were included. The C-section rate was 4.4%, and the infant death rate was 1.3 per 1000 births, comparable to hospital rates. The authors concluded that for women without risk factors, "birth centers offer a safe and acceptable alternative to hospital confinement." In a matter of a year, three major research endeavors called into question all aspects of conventional maternity care: the methods, the setting, and even the attendant.

THE BUSINESS OF BIRTH

A common theme emerges in the history of obstetric care: procedures and devices developed for the treatment of abnormality rather quickly became routine practice in the name of prevention, and then simply in the name of speeding up and ordering an unpredictable, at times tedious, process. Under O'Driscoll's protocol, speed and efficiency were themselves thought to be protective. Call it better birthing through preemption.

Induction of labor—starting labor rather than merely expediting it—followed the same pattern. It was written about in the 1800s as a medical strategy to stave off obstructed labor in women with "contracted" pelvises, a relatively common deformity at the time (the idea was to induce a premature birth while the infant was small enough to fit through the pelvis) and to resolve prelabor hemorrhage with a live mother and child. Another indication was preeclampsia or eclampsia—diseases that are still poorly understood today, in which the pregnancy becomes increasingly toxic to the mother. They are marked by high blood pressure and protein in the urine. But induction was for years a risky proposition, frequently ending in maternal death from infection or uterine rupture and hemorrhage. For induction to be justified, the risks of continuing the pregnancy had to outweigh the risks of inducing.[114]

Pitocin, however, promised safety and success. Around the same time of DeLee's call for prophylactic forceps and Pomeroy's call for prophylactic episiotomy, another physician, by the name of Reed, called for prophylactic induction: "[W]hen the child becomes demonstrably mature, labor should be induced at the first convenient opportunity." The tools to determine maturity were crude. Reed suggested measuring the belly and inducing at 35 centimeters (it is now accepted that the height of the belly roughly corresponds with the weeks of gestation, so 35 centimeters from pubic bone to breastbone is assumed to be normal at 35 weeks, which is premature). Reed went on: "Whether or not the maturity of the child be generally accepted as a satisfactory and legitimate basis for bringing on the labor, at all events our ability to produce the delivery at will is an important addition to our obstetric armamentarium."[115]

Reed was no DeLee, but his words were prophetic. The addition of Pitocin to obstetricians' "armamentarium" was indeed revolutionary, affording the obstetric profession an effective tool by which to schedule birth, and the shift from expectant management to active management tracks the development of pharmaceutical-grade oxytocin.

Some have observed this shift as an extension of industrialization. As Barbara Bridgeman Perkins argues in *The Medical Delivery Business*, there was a direct tie between the rise of the assembly line—of mass production—and the rise of standardized, mechanized birth. Pituitrin itself "owed its commercial availability to the centralization of the meatpacking industry. One pound of dried extract became the profitable by-product of pituitary glands from twelve thousand young cattle. The assembly line in slaughterhouses thus contributed to assembly line obstetrics."[116]

It is clear from reading early papers and symposia on labor induction that the desire to prevent complications was not the only motivation driving research and development. Streamlining birth also held enormous possibility for the profession. The desire for control wrought sundry experimental methods during the nineteenth and twentieth centuries, "too numerous to mention and very difficult to categorize," as the 1965 medical text *Induction of Labor* put it. In addition to administering derivatives of ergot, these methods included inserting into the cervix "bougies, various tubes, catheters, packs, bags, and other instruments" or even "small rubber balloons" and "animal balloons made from pigs' bladders." Also prescribed were sit-ups, fasting, soap-and-water enemas, intrauterine douches alternating tepid and chilled water, and ingestion of quinine, castor oil, calcium gluconate, and estrogens. Other techniques included intravenous lipids, air or carbonic acid pumped into the uterus, and even electricity (mentioned four times in the literature during the 1800s). A "bag or forceps with a 200- to 500-gram weight attached," was recommended by doctors Diekmann and McCready in 1947. Manual dilation of the cervix with fingers, "until two, three, and finally four fingers could be introduced" was proposed by doctors Koster and Perotta in 1943.[117] Reed, for his part, preferred a bag.[118]

"The operation may be brought entirely within the control of the operator," wrote a London obstetrician in 1871. "Instead of being the slave of circumstances, waiting anxiously for the response of nature to his provocations, he should be master of the position."[119] The time saved by inducing had in fact been recognized immediately. In 1808, the Albany physician John Stearns wrote that since discovering ergot, the use of which he had learned from a German midwife, "I have seldom found a case that detained me more than three hours."[120] Even O'Driscoll and colleagues in Dublin cited housekeeping as a perk of active management: "The newfound ability to limit the duration of stay has transformed the previously haphazard approach to planning for labor," they wrote.[121]

With forceps, physicians already had the ability to extract the child at will, but they still had to wait some length of time for physiological labor to work the baby down through the birth canal before they could apply the instruments. With Pitocin, they could hasten the baby's descent. "The advantages of this technique were obvious, and 'controlled labor' was the exciting new expression in obstetrics," wrote the authors of *Induction of Labor*, which outlines a regimen of amniotomy and intravenous oxytocin. Among the medical indications was "Maximum Utilization of Physical Facilities." "Labor by appointment," they wrote, could avoid maternity ward traffic jams.[122]

"Elective induction of labor is well on its way to becoming an established part of American obstetrics," the authors continued. "As more successful reports appear in the literature, its justification will become more widely accepted." The book was dedicated to the 7000 women who gave birth at the Hospital of the University of Pennsylvania between 1950 and 1965, "who had the advantage of induced or stimulated labor."

By the 1950s and 1960s, casual use of induction can be found among private patients in several hospitals—rates varied widely—with convenience an acceptable justification. A physician at Sloane hospital for women in New York noted in 1961 "considerable convenience to the doctor," "ample evidence of the safety," and "obvious" advantages to the patient, adding, "I think it is high time we shed our shame over preferring to practice obstetrics in the daytime."[123] In 1999, ACOG modified its policy on labor induction, sanctioning it for "psychosocial" or "logistic" reasons.[124] Although Gary Hankins says the intention was never to "loosen criteria and to massively increase inductions," that seems to have been the effect. "This was the watershed," says Kathleen Rice Simpson.

As Lethbridge observed in Florida, and as national birth data suggest, Pitocin makes possible what Marsden Wagner calls "daylight obstetrics." He explains it this way: between managing the country's 4 million annual births, family planning needs, preventive screenings, gynecological surgery and menopause, "obstetricians have a plate that is full to overflowing," he says. "They've got to try to get some control. The biggest problem in their practice? Birth. Why? It's 24-7."

Pitocin is used to speed up labor because "Physicians want to get done," says Simpson. "They don't want to stand around waiting." In her study of physician–nurse communication, nurses spoke of physicians trying to "hurry labor" and have birth occur "at a convenient time." They even spoke of keeping conversations with doctors to a minimum in order to avoid conflicts. One nurse said, "You just want to update them, 'Everything is just fine . . . she's progressed another centimeter,' and keep them away from the patient."

With induction, doctors don't need to wait for their patients to go into spontaneous labor, says Simpson, which "is not in their best interest. Think about it from the physician's perspective," she says. "Let's say you have a very busy practice, and you're trying to have a quality of life, maybe you've got a young family, you don't want to be running out every night to deliver a baby, or not coming home in time for dinner, missing everything that your child is doing. So what happens is you try to get all the births in between 9 and 5, and to do that, you have to make sure nobody goes into spontaneous labor; and to make sure of that, you have to induce them all early. Or let's say this is the day you have to be on call, it's best then for you to induce three or four people on that day because you can get them all done at once. Those three or four people aren't going to call you on the weekend, they're not going to call you in the middle of the night, they're not going to interrupt your office hours, they're not going to give birth at any time that's inconvenient."

When I called Jacques Moritz in New York, who has a reputation for being a noninterventionist, to talk about the frequency of labor induction, he feigned surprise at the question, "That's our dirty little secret! How did you know about that?" Painting a near facsimile of Simpson's scenario, he says doctors in solo practice, those who do not work with a group of physicians, will often induce a slew of patients the day they're on call. "They almost don't have any choice. It's actually pretty standard even in some group practices."

"There are pressures for a doctor to say, 'I don't want to be in the hospital every night this week.' I think it happens more than we even acknowledge—it's just that it's not talked about," says obstetrician and researcher Peter Bernstein, MD, associate professor of obstetrics and gynecology and women's health at Albert Einstein College of Medicine and Montefiore Medical Center in New York, who has criticized elective induction. Some say scheduling births is all doctors can do to maintain their level of income while larger and larger portions of it are earmarked for malpractice insurance premiums. If a doctor misses a birth, he loses revenue. Even if an induction doesn't work, a cesarean is waiting. And from incision to sutures, a cesarean takes less than an hour.

In addition to time management, the looming fear of lawsuits drives doctors to act rather than to wait. "Doctors are practicing more defensively," says Bernstein. It's irrelevant that an induction might lead to a cesarean. "To be blunt, you don't get sued when you do a cesarean," he says. "You get sued when there's a damaged baby. And if they can find any reason that the woman should have been delivered earlier, then it doesn't matter whether the damage had anything to do with how you managed the baby. All that matters is did you do everything that you could have possibly done? And that causes doctors to say, 'Well, it's got to look like I've tried my best. And trying my best would be to deliver the baby.' So you explain to the mother that the fluid's a little low."

Malpractice insurers often organize talks with physicians and attorneys, brown-bag seminars in self-protection. "They give us scenarios of cases that are 'unwinnable,'" says Richard Fain, MD, an OB in Livingston, New Jersey. "They tell us, if a baby looks big, and there's a shoulder dystocia, and the shoulder dystocia leads to Erb's palsy, then that doctor will be sued, and that doctor will lose. And that doctor might be faced with the possibility that she or he will never be able to practice obstetrics again." Fain and his colleagues can even get continuing medical education credits, which they need to maintain their licenses, for attending such "risk reduction" seminars.[125]

The effect, not surprisingly, is to gently steer doctors away from allowing spontaneous labor at all. If a bad outcome occurs, it has to look like the doctor has *done everything* she or he possible could. In other words, physiological birth doesn't look good in court; getting the baby out earlier, faster, and with as many medical interventions as possible does.

CHAPTER 2

The Short Cut

I T IS JUST AFTER DAWN on a dewy September morning, and a young couple expecting their second child checks in to St. Barnabas Medical Center in Livingston, New Jersey. After triage nurses draw blood, check vital signs, and confirm the baby's position with an ultrasound, the two are admitted. She is given a jonnie, he, turquoise scrubs. At 9 a.m., the pair make their way down the hall of the labor and delivery ward, pass the nurses' station, and sit by a wide wooden door with a red DO NOT ENTER sign. A nurse meets them and gives a hair net to her; blue shoe booties and a white surgical mask and headdress to him. The doors open automatically and the two are ushered into a large, bright room with a padded table in the center. The sun illuminates thick block glass windows that stack up to the ceiling. A radio hums. One nurse is setting up instruments on a tray; another lays out color-coded paperwork on the tiled counter beneath the window.

The young woman sits on the table, hands folded—a clinic patient, I am told several times by residents and nurses, meaning she's on Medicaid. A tall anesthesiologist introduces himself. He asks her to sit forward as he exposes her lower back, swabs with brown antiseptic, marks

45

a point of entry, and injects anesthetic that will block sensation from the waist down while allowing her to remain awake.

The obstetrician, a resident, and two medical students scrub in a side room and flow in through a swinging door one by one. A "circulating nurse," so called because she is not bound to the sterile field, and a scrub tech, garbed in blue and responsible for instruments and suction, make final preparations. The patient is asked to lie down and extends her arms cross-like on padded supports that one of the residents clicks into place on both sides of the table, though the staff do not strap her arms down as they often do with women undergoing unplanned cesareans. They lather her prominent belly with more antiseptic, and the circulating nurse inserts a urine catheter and intrauterine catheter between her legs. Beeping fills the room. The surgeons set up what looks like black vacuum cleaner tubing in an arch over the patient's chest and hang up a blue plastic drape, blocking her belly from view.

The expectant father sits in a chair by his wife's side, holding her hand. The nurses cover the woman's legs with a clear plastic and then a blue drape, and the surgeon begins marking the belly with what looks like a pincher. The patient doesn't flinch. The surgeon, a woman, then switches out the pincher for a scalpel and without fanfare starts to cut. The patient speaks up. "Are you feeling pain or is it just pressure?" asks the surgeon. She says it pinches. "Ok, Ok, I'll stop," says the surgeon, blotting the blood and holding the incision together for a moment, looking up toward the ceiling. After a beat, she turns to the patient. "Are you expecting a boy or a girl?" A boy. The surgeon nods.

In another minute she tries the scalpel again, glancing over at the patient, who stares off to the side. The scalpel is drawn crosswise low on the woman's belly, repeatedly from left to right, leaving a bright red streak as if applied with a dripping watercolor paintbrush. The surgeon continues to cut and cauterize with a pen-like device, smoke rising and blood soaking white gauze cloths as she excavates through human layers—skin, then fat, then a sinewy sheet of white fascia, or connective tissue, and finally muscle a color between brick and mashed raspberries. From my vantage point on the patient's right side, the round belly splits along the incision like a hungry Ms. Pac-Man. The residents insert curved metal spatula-like instruments, pulling back the layers to create a round opening into the belly, bringing the amethyst-colored uterus into view.

I've never seen abdominal surgery before, but in this context, a cesarean operation, I am immediately struck by the resemblance to vaginal birth. Mere inches above the vagina, surgeons have created what seems to me a misplaced double, like an extra mouth where one's nose should be. Here is this oval opening, about the diameter of a baby's head, red and ripe against the patient's skin with folds of tissue and muscle not unlike folds of labia. As the doctors' gloved hands feel and probe inside, they look not unlike an attendant's hands stretching a bulging perineum.

The surgeon works gingerly on the uterus, which has developed scar tissue and adhesions (places where it is sticking to the peritoneum, the thin membrane encasing the abdominal organs, and muscle) from the patient's previous cesarean. This is common with repeat cesareans, I'm told, and the surgery is taking longer than it would with a "virginal abdomen." When the uterus is finally opened, amniotic fluid and blood bubble out, and the scrub tech suctions, sending the red fluid cascading through a clear tube into a small bucket.

The baby's head, covered with dark hair, comes into view within the abdomen, and four hands work quickly to maneuver it up and out, tugging this way and that with great effort. Finally, the surgeon asks for a vacuum and is given a white plastic cap attached to a cord and gauge of some sort—the nurse tells me it's called a Kiwi—and places it on the baby's head. The cord retracts like a lawnmower string, effectively sucking the baby out up to his chin. The four hands resume the extraction, a resident leaning back on the metal retractor with all his weight, stretching the ersatz birth canal as the others twist and turn and finally shimmy the baby out. The birth is called at 9:30. "Still a boy!" says a nurse.

The cord is cut, and the baby, crying, is taken across the room by more nurses and a neonatologist, who have materialized without my noticing. The baby is put in a warmer, and a tube is guided down his throat to suction out fluid, as the surgeons set about retrieving the placenta from the uterus. The disc-shaped, veiny organ is soon deposited in a blue plastic container the size of a brownie pan. I'm told that normally the uterus would now be "exteriorized"—that is, lifted entirely out of the body cavity and onto the abdomen for suturing—but because of the adhesions, the surgeons have decided against it. They spend several minutes resealing the uterus as more blood and fluid flow through the siphon. There's a blue plastic cover spread out on the floor by the window with ten balled up bloody cloths, neatly arranged by the circulating nurse, easily countable. Over the next half-hour, the collection grows to 27, laid out in rows of 5.

While the surgery continues, the squalling infant is diapered, weighed, measured, and footprinted. The father walks over to the warmer and takes a picture with his digital camera. He returns to his wife and excitedly shows her the picture in the camera's viewer. The pixilated image is this mother's first glimpse of her son.

At 9:38, the baby is swaddled in a pastel blanket and presented to his mother; she kisses his forehead. She turns her head toward her husband, and the rosy bundled baby is laid down briefly cheek to cheek, where he puckers his lips and forehead and gives out a big cry, then settles into silence for the first time. Dad takes another picture and the nurse takes the baby away, puts him on his back in a glass cart, and, over his resumed cries, smiles at mom, "Congratulations! We'll see you in about 3 hours." Dad gives his wife a kiss and follows to the nursery.

The circulating nurse goes to change the radio station. "If we stay with classical we'll be here all day," she says, and the tenor of the operation changes. Over the static, we hear a loud "It's a booooooooooooooyyyy-eeeeeeeeeee!" echoing from an adjacent operating room. Another doctor's shtick, apparently; the nurses chuckle and roll their eyes. The beeping sound I heard in the beginning, I notice, is gone. "Dancing Queen" comes on the radio.

It is now 9:55 a.m. and the stitches are up to the muscle layer. The surgeon looks down over the drape at mom, "You had a lot of scar tissue from the last C-section," she tells her. In another 5 minutes they'll be up to the fascia, and the surgeon leaves the rest for the resident. Gloved hands held up in front of her, she backs up from the sterile field, removes her blue smock, and drops it into a bin. She then takes off gloves, mask, and hair net and tosses them into the bin as she pushes through the side door. "Thanks everyone," she says on her way out.

Now bringing together the skin, the resident explains the stitching technique to the senior med student and has her try a few. The needles look like large metallic eyelashes and are inserted and retrieved with surgical clamps. "There's a lot of scar tissue," the resident reiterates to the patient. "So next time you want a C-section, just know it's going to be a . . . challenge."

Finally, the woman's abdomen is sealed and bandaged, and the nurse brings the soles of her feet together, bending her knees outward. The resident comes around, facing her pelvis, and inserts two fingers into her vagina, places his other hand on her belly, and summons a gush of blood into another plastic blue container. "Celebrate" plays on the radio. The scrubbed nurse washes the patient from belly to thighs, and then she and the resident transfer the woman onto a gurney. It is 10:17 a.m., and as the patient is being wheeled out the door, the resident takes off his mask and says, "Congratulations, Mom."

For roughly 1 in 3 women in the United States, this is childbirth. For 1 in 3 American babies born each year, this is their entry into the world. At St. Barnabas, which hosts some 7000 births a year, 44% were cesareans in 2004, and more than one-third were planned beforehand, like this one.[1]

I came to St. Barnabas because I wanted to understand how the cesarean rate got to be that high. The World Health Organization maintains that in a developed country, the proportion of cesareans should not exceed 15%; beyond that, the maternal injury and death consequent to major abdominal surgery begins to eclipse the lives and health saved.[2] And there is mounting evidence that babies are not, as is widely believed, better off skipping the birth canal. A CDC researcher's 2006 study of 5.7 million U.S. births found that infants born by cesarean with no medical risk factors were nearly three times more likely to die within the first month of life than those born vaginally.[3]

New Jersey leads the United States in surgical birth, with a 35% cesarean rate.[4] In response, Governor Jon Corzine declared April 2006 "Cesarean Awareness Month," saying that "maternal-child health is improved by preventing unnecessary cesareans."[5] St. Barnabas is among the institutions leading the state. What a 44% rate looks like on the labor and delivery ward is six scheduled cesareans, plus four to six more "add-ons" each weekday. And to accommodate the growing volume, the hospital recently began scheduling two C-sections on Saturdays. One reason for the high rate is that, like many other hospitals, St. Barnabas strongly discourages vaginal birth after cesarean, called VBAC (see Chapter 3). Most of the obstetricians there will not attend a VBAC, and most women are not offered VBAC. This means that the more primary cesareans they perform, the more repeat cesareans will be scheduled.

This large teaching hospital is not necessarily representative of the rest of the country, and the routines I saw in the operating room may not even be representative of other physicians at the hospital, but it offers a glimpse, and perhaps one into the future. Historically, St. Barnabas has been the harbinger of obstetric technology to come. In the 1970s, it was the first hospital in the area to make routine use of electronic fetal monitoring. In the 1980s, it was augmenting and inducing routinely, long before ACOG sanctioned it—"You were lucky if you got away without any Pitocin," a nurse who worked there in the late 1980s told me. By 1992, the cesarean rate was already 29.7%, more than a decade ahead of the rest of the country.[6] If cesarean births continue to increase as they have been, the rest of the country might look like St. Barnabas in 10 more years. Plans for a new hospital at the University of Michigan, for instance, include a maternity ward with the capacity to handle 50% cesareans.

Over several conversations in Livingston, I was able to talk with obstetricians and nurses about the high cesarean rate. Not one practitioner cited medical necessity as the reason, but many cited the patients.

"It's our population mix," one doctor tells me. "Think of New Jersey as one big suburb. The women tend to be older, with more money, they've delayed childbearing—they're more uptight. They tend not to want to push. All their friends have C-sections and did fine, so they say, 'Why can't I have a C-section?'" Updating century-old concerns about "civilized" women, the doctor presses the point further, revealing some decidedly unscientific stereotypes, particularly for a women's health professional. "The young black women have no problem pushing," he says. "They push when you want them to push." He plunges even deeper in this vein: "I should say young women, really. Maybe women who are pregnant at 19, 20, 21, are just more comfortable with their bodies. They're obviously involved in sexual relations younger. . . . They just seem more comfortable with their sexuality, much more so than some of these women who are older, who maybe delayed relationships until they were 30. That group of women tends to be much more uptight."

Another doctor, a woman, explains it a bit differently. Many of her patients are older, she says. They have gone to fertility specialists and been through repeated in vitro fertilization procedures to conceive. This puts their pregnancies at a slightly higher risk, but that's not what she attributes the cesareans to. "I think it's control. Their entire lives they've been in control. They're in control of their careers, they're in control of their husbands, they're in control of getting pregnant, and they don't like the idea that they don't know when they're going to go into labor, how it's going to go, how their body is going to react to it. It is a huge unknown. It's scary for all women going through it, but these women would rather choose something where they can say, 'OK I'm planning on this day at this time.'"

The day we talked, she had performed an elective cesarean on a 37-year-old woman who conceived with assisted reproductive technology. "This was a very sought-after pregnancy. She was going to all these specialists, getting ultrasounds every week. She's a very high-strung, nervous woman. All she wanted was a healthy baby, and she didn't care that she took the risk on herself of the cesarean section."

Nervous and high-strung, perhaps, but the woman was told by another OB in the practice that her amniotic fluid looked low and that the baby was measuring small—cause for some measure of alarm. The woman was clearly given reason to worry and was led to believe that a cesarean would guarantee a healthier baby. "She came in today, got a scan, and said, 'OK, I'm ready for my C-section,'" says the doctor. The pregnancy was a few days shy of the due date. "She didn't want to be induced, she didn't want to hear about anything, so that's what I did. I went and did a primary section." How was the fluid, I ask. "The fluid was great! Totally normal." And the actual weight of the baby? "Six pounds."

"Some women are pushing with all sorts of verbal and nonverbal communication that they don't want a vaginal birth," says Richard Fain, MD, recalling a recent patient who ended up having a cesarean. Fain has been an OB for 30 years and has practiced at St. Barnabas since he was a resident. "She was letting me know with her body language, 'Dr. Fain, I don't like this business of labor, I don't want to push a kid through my vaginal opening, I don't want you to take liberties with my body in getting this baby delivered'—you know, doing an episiotomy, which I try not to do. Years ago we stonewalled this kind of thinking, but in the year 2006 that's harder to do. We're more inclined to say, OK, doing a C-section isn't so bad an option."

From his point of view, it's not so much control as fear. He says that more and more of his patients are going to perinatologists, maternal-fetal medicine specialists, and getting sophisticated ultrasounds to measure the size of the baby. "The perinatologist does a growth scan and says that the baby may be large for dates. I can show you one-page paragraphs where they document that they've discussed with the patient the risks of being in labor, including shoulder dystocia and Erb's palsy. And that patient is back in my office worrying, 'Dr. Fain, maybe you should do a C-section. I don't want to have a baby that's too big.' Already her mindset is, 'Labor could be dangerous for the baby and dangerous for me.'"

And there are women who bring up elective cesarean without any prompting, say the physicians. One group of OBs I spoke with at St. Barnabas agreed that they get one or two unprompted requests for an elective cesarean each month—1 out of every 60 patients, they estimate—whereas just 5 years ago this was unheard of. This may be a site-specific trend; physicians in the heartland, and in the Bronx, still say it's unheard of.

HealthGrades, a company that rates the quality of hospitals and doctors, reviewed birth data from 2001, 2002, and 2003 in 17 states, looking into the question of the patient-requested cesarean.[7] They used the term *patient choice* to describe preplanned, first-time cesareans absent a medical indication, and they reported that this subset rose each year, to 2.5% of all births in 2003, with Florida, New York, and New Jersey leading other states. Samantha Collier, MD, a vice president of HealthGrades who spearheaded the study, told me it was in part prompted by obstetricians, who elect cesareans for their own births in high numbers. A 2003 ACOG/Gallup survey found that 22% of female OBs who had at least one C-section said it was elective;[8] a 1997 survey in Britain found that 17% of obstetricians, and nearly one-third of female OBs, would choose a preemptive cesarean for themselves or their partners. When asked why, 88% said they feared rectal damage, and 58% said they feared sexual dysfunction.[9] "For a lot of women, it's about avoiding complications that they perceive as being associated with vaginal delivery," says Collier.

But there is little evidence of a significant "patient-choice" cesarean trend outside of physician circles, the HealthGrades data notwithstanding. To get their findings, HealthGrades investigators used a methodology developed by researchers who studied birth trends at Cedars-Sinai Medical Center in Beverly Hills—where Hollywood has its C-sections—and applied it to a much larger patient population.[10] They looked at maternity patient data for some 1500 hospitals. They sorted that data for cesareans that were performed before labor or without labor; then they factored out repeat cesareans, breeches, and multiples. They also discarded medical complications that warrant surgery, such as preeclampsia, placental abruption, and active herpes. The cesarean births they were left with had previously been labeled "no indicated risk" or "unspecified" primary cesarean in the literature. "We called those 'patient-choice,'" explains Collier. In other words, the company arrived at "patient choice" not by asking women, but by the process of elimination.

Are patients responsible for the 44% cesarean rate at St. Barnabas? Can, or should, patients be responsible for *any* medical trend outside of plastic surgery? Next in line for the OR after the cesarean I observed was a first-time mother with a "macrosomic" baby. Over a sushi lunch in the conference room provided by the maker of the anticlotting drug Lovenox ("Lovenox is not for *all* your patients . . . " the rep's spiel began), I asked the surgeon how much she thought the baby weighed. "Probably 8 pounds," she said, then paused. "Well, that's not really macrosomic. But we're just going to do the C-section anyway. She's 38 weeks." (The baby was born 8 lb, 5 oz). By HealthGrades standards, this would have been labeled a "patient-choice" cesarean, but it was not at all clear who was requesting it.

At the hospital I felt a casual resignation in the air. When I met the charge nurse and told her I was there to observe a cesarean, she said, "Oh, well, C-sections we do all day. If you want to see a vaginal birth, though, there's a woman in room 5 who's at 7 [centimeters dilated]. You might want to catch *that*." In a conversation with one of the nurses, pregnant 28 weeks, she told me that her placenta is lying low and she might end up needing a cesarean, even though 28 weeks is considered too early to tell. "I'm getting used to that idea, of just planning it," she said. In Mineola, New York, at Winthrop Hospital, which had a 41% cesarean birth rate in 2004, the nurses breathe the same sighs. "The doctors are not really pushing labor as much anymore," says Jane Haley, the nurse manager there. "They're fearful of malpractice." And the patients? "I don't see a strong desire to deliver vaginally," she says. Winthrop now does so many cesareans that the hospital is scheduling them in the ambulatory surgery unit, with blueprints for a third OR.

In Mineola, I met with Gary Levine, MD. Levine throws the notion of "cesarean on demand" into question, because he offers the option to all his patients. "At some time during the pregnancy, I'll say to the patient, 'Have you thought about how you want to deliver this child?'" he says. "And if she doesn't know what I mean, I'll tell her, 'Well, it's 2006, if you want you can have an elective cesarean section.'" Levine says he feels like he has to put it on the table; some patients have brought in magazine articles warning of incontinence down the road. "There's this whole new movement of 'perineal sparing,'" Levine tells me. "The urogynecologists [who specialize in pelvic floor disorders] are saying that with vaginal birth there are risks of bladder prolapse, urinary and rectal incontinence, and sexual dysfunction, and by doing the cesarean, you're avoiding that whole phenomena." He pages through an old obstetrics book he's dug out on my account, arriving at a grainy, black-and-white image of a baby crowning on the perineum. "Look at that stretching," he says.

Levine adds that vaginal birth may not even be to blame. "Just having a cesarean doesn't mean that you're going to avoid problems later on in life—there's genetic predisposition. There's just being pregnant. And there's gravity. We're the only mammal that stands erect, and I'd venture to say we're the only mammal that has problems with urinary stress incontinence," he says. The data do show slightly more short-term "stress" incontinence—a small amount of urine escapes during a cough or a laugh—following vaginal birth as opposed to cesarean, especially among first-time mothers. Severe incontinence following delivery among either group is rare—about 2%.[11] Later in life, about 30% of women have problems, ranging from "stress" to adult diapers, but giving birth doesn't seem to be the cause. A study of postmenopausal nuns and mothers found similar bladder issues,[12] and a 2005 study of biological sisters found that heredity was the predictor, not vaginal birth.[13] What remains open to question is the degree to which directed pushing, lithotomy position, and laboring supine as artificial oxytocin drives the baby down might be what is stressing women's bladders, rather than vaginal birth per se. Studies have implicated each practice in contributing to pelvic floor ailments.[14] And the research is clear that episiotomy is a direct cause.[15]

Levine does warn his patients of the risks of cesarean: hemorrhage, infection, organ damage, and threats to future fertility. "I say, 'Let's talk about how many babies you want to have,' because we're seeing complications with repeat cesareans," he says. Those include scar tissue, adhesions, uterine rupture, and catastrophic placenta implantation problems, where the organ grows into the uterine scar or through the scar—grave threats to both mother and baby. "We've seen where the placenta grows through the uterus and into the bladder. You're talking about blood loss, hysterectomy, bladder repairs. . . . You know, for everything you do in medicine that you think is going to be terrific, there's a whole other ball game that comes to the forefront," says Levine. Still, he says, elective cesarean is a "very hot number," and his patients are a hip, savvy crowd. If he doesn't bring it up, they will.

THE VAGINAL PRESERVATION SOCIETY

Joseph DeLee predicted this moment. Just as he called for the forceps to go "prophylactic" in 1921, which was followed by Pomeroy's episiotomy for every first-time mother, Reed's routine induction of labor, Corometric's continuous electronic fetal monitoring, and O'Driscoll's "prevention of prolonged labor," the term *prophylactic cesarean* first appeared in the *New England Journal of Medicine* in 1985.[16]

The authors of the *Journal* article used a recent malpractice suit as a springboard for discussion, though the suit had been dismissed. The plaintiff had been in normal labor when her placenta suddenly detached from the uterine wall (such an "abruption" shuts off the baby's oxygen), a crash cesarean ensued, and the infant survived but with profound brain damage. Her lawyer asked the court, "Would this baby be alive, healthy, and undamaged today if it had been delivered by cesarean section one week earlier?" Inspired by the argument, the authors wondered aloud what a "universal switch to prophylactic cesarean section at term" might look like.

They concluded that "patients ought to be given a definitive opportunity to consider electing prophylactic cesarean section" and asked physicians to consider the possibility of being sued down the road for failing to inform a patient of the option—even though the argument was legally untenable. They carried it one step further and asked if an informed patient were to opt out of a prophylactic cesarean, "must she then be required to sign a consent form for the attempt at vaginal delivery?"

The authors were roundly criticized and ignored by the obstetric leadership of the time. But when W. Benson Harer, Jr., MD, president of ACOG from 2000 to 2001, argued in speeches, on *Good Morning America*, and in ACOG newsletter editorials in 2000, 2002, and again in 2005[17] for the "elective prophylactic cesarean," it was a new era. Harer calls the cesarean a "life-enhancing" procedure and vaginal birth "the most dangerous trip that any of us will ever take." He argues that a cesarean will reduce "problems with incontinence of urine, flatus or feces," and he told me in a reverse logic that "There's no evidence to refute the statement that the safest way for the baby to be born is by the elective cesarean section at 39 weeks."

In 2003, ACOG came around to thinking prophylactically, issuing an ethics opinion that gestated during Harer's tenure. The opinion, obliquely titled "Surgery and Patient Choice," green-lights the patient-chosen cesarean.[18] In 2006, the National Institutes of Health sponsored a State-of-the-Science conference on "Cesarean Delivery on Maternal Request," which concluded that until further data could be collected, and provided there is thorough doctor–patient communication, "cesarean on maternal request may be a reasonable alternative to planned vaginal delivery."[19] In the last 15 years, the American obstetric profession, facilitated by government health agencies, has recast major intra-abdominal surgery as potentially superior to vaginal birth.

The Healthgrades surveys and later the NIH conference have generated predictable headlines about women and their demands. "More women are demanding Caesareans," was one.[20] But the hullabaloo over women's choice may be a canard. The researchers who developed the methodology used by HealthGrades have since bemoaned the extrapolation of "unspecified" to "choice." Kimberly Gregory, MD, the lead Cedars-Sinai researcher, urged the NIH conference to respect the distinction. "Maternal request is likely a very, very small subset of non-indicated procedures," she told the panel charged with drafting the final recommendations. Our only measure of what women really want is the 2005 *Listening to Mothers* survey, which surveyed 1500 women directly and found a much smaller rate than HealthGrades: just one woman said she requested a cesarean.[21] Those data were absent from the NIH's final report.

Eugene Declercq, PhD, professor of maternal and child health at Boston University and lead author of the *Mothers* survey, admonished the NIH for titling the conference as it did. "We don't have measurements of maternal requests, and to suggest that these are maternal requests is a leap of faith that goes beyond what the data justify," he told the panel.

The NIH conceded in its final statement that maternal request is only "a component" of the rise in primary cesareans, for which "the magnitude . . . is difficult to quantify." Others argue that choice itself is hard to quantify in the context of medical care, and especially maternity care, because any decision is strongly informed by the care provider. On the whole, patients trust their doctors. If Levine tells his patients that they can prevent vaginal stretching and resulting dysfunction by having a cesarean and they agree to it, should that be considered "maternal request"?

And women are being led to believe that vaginal birth harms. One of the nurses at St. Barnabas told me, "I'm all for the vaginal preservation society." Another is recommending that her childbearing-age daughters go for primary cesareans. "If I were a woman, knowing what I know, my first choice would be a cesarean," a Pennsylvania obstetrician told the *Philadelphia Inquirer* in 2001.[22] Well-known sex therapist Laura Berman—as seen on the Discovery Channel with her sister Jennifer Berman, a urologist—touts her own elective C-sections. "Why undergo a process that is strongly associated with later problems, when another option is available?" she wrote in a column for the *Chicago Sun-Times*. "Or, as I like to put it to my friends, why ruin a perfectly good vagina?"[23]

The patient may not only fear for her bodily integrity, she is given more things than ever to worry about concerning her baby. The typical obstetric patient now goes through a battery of tests, screens, and ultrasounds during pregnancy. She meets with genetics counselors and weighs whether to get amniocentesis. She is put through sensitive glucose challenges and increasingly diagnosed with gestational diabetes, although such diagnoses have not improved outcomes.[24] There's new worry over Group B streptococcus (a bacterium commonly found in the vagina) causing infection in the baby—a 0.01% chance.[25] Though screening for such conditions results in more false-positives than accurate diagnoses—

and in unnecessary intervention—all women are tested. Obstetrician-gynecologists order more diagnostics than any other medical specialty.[26] "The focus is no longer on birth as a normal life process, but an accident waiting to happen," says Maureen Corry of the Childbirth Connection. Women are so worried, in fact, that there's a new psychiatric diagnosis: tokophobia, the fear of giving birth.[27]

Meanwhile, the focus on "patient choice" ignores the larger issue, which is that the vast majority of women do not ask for cesareans, and two-thirds are still unplanned and performed during labor. Socioeconomics doesn't explain it. At Mississippi Baptist Medical Center in Jackson, which like St. Barnabas is a level III hospital, with 24-hour on-site anesthesia and a NICU (and can therefore take high-risk cases more likely to require a C-section), the cesarean rate in 2005 was 48%.[28] Like St. Barnabas, it has been ahead of the rest of the country for decades; in 1992, the rate was 33.6%.[29] But unlike northern New Jersey, where a high proportion of childbearing women are over 35 and white, in Hinds County, Mississippi, the bulk of maternity patients are in their twenties and black. Among the 2005 *Listening to Mothers* respondents, the cesarean rate among black first-time mothers was 49%.[30]

Some argue that the general ailments facing the U.S. population are to blame (the diabetes, the obesity, the hypertension), but C-sections are rising among women with no risk factors as well, and rising at a clip that has outpaced the relatively small increase in medical conditions.[31] "Women aren't changing all that much," says Declercq. "The only demographic change we're talking about here is more older mothers." Women are more likely to give birth by cesarean as they get older, but Declercq says this doesn't account for the rapid cesarean rise either. "I think this is more about changes in provider behavior."

The strongest predictor of surgical delivery is not health status or age, but where and with whom a woman gets care. In Milwaukee, a level III hospital has a 19% cesarean rate; in Boston, a hospital similar in size and capability has a rate twice as high, at 37.4%.[32] A small hospital in Indianola, Mississippi has a rate of 66.9%, while a small hospital in southern New Jersey has a rate of only 17.8%.[33] A birthing center in Taos, New Mexico boasts an 8% cesarean rate; the nurse-midwives at the University of Wisconsin hospital in Madison advertise a 4.7% rate. One 2006 study concluded that "a geographic variation in the number of

C-sections performed is driven by mostly nonmedical factors, such as provider density and local medical malpractice pressures, and is mostly unrelated to the mother's medical condition."[34]

CUTTING LOSSES

Cesareans are labeled either "elective" or "emergency." But most are done in more of a gray zone; it's neither a clear emergency, but nor are things progressing smoothly, and what happens next is a judgment call. "Will the woman dilate and push the baby out efficiently and easily in the next couple of hours?" says Richard Fain, offering a typical scenario. Or will she not progress, will the baby not descend, will a cesarean happen anyway—"I don't want to say at four in the morning, but that's what comes to mind,"—and will there be an unfavorable outcome, like a baby that spends its first 3 days in the NICU getting IV antibiotics because the mother developed a fever? "The question is, should we have just cut our losses at midnight and done the cesarean?" More and more, he and nearly every other physician say, OBs are erring on the side of the scalpel. "We'll move to C-section a lot quicker than we would have 30 years ago," says John Marcus, MD, director of OB/GYN at the Valley Hospital, 25 miles north in Ridgewood, New Jersey (cesarean rate: 42%).[35] "And that's a lot due to the malpractice crisis."

The doctors at St. Barnabas were candid about the economic and litigious pressures influencing this trend. Back in the conference room, while the Lovenox rep answered questions about dosage and indications ("More people are dying of thromboembolic events [blood clots] than breast cancer and AIDS combined!" she said), my end of the oblong table turned into a salon on the obstetrics profession. Three graying male doctors hung on to continue the conversation even after the rest of the room, mostly younger female OBs and residents, headed out. One of them was Thomas De Angelis, MD, who didn't think twice about being quoted. "I'm getting out of this in the next couple of years," he said.

De Angelis is called "a car mechanic who does OB on the side," and some joshing about female parts and car parts ensues. The ID, however, works. De Angelis has the look of a guy whom you'd be just as likely to find fixing a muffler or propelling pizza dough. He's a short man, with thick salt-and-pepper hair that he's obviously been running his hands through all morning, and two days of stubble. "You'd be crazy to do obstetrics now," he says, nodding toward the young women filing out of the room. "It's all about volume. You have to do volume now to survive."

De Angelis was a chemist for 5 years before he went to medical school. He found the lab lonely. "I went to medical school because I wanted to work with patients, I wanted to work with people," he says. Now he finds obstetrics lonely, and stressful in ways he didn't imagine. A solo practitioner, to maintain his standard of living in suburban New Jersey, send his son to a 4-year private college, and pay out an annual $90,000 in malpractice insurance, he's had to double his case load. Which means halving the time he spends with patients in an office visit. And he's irate about it. "You tell me what other profession has to pay $300 just to go to work every day! The bottom line, the bottom line is the care for patients. And as a consumer," he says, pointing to me, "the consumer right now doesn't get a good evaluation. She gets 5 minutes in the office." And when the consumer is in labor? "It's a vicious cycle. I can't sit with that patient. I have to go back to the office."

"OB is a business. It's a volume business," chimes in another doctor, Stephen Crane, MD. "If you get paid $2400 to deliver a baby and you pay out $90,000 in malpractice insurance, you have to do a lot of deliveries to pay that fee." Sheldon Wasserman, MD, an obstetrician in Milwaukee, on the other hand, pays out an annual $34,000 in malpractice insurance and maintains a more low-key, midwestern lifestyle (his kids will go to state school). He isn't subject to the same pressures. Wisconsin is also the only state in the union with a law that prevents a damage judgment from taking a physician's property and assets. Wasserman rarely induces or uses Pitocin, and his cesarean rate is 12%. He's also serving his seventh term as a state representative (an OB who does politics on the side), and is introducing legislation called the "I'm Sorry" bill, which would allow physicians to console their patients without it being legally incriminating.

"This is not the way to practice medicine," says De Angelis. "Why do women put up with this? I have no idea. You know, back in the 80s, when I was in residency, there was a feminist movement. The women back then would never have tolerated this."

The discussion turns to the cesarean rate, and the 8-pound "macro-somic" baby about to be extracted. "Everybody covers themselves in this profession," says Crane, shrugging. "Unfortunately, this profession is outcome-based." He cites a colleague who is 36 and will never practice medicine again because she's already had four lawsuits and is uninsurable. "If that kid has a shoulder dystocia, and there's damage, that case will go to court, and that doctor will lose," he says. This same fear is behind the doctors refusing to attend higher-risk breech births, vaginal births after cesarean, and twins, opting instead to schedule a cesarean, even though a cesarean also makes the birth higher-risk. Over the course of the day, I survey the OBs on their willingness to attend these births, and the answer is repeatedly no. "We learned 20 years ago that if you got a lawsuit for a breech in labor, then it was indefensible," says Crane. "Now that's true of VBAC and twins and shoulder dystocia. Those are the cases that can make you unable to practice obstetrics."

That said, "a cesarean isn't always an easy way to get the baby out," one OB explained to me. Breech babies are still tricky to deliver abdominally, and after hours of labor, a baby may be so far "engaged" in the pelvis that it requires what's called a "push up": a practitioner who's not operating inserts a hand into the vagina to push the fetus's head *back* into the uterus as the surgeon pulls it out from above.

The same impulse that pushes a gray-zone labor toward a cesarean pushes a gray-zone pregnancy toward an induction, which increases the woman's chance of having a cesarean. On one of my early-morning visits to the hospital, a doctor was inducing a patient because she had reached 41 weeks. In the elevator, I asked whether he thought the induction would work. "No," he said. On the third floor, we walked into the patient's room. She was lying on her side with an oxygen mask over her face, clutching the rails on the bed. She had been admitted the night before and was induced with a Cervidil suppository and a rubber "balloon" inflated into her cervix. Staff started Pitocin overnight and an epidural at around 6:30 a.m., but she was still uncomfortable. The nurse and resident showed the doctor some "scary" decelerations on the electronic fetal monitor tracing, which had then picked back up. The paper strip streamed and gathered on the floor like a wide ribbon. The doctor broke the woman's water bag and retrieved the Foley balloon, holding it up for me to see. "The reason she has the oxygen mask is because the nurses are worried about the baby's heart rate," he told me, then turned to the patient. "M_____, I don't care what anyone says, you're doing beautifully!"

The physician said he now had some hope for the patient—the balloon had "done its job," and the patient was in a "good labor pattern." Residents and nurses kept the Pitocin flowing all day, and at around 9 p.m., the doctor manually rotated the baby's head as it descended—it was turned such that it would have come out sunny side up, which is much more difficult—and held back the remaining "lip" of cervix while the woman pushed. The baby was born vaginally, weighing 9 lb, 5 oz. "With another OB, there's a good chance she would have had a C-section around dinner time," said the doctor.

When I asked the doctors what worries them, the actuality of having a bad outcome or being sued, they shrugged. "That's a good question," said Fain. "I know that we should not be inducing so many patients; I know that we should be giving patients more time to be overdue; I know that as we speak, somebody pregnant with twins is being told that she can't have vaginal birth, and someone else is being told she can't have a VBAC," he said, clearly frustrated. Fain is an elder now at St. Barnabas. His first impulse isn't a cesarean for "failure to progress," but more time—or possibly forceps. His first impulse with twins is to try for a vaginal birth and see how things go. But the younger doctors won't back him up, and some of the residents he's training have actually refused to participate in cases they perceive as risky. "Here's the thing," he said to me. "Why fight it? People tell me I'm crazy, I'm a cowboy." Meanwhile, the insurance company is "teaching me how not to get sued," which means not taking vaginal twins or VBACs, abandoning the forceps, and wheeling more patients to the OR at the first sign of difficulty.

A physician in Cleveland, the city with the second-highest malpractice premium rates in the country, put it to me this way: "You can't have a 10% cesarean rate and be staring at $120 million judgments."

There is so much risk aversion on labor and delivery wards that hospitals have dedicated "risk management" departments. The anxiety in fact has created a competitive market. A Canadian company recently released a computer system called CALM (it stands for computer-assisted labor management), and its purpose, essentially, is to calm doctors down. Nurses punch in several criteria, and the software churns out a graphic representation of neonatal risks, such as shoulder dystocia and fetal distress. In a study of 11,000 first-time mothers, CALM contributed to a decrease in cesareans from 19.5% to 16.6%, according to company literature.[36]

The solution often proposed for the malpractice crisis is "tort reform." But in states with judgment caps, such as Texas and Nevada, insurance premiums have not decreased, and neither has the cesarean rate. The American College of Obstetricians and Gynecologists supports "tort reform" via its political action committee Physicians for Women's Health, which is housed within ACOG's Washington, DC, headquarters. During the 2006 election cycle, 78% of the PAC's $230,000 campaign contributions went to Republicans; nearly $10,000, it should be noted, went to the anti-abortion, anti-stem cell research Pennsylvania senator Rick Santorum.[37] The 2006 ACOG conference, also in DC, happened to coincide with a Senate vote on President Bush's medical liability reform bill; companion legislation, sponsored by Santorum, would have specifically limited what women could collect in damages from obstetricians. ACOG sent a busload of doctors in lab coats to the Capitol to show their support (the measure was defeated).

Calling the liability situation a "crisis" is itself debatable. Tort filings and judgment awards are both actually down, and a 2006 Harvard study of 1500 lawsuits found that the vast majority were not frivolous; most cases were settled out of court, and of those that went to trial, plaintiffs lost 80 percent of the time.[38] A 2003 report by the General Accounting Office found the so-called exodus of physicians from practice to be unsubstantiated.[39] Physicians claim that although most cases don't make it to court, out-of-court settlements are frequent and astronomical. Whatever the actual threat, the annual premiums reach dizzying heights in some states—$200,000 in Florida, for instance—and fear of a suit seems to weigh heavily in clinical decision making. Every patient is a potential plaintiff, every less-than-perfect fetal monitor strip potential evidence. Most doctors have dealt with more than one suit.[40] One physician explained the phenomenon this way: "The minute you see a deceleration on the heart monitor, you say maybe it's fetal distress, better to do a cesarean. You see the ultrasound and think maybe it's too big, maybe we'll have a shoulder dystocia, better to do a cesarean. A lot of that is driven by fear of liability."

De Angelis calls it the monkey on his back. "Society is not accepting of one bad outcome," he says. "I can't afford to have one bad outcome." Sitting in the central nurses' station later that afternoon, filling out forms, De Angelis points to the tic-tac-toe board of monitors behind him, like a wall of TVs in a department store, which display the fetal heart rates and uterine contractions for all patients on the ward. (There's another wall of monitors, next to a TV, in the OB lounge/men's locker room). "You want to know why the C-section rate is so high?" he says, gesticulating toward the wall. "Right there. The electronic fetal monitor." Nearly every doctor I talk to acknowledges that the monitors only increase the chance of a cesarean but are required by the hospital for its legal protection, although it doesn't seem to work for that either, because an expert can read a strip any which way in court. "You know, there's a term in psychology, *learned helplessness*," says De Angelis. "That's what's happened in medicine."

The doctors at St. Barnabas admit that a cesarean does not guarantee a good outcome and that surgery is more likely to result in a complication for the mother. Crane is arrestingly blunt on this point. "The risks are maternal, and maternal risks are much smaller to us as obstetricians," he says. "There's no doubt in my mind that there's more maternal morbidity with a cesarean. But a hole in the bladder, a post-operative infection—that's not going to ruin their lives. A bad baby is going to ruin our lives."

PATIENCE

Thirty-two miles south on the Jersey Turnpike, Andrew Garber, MD, is the director of maternal-fetal medicine at Pascack Valley Hospital. "We're one of the rare specialties where patients require 8, 10, 12 hours," he says, sympathizing with his peers to the north. "And in the HMO climate you don't get paid any more for spending 12 hours with a patient than you do for 45 minutes. You're not being reimbursed by the hour; it's by getting the baby delivered and getting yourself out of there." Garber's mother was an obstetrician in New York City; she knew her patients and what was going on in their lives. He entered medicine thinking he'd do the same. But the climate, both legal and economic, encourages inductions, cesareans, and drive-through office visits. He repeats the word *convenience* over and over. A cesarean "takes 45 minutes. They come in, they do their C-section, and they go back to their offices or back to the rest of their lives."

In 2002, Garber felt he had a solution to this problem. "My personal feeling is that physicians should work with midwives. This is my answer," he says. "The American system in my opinion is faulty. It tries to get physicians to be in two places at once. In the European system, midwives run the labor floor. And they call the surgeon when they feel that a patient needs surgery."

Garber approached Lonnie Morris, a certified nurse midwife who had been practicing in the area for 30 years and could no longer deliver at her birthing center—her malpractice insurer, Princeton Insurance Company, jacked up her premium from $30,000 to $300,000 in one year. Morris and two other midwives now attend 20 percent of the 1000 yearly births at Pascack. The overall C-section rate at Pascack is still high, 36.7% in 2004,[41] but among the midwives, the rate is 11%, and that number includes women having VBACs and twins—births that are considered higher risk. I asked Morris what her secret is: "Waiting," she told me. "The tincture of time." She also encourages women to stay mobile during labor and push in advantageous positions. "I do water births, I do side-lying, I do all-fours. We have birthing stools," she said. "I do it anyway they want—however they're comfortable."

"Midwives are committed to labor. They're not committed to C-sections," says Garber. "They will spend 8, 10, 12 hours with a patient. And that allows me to go back to the office, see my patients, or take care of my life, my children, my family." Garber told a local newspaper that he started the midwifery program because "We thought it would give us an opportunity to continue to have some vaginal births."[42]

"The numbers are out of control," he says of C-sections, and he points out that maternity wards seem to be held to lower ethical standards than other specialties. "If you do major intra-abdominal surgery for no good reason anywhere else in any major medical center, somebody is going to come and talk to you about it. The only other area like this is plastic surgery," says Garber. "I think the medical community is not taking this as seriously as it should."

The midwives are not necessarily a financially attractive solution, Garber concedes. "You have to pay midwives, but you don't get reimbursed any more [money]." Nurse-midwives cost less, earning a fraction of an obstetrician's salary, but they still require malpractice coverage. They also spend more time with fewer patients, and their patients receive fewer billable procedures, which brings in less revenue. "The system doesn't support midwifery, but it seemed like the right thing to do," says Garber. "I realized that I couldn't give patients an appropriate level of commitment. So I came up with the idea of who could. Either it's going to be a resident, whom they've never met, or it's a midwife whom the patient knows. I'd prefer the midwife." I ask him if in working with midwives he'd learned anything new. "Patience," he says.

When I first spoke with him, Garber was also supporting several home-birth midwives by signing what's called a practice agreement. By law, licensed midwives in New Jersey must have a documented relationship with a physician who agrees to provide consultation and urgent care if a transport is required. But in the fall of 2006, his insurer, Medical Malpractice Insurance Pool (MMIP), told him surcharges would apply for each independent midwife he backs up. "According to them, you get what's called vicarious liability for anything they do," Garber tells me. That is, he could be sued by a midwife's patient, even if he never once treated her.

Susan Jenkins, former general counsel for the American College of Nurse Midwives, has been litigating on behalf of health professional for forty years—one of her clients was Bill Clinton's mother, Virginia Kelley, who was a nurse anesthetist. Jenkins says vicarious liability is a myth. Jenkins explains that insurance companies set premiums based on the number of claims and the severity of claims filed previously against a particular specialty. But vicarious liability claims are not recorded separately; if there were any such claims they would just be counted with all the rest. "So if you impose a surcharge on the subset of those claims that involve vicarious liability, you're double dipping," says Jenkins. "Insurers have no empirical basis for doing that and no actuarial basis for doing that, which makes it an unfair insurance practice."

After Garber got the call from MMIP, he decided to sever the practice agreements with midwives who are not based at the hospital like Morris. I ask him how those midwives will practice now. "They're in trouble," he says. "I'm telling you, it's a disaster, this whole situation. You try to do the right thing, and you may not get covered if you do the right thing, even if it's accepted medical practice."

WE'RE VERY PRO-EPIDURAL

At St. Barnabas, each nurse handles at least two patients, and nearly all the labors are actively managed. That means patients are admitted in early labor, given amniotomies if their water hasn't already broken, and given an epidural usually followed by Pitocin. The nurses estimate that 90% of the patients are induced or augmented. "There's no reason not to do the Pitocin," said one doctor. Another called expectant management "babysitting." "I don't do the expectant management thing," she said. The hospital is also crowded, which determines the type of care given. Just as Lethbridge described in Florida, beds need to be kept free. "This is not the kind of place you come to if you want to sit in a bathtub or roll on a ball," the charge nurse told me. "We have a high volume of deliveries. We can't have people just sitting around, taking up labor beds, and walking the halls. We're very pro-epidural."

"A lot of times we'll get a call from a resident," says Richard Fain. "The resident says, 'Listen, we have a bed situation here. We've got to get your patient going.' Sometimes that will happen, and you're in the office and it's 10 in morning, and you say, 'Well, I can't be there until dinner time, leave her be.' And they'll call back up. Usually it's a second-year resident saying, 'I've got to get her delivered. We've got to get something going.'" If the going doesn't happen, the operating room is down the hall, just past the nurses' station. A patient would just need her epidural "topped off," and she's ready for surgery.

Cesarean section is, after all, the doctrine of active management taken to its logical conclusion, the replacement of the physiological birth sequence in its entirety, and it can be achieved in a tiny fraction of the time. In some places, physicians who wait for vaginal birth have actually been told that they are a drain on too many resources. Helen Sandland, an obstetrician in Wilmington, North Carolina, resigned in June 2005 after hospital administrators told her to increase her cesarean rate, which was a modest 10%. "Quite a lot of C-sections are being done for so-called failure to progress," Sandland told the *Wilmington Star*, "If you haven't progressed in a couple of hours, a C-section's waiting. There's certainly a pressure to keep patients moving through."[43] In the 2005 *Mothers* survey, a quarter of the women who had cesareans said they were pressured into it.[44]

The charge nurse at St. Barnabas guesstimates that 40% of the women who labor end up with cesareans. "Some women just aren't willing and active participants in the labor process," is how one doctor explains it, "including pushing." Then again, once a woman is fully dilated, she is likely to have been immobile for hours, with a paralyzing agent and narcotics streaming into her spine and artificial oxytocin pumping her uterus, and she hasn't eaten or had anything to drink since she got to the hospital. Her body's own labor sequence has been hijacked, for all intents and purposes. She has been made passive, yet she is expected to be active.

In the case of a shoulder dystocia—the complication that every doctor dreads—a simple position change to hands-and-knees is the least invasive and often the most effective remedy. It can also resolve fetal distress because it takes pressure off the umbilical cord. Studies have shown the efficacy of this age-old birthing position, which has come to be called the Gaskin maneuver after the Tennessee midwife, Ina May Gaskin, who reintroduced it into practice in the late 1970s.[45] With an anesthetized patient, however, the maneuver is difficult, if not impossible. The patient is physically no more capable of being an "active participant" than the Victorian women passed out on chloroform.

On my visit to Barnabas, I did get to see the vaginal birth in room 5—an actively managed birth. I introduced myself to the woman, who had the likeness of an exhausted, swollen Penelope Cruz, and asked her how she was feeling. "I just want to get this over with," she said. She'd come in at 4 a.m. and was quickly set up with an epidural. At 9 a.m. they gave her Pitocin. "I stalled at 7 centimeters," she told me.

It was about 10:45 a.m., and the doctor sat at the foot of the hospital bed to check the woman's cervix. It was fully dilated. "OK, try and push for me. Let's see if this baby is coming," she said, her fingers still inside. "That's great!" she said. "Really?" asked the woman. "I can't feel anything." "Don't worry, you just need to follow directions," said the doctor.

The nurse lowered the head of the bed so that it lay flat, helping the woman to shift herself farther back and bend her knees open. The doctor flipped up pedals on either side and told the woman to rest her feet on them. "I can't, I can't," she said. "Come on, just try," said the doctor. "They will help to brace you."

The nurse, a slight woman with the voice and vocabulary of a track coach, stood at the patient's left side, turning between her and the flat-screen monitor. When the monitor showed a contraction approaching, she had the patient hold her breath and push for 10 full seconds. "Pick your head up! Chin to chest!" yelled the nurse, counting out loud to 10. "OK, catch your breath." This went on twice or three times, and then the nurse grabbed an extra pillow to help the woman keep her head up. The OB checked her again. "You're doing great, the baby is coming down!" "Oh, so you don't think you're going to need to cut me?" asked the patient. The doctor shook her head. "Oh good, because last time that was even worse than the birth," she said.

The doctor then asked whether "Dad" could come over to the bed. He had been sitting with the patient's mother—who was looking slightly green—in chairs to the side. The doctor had him hold his wife's right leg, knee to elbow, and the nurse held the other. The woman was now essentially in lithotomy position, with human stirrups. "OK, deep breath. Ready? Go!" shouted the nurse. "One! Two! Three! Four! Five! Six! Seven! Eight! Nine! Ten! OK, rest." The baby's head was now bulging, and the OB's gloved hands were stretching the perineum around it as the mother pushed. "OK, catch your breath, you're doing great," said the doctor. The cycle repeated again, and out came the head with the next full push. "Push again! Harder! Go again!" yelled the nurse. The baby slid out into the doctor's hands, and she immediately cut the cord and carried the crying infant to the warmer. "Happy Birthday," she said. Two nurses and a neonatologist hovered over the warmer, rubbing the baby with towels and suctioning with a long plastic tube they repeatedly threaded down his throat. The birth was called at 11:18.

The placenta was summoned immediately by the OB, who steadily drew the cord out with a surgical clamp. While the baby was being measured and weighed, its eyes smeared with antibiotic ointment, and its arm injected with vitamin K, the physician drew the blood out of the cord for preservation. After she'd sealed the blood pouch and packed up the kit, she returned to the mother to examine her vagina, noting a second-degree laceration along her episiotomy scar. She asked the nurse to call in a resident, a young man with glasses and the build of a linebacker, who broke down the lower third of the bed to get closer to his patient and pulled up a stool. Over the next 20 minutes, the OB stood by directing the perspiring resident in the repair. On the television near the ceiling, which had been on the entire time, Rosie O'Donnell was waving her hands at the audience. The mother and the physician were both glancing up at it. At 11:36, the nurse brought the bundled baby to its smiling father, who held it up to mom for a kiss on the forehead. At 11:55, 37 minutes after she gave birth, the baby was laid in her arms.

AN UNFAIR COMPARISON

At the NIH conference titled "Cesarean Delivery on Maternal Request," which took place over 3 days in an auditorium on the NIH campus in Bethesda, Maryland, in March 2006, a graphic was projected onto a wide screen several times: the scales of justice, with elective cesarean on one side and planned vaginal delivery on the other. The scales were balanced.

A panel of 18 professionals, handpicked for their impartiality by the NIH, sat in two rows of nine on the stage. The audience was packed, orchestra to balcony, with all manner of stakeholders: obstetricians, family practice physicians, pediatricians, nurses, midwives, doulas, childbirth educators, journal editors, public health researchers, authors, academics, and activists. They came from England, Canada, Texas, Michigan, Florida, Tennessee, New Mexico, and several other faraway places. They clapped, they laughed, they moaned, they hissed. The research presentations were bundled by several topics and presented two or three at a time, after which a 20-minute period was allotted for audience questions and comments. That period proved inadequate for the number of comments. Attendees would begin lining up at the two microphones, set up in both aisles of the auditorium, as the last word of the last presentation was uttered (some would arrive 30 minutes early each day to save seats next to a microphone).

Even if it was not clear to the NIH prior to the conference, the energy in the auditorium hinted at the social and political dimensions of the topic at hand and at the perceived impact the conference would have, even beyond U.S. borders. The audience seemed to feel that this wasn't just about whether an uncertain minority of American women should be able to choose a C-section if they so desire; it was a referendum on the cesarean trend itself.

At times, it felt like the audience, dominated by critics of obstetric care, and the panel, dominated by ACOG members, were coming from two distinct and isolated cultures and were speaking two different languages. What the panel was calling a "planned vaginal delivery," many of the audience members were calling "poorly managed childbirth." The scales, the audience was saying, cannot be balanced, because the outcomes of medically unnecessary cesareans were being compared to the outcomes of *typically* managed vaginal birth, not optimally supported, physiological childbirth.

"This was an unfair comparison," explains Michael Klein, MD, a professor emeritus at the University of British Columbia and chair of the Department of Family Practice at British Columbia Women's and Children's Hospital. Klein was asked by NIH to participate as a research reviewer. "The vast majority of hospital-based births that were being used for comparison are what we call unphysiological births—that is, births that involve a lot of technology, a lot of electronic fetal monitoring, usually the more conventional birth positions, such as the lithotomy, episiotomy rates way above what should be the accepted norm, and heavily coached pushing that is damaging to the pelvic floor. That's the norm in America. And you're comparing that against cesarean sections, which are probably conducted reasonably well."

The point was made at the microphone over and over. Why not look at planned vaginal delivery that is physiologically supported and compare *that* to planned cesareans, they asked. Some referred the panel to specific studies that were not included in the presentations and that showed that low-risk women planning to support the normal birth process, often with midwives, experience fewer interventions. At times, the panelists appeared genuinely confused by referrals to literature on midwife-attended births. "I don't see the utility of this design with respect to cesarean delivery on maternal request," rejoined one panel member, dismissing the point that actively managed childbirth should not be synonymous with "normal."

Then again, traditionally managed, unphysiological childbirth—the kind I saw at St. Barnabas—*is* the norm, and most women, especially first-time mothers, face a significant risk of a long labor followed by cesarean or trauma to the perineum. This leaves women "choosing" between poor labor management and major surgery. One physician made this point clearly during her presentation. She blamed the "subtle infusion of technology into obstetrics . . . the numerous tubes, drugs, and attachments. . . . No wonder some women may choose cesarean delivery," she said. Peter Bernstein in New York sees this not as a reason to sanction and encourage surgical birth, but rather as cause for professional introspection. "Part of problem is the way we're managing labor," he told me. "And I'm part of the problem. I can't do a labor without continuous electronic fetal monitoring; the number of patients I'm inducing for this, that, and the other reason is increasing." In an essay, Bernstein called the desire for a medically unnecessary cesarean a "failure of modern medicine and society at large."

DeLee could not have predicted the malpractice climate, but he manifested the notion of "patient choice" back when women had just won the right to vote. After all, DeLee wasn't just calling for prophylactic forceps; he was calling for a transformation of childbirth from a sequence the woman's body executes into a procedure the physician performs. And he saw this procedure evolving from forceps and episiotomy into the cesarean, and he recognized that women would have to be on board for the transformation to be complete: "Many women are ready to undergo the slightly increased risk of cesarean section in order to avoid the perils and pain of even ordinary labor," he said in 1921. "I am confident that if the women were given only a little encouragement in this direction, the demand for cesarean section would be overwhelming."[46] Critics charged the NIH conference with giving such encouragement. As one attendee, a journal editor, put it, the NIH effectively "put cesarean section over the counter."

CHAPTER 3

Denied Birth

JANE EVANS IS ABOUT TO CATCH a breech baby. The woman she's attending is on all fours, and the baby's buttocks are emerging: one cheek, then the crease demarking two; then one chubby leg plops down, then the other. The baby—a girl—is now dangling from her mother. "Most women left to their own devices will get on hands and knees," Evans explains, clicking to bring up the next slide. "The baby needs to turn its pelvis, which is really hard to do if mum is on her back." We next see her gloved hands gently bringing one of the baby's elbows down, then the other. "Remember, you're assisting progress—you're not pulling," she says. More of the baby hangs free—she's jerking her knees up in midair. Evans explains the mechanics at work: the head needs to be flexed chin-to-chest to be born safely. There are maneuvers an attendant can use to facilitate this; one is to reach up with a finger, find the baby's mouth, and draw the chin down. But here, the baby is doing it herself. "What happens when you lift your knees?" Evans asks rhetorically, as members of the audience bob their heads. "You drop your chin to chest." She clicks to the next slide. The mother has now sunk to chest and knees, butt to ceiling, with arms extended as if supplicating before royalty. "When the baby hits the G-spot, mother drops to the floor and goes

73

Muslim," says Evans. Laughter in the audience. She grabs a skeletal pelvis and fetus doll off the podium, modeling how on supplication, the mother's pelvis pivots around the baby's head like a visor, setting it free. "And look," she says, moving to the next slide. "The baby practically falls out."

Evans is a British midwife who has been in practice for 30 years. She has a slight Martha Stewart look about her—mainly the silvery bob and exacting, lashy eyes—but also a playful, saucy air. We are in a low-lit auditorium at the Women's Hospital in Vancouver, British Columbia, and she is teaching vaginal breech birth 101. Not to the doctors at the hospital, though. Like nearly all obstetricians in North America, they no longer attend vaginal breech birth, instead performing a cesarean section. Evans's audience is mainly midwives from the United States and Canada who have come for a 2-day conference on the subject. Evans has flown in from England; Maggie Banks, midwife and author of *Breech Birth Woman-Wise*, has come from New Zealand; physicians from Belgium, Germany, Norway, the Netherlands, Australia, and across Canada have come to present research. Evans is introduced by Philip Hall, MD, the Manitoba perinatologist and professor of maternal-fetal medicine, who bemoans the current standard of automatic cesarean. "Can't we offer something better to women? Can we do anything to turn the tide?" he asks.

The breech baby greets the world with his bottom rather than his head, his first hello often a poop instead of a cry. It is difficult to visualize, but imagine the Olympic diver doing a perfect pike; he jumps straight up off the board and brings his feet up to touch his hands. The frank breech, the most common breech position, is the pike dive. The baby, even more flexible than the world athlete, is essentially folded in half, and instead of a head crowning on the perineum, it will be a right or left buttock. A "complete" breech, almost sitting cross-legged, might drop knee-first. And if the baby is a footling breech, she will greet the air first with her toes.

Fetuses grow sitting up, but by 33 weeks, 85% to 90% have turned head down, or vertex.[1] A head-down presentation is easier on all parties, and the shape of the uterus and abdominal muscles usually make it so, crowding a growing fetus's body so its head is drawn toward the exit. But there are stubborn babies, who at 34, 35, and 36 weeks still haven't flipped. As time goes on, they get even more set in their ways, and the chances of their turning plummet. Practitioners have ways of coaxing fetal gymnastics—there's the Webster technique, a chiropractic adjustment; there's manipulating the fetus via belly palpation, called external version; there's acupuncture, acupressure, and even a Chinese practice called moxibustion, in which a cigar roll of herbs is burned near the outer edge of the mother's pinky toe. This technique showed a 75% success rate in a clinical trial and made headlines in the *Washington Post*.[2] Most of these methods are never tried in the United States, however, and at term, about 3% of fetuses insist on diving pike rather than swan.

What are we to do with these babies? The vaginal breech birth poses some additional risk, the footling much more so than the frank or complete. "What's highly debatable," says Andrew Kotaska, MD, a Vancouver physician who spoke at the conference, "is the magnitude of that risk." With a vertex presentation, the widest part of the baby, the head, leads the way, thereby ensuring the rest of the body passage. What complicates the breech birth is that this does not work in reverse: the baby's body can clear a partially dilated cervix, but its head cannot. If that happens, it is called "head entrapment," and it's as threatening as it sounds. The other complicating factor is the umbilical cord, still the baby's lifeline until it takes its first breath. As the breech baby backs out, the cord is between his head and the cervix. The baby is equipped to withstand some cord compression, but only some. One of the main charges of the breech attendant is to ensure that the cervix is completely dilated before the mother pushes, because once the body is out to the navel, the head needs to follow within minutes. For the woman giving birth, the process is counterintuitive: at the first urge to push, she should resist.

The breech birth is counterintuitive for the attendant, as well, and has been called the "hands off the breech" approach. Maggie Banks tweaks it to "hands off, brains on." A breech birth, Jane Evans explains to her audience, can't be induced. It can't be rushed with artificial oxytocin or rupture of the membranes. Forceps can be deadly, and episiotomy risks the baby inhaling blood. For the most part, the tools of obstetric labor management are off limits. The breech baby demands patience; she rejects active management; she demands normal, physiological birth. "The mother has got to be very, very aware of what's going on in her body. You must not give any direction whatsoever," Evans tells her audience. "No, 'Push! Push! Push!' You never even wipe the poo away," she says, referring to the maternal bowel emptying that often happens during childbirth. "What happens when you wipe? The sphincter closes. Now you try closing your anal sphincter without closing everything else down there."

Evans and her midwifery partner Mary Cronk have attended numerous breeches and twins over the past 7 years. They are now England's resident experts on breech birth, conducting trainings and breech simulations—called "A Day at the Breech"—with midwives, who are the primary maternity care providers in the UK, just as in the rest of Europe. Evans is in the process of publishing her observations on the mechanics of breech birth. Little has been written in the English-language medical literature about the hands-off method. Breech delivery has typically been managed like a head-down birth but even more proactively. One approach is to lift the baby's body toward the ceiling as it is emerging, exert pressure on the mother's abdomen, and apply forceps to release the head. Epidural anesthesia is often mandatory.

Evans and Cronk previously worked for the UK's National Health Service, which is supposed to provide the option of midwife-attended home birth to maternity patients. Both midwives left the service in 1991. They found that women with breech babies were being denied home birth and encouraged to schedule cesareans. "In the UK, choice rests with the woman," said Evans. But if the choice is between surgery and a hands-on breech delivery, they aren't given much of a choice. So Evans and Cronk went freelance to care for those women pushed outside the system. Evans told the audience at the conference about one woman who lived clear on the other side of Great Britain and took an overnight sleeper train to deliver near Evans. "She was contracting the whole way," said Evans, and arrived ready to push. "The dad likes to say, 'The first time I saw my daughter, she was wearing her mother as a hat.'"

"Choice has been removed from women," said Kotaska, who was a general practitioner in rural British Columbia before becoming board-certified in obstetrics. ("I realized that I needed to have surgical skills, since there is no backup care for miles," he told me.) During his obstetric residency, he wanted breech experience but found no North American program that could accommodate him. Instead he traveled to Germany's

Klinikum Nürnberg, where 62% of women carrying breech babies give birth vaginally. He studied under Michael Krause, MD, author of the German medical text on breech birth *Beckenendlage*. "One of the reasons a lot of us are here is to figure out how to reestablish choice for women," Kotaska told the conference.

Women in North America who want a vaginal breech birth are often denied it outright. The same is happening for women carrying twins—one or both babies may be breech—and women seeking a vaginal birth after cesarean, or VBAC. These births carry some additional risk, but these risks must be weighed against the risks of cesarean section. In 2004, the *New York Times* reported that some 300 U.S. hospitals had banned VBAC,[3] and the 2005 *Listening to Mothers* survey found that 57% of women who sought a VBAC were denied the option by either the hospital or their caregiver.[4] Few women have breeches or twins, but as the primary cesarean rate continues to climb in the United States, the VBAC climate affects a large segment of the population; there are millions of American women in their childbearing years who have at least one cesarean scar. And it is a further burden on a woman with a breech baby that undergoing a primary cesarean predisposes her to an unwanted repeat.

Ironically, it is independent home-birth midwives, some of whom practice illegally, who are left attending these higher-risk vaginal births. And they are surpassing physicians in experience and expertise in the delicate matter of vaginal breech delivery. What has become a lost art in the delivery room is kept alive in women's homes by care providers who are largely unrecognized by the obstetric profession and even criminalized in several states. The conference in Vancouver was organized by a British midwife, three of the presenters were midwives, and not one speaker, physician or midwife, was American. Many of the midwives in the audience wouldn't sign the roster because they practice illegally in the United States.

Evans's talk ends with a final slide of the mother (the one who "went Muslim") sitting at the edge of her bed with the baby on her breast, a streak of blood on her thigh, and a smile that is pure, flushed joy. "This is one very proud mother, and she was told that if she went to the hospital she would have to have a cesarean section, because she was a first-time mother, a primip breech," says Evans. "She was forced to stay at home. And that's why we have to keep our skills up. She had no other options."

THE ART OF WAITING

Breech babies were always more problematic. They seemed to get stuck more, they seemed to get hurt more, they seemed to die more. In the 1940s, about 1 in 20 American breech babies died, or 13,000 each year.[5] Today, we know that breech babies are more likely than vertex babies to be compromised in some way. We also know that their high death rate in the first half of the century was due to the "assisted breech" delivery technique of the day: heavy anesthesia, manual pressure on the uterus, traction on the baby's body, and routine forceps to extract the head. This was demonstrated in a landmark 1953 review by two Columbia University obstetricians. They found, "The more manipulation is performed and the earlier this manipulation is instituted, the greater is the fetal mortality and morbidity, to say nothing of maternal injuries."[6]

The review cited the dramatic benefit of the Bracht maneuver, developed by a German obstetrician, which was as close to "hands off" as one could get with the mother flat on her back. The key to the Bracht maneuver was "the art of waiting" for spontaneous delivery with minimal manipulation, mainly supporting the baby's body with a force "equivalent to the force of gravity; that is, equivalent to the weight of that portion of the baby which has already been born" (in other words, equivalent to the gravitational pull on the baby were the woman upright). Bracht presented a film of the technique to a meeting of physicians in Amsterdam in 1938, along with analysis of 206 successful breech deliveries, without one fetal injury or death. "Bracht's work represents the largest reduction in breech-related infant mortality in obstetric history," says Kotaska. At the time it led to more than 30 trials in Latin America and Europe, showing dramatic reductions in breech-related mortality. Not one of those studies, however, was translated into English.

In Europe, breech technique continued to improve; in England and North America, it gradually fell out of fashion. Surgery itself was becoming safer, and the more obstetricians performed the cesarean, the better they got at it. By 1978, 60% of breech babies were born by cesarean.[7] By 1990, that number was 85%.[8] The practitioners who continued to deliver breech in the 1990s were considered at best quaint, at worst dare devils, even though the true risk of vaginal breech birth, as compared to the risk of cesarean, was still up for debate.

Then a large study seemed to settle it. Led by Toronto epidemiologist Mary Hannah, MD, highly respected in the obstetric research world, this randomized controlled trial—considered the gold standard of clinical research—involved more than 2000 women in 121 centers around the world.[9] The women, carrying singleton babies (i.e., not twins or multiples) presenting breech, were assigned to plan either a vaginal birth or a cesarean. The study, published in the *Lancet* in 2000, reported a statistically significant difference in the number of poor infant outcomes—babies that died or suffered "serious neonatal morbidity." The rate was 5% among the vaginal breech group and 1.6% among the planned cesarean group.

Hannah concluded that a policy of planned cesarean for a term fetus in the breech position "is substantially better" than vaginal birth. And the standard of care changed overnight. Women were told they'd be risking their babies' lives if they didn't plan a cesarean, ACOG released a new recommendation,[10] and the debate was officially over. The effect was worldwide: a 2003 survey found that among 80 centers in 23 countries that had previously been offering vaginal breech delivery, 92% had declared a moratorium on it.[11] Even in the Netherlands, where half of women carrying breeches had delivered vaginally, the proportion dropped to 20% within just 2 months after publication of the study.[12]

Then people took a closer look at the data. The study comprised subjects from 26 countries, some with high infant mortality rates—among them Brazil, Egypt, India, Mexico, and Zimbabwe—and some with low infant mortality rates—among them Australia, Chile, Finland, Portugal, and the United States. Overall, it appeared that breech babies were three times more likely to die if born vaginally. But among the countries with good track records of infant mortality, there was no significant difference in the numbers of deaths, indicating that the standard of care in certain countries was likely to blame, not the route of delivery. What remained more prevalent among the babies born vaginally in developed countries was "serious neonatal morbidity," an umbrella term for several unfavorable outcomes, but the long-term significance of that diagnosis was yet unknown. Citing these criticisms, two U.S. obstetricians with successful breech experience, including the lead author of *Williams Obstetrics*, published a 2002 letter urging ACOG to revise its "didactic" policy.[13]

Others argued that Hannah's methodology was inconsistent. As is standard, babies with lethal congenital anomalies were excluded from the results, but several questionable deaths remained, including a baby with a large head, low-set ears, and deep-set eyes and another baby with an exposed spinal cord—both features consistent with lethal anomalies—as well as a 2.5-pound stillborn twin and a baby who presented head-first. Each scenario violated the study's criteria. "We are left wondering whether there are similar irregularities and violations of the inclusion criteria elsewhere," wrote Peter Bernstein, MD, of Albert Einstein College of Medicine in New York City. The Hannah study "should not be the last word on vaginal breech deliveries."[14]

Others questioned the study's design. Researchers intended for an "experienced clinician—i.e., someone who considered himself or herself to be skilled and experienced at vaginal breech delivery" to attend the births. But many of the most experienced centers did not participate, including Southwestern Medical Center in Dallas, Texas, the U.S. hospital with the highest number of vaginal breech deliveries, at 19%;[15] the University of Alabama at Birmingham Hospital; and Klinikum Nürnberg in Germany, where Kotaska studied. Michael Krause said his center declined because they didn't think the protocols were either safe or ethical, particularly the directive to randomize women to vaginal birth or cesarean section. "Why would we randomize women to a cesarean that they don't need?" he said. An OB/GYN chair from Australia who also opted out said that hospitals "had to be dragged kicking and screaming to be in the study. They were scraping the bottom of the barrel to get participants."

The researchers expected the participating centers to achieve a 50% rate of vaginal breech delivery or they would be excluded from the results (they needed the numbers to achieve statistical significance). If Southwestern had decided to participate, for instance, it would have had to more than double its rate overnight. That's not an ideal study cohort, explains Andrew Kotaska. In a paper published in the *British Medical Journal*, he argues that breech delivery requires "considerable skill." If you ask inexperienced physicians to start performing with "considerable skill" overnight, you will get poor outcomes because they are at the bottom of their learning curve. Further, protected from liability by participating in a randomized controlled trial, physicians were given license to push their comfort zones.[16]

Kotaska offers an analogy. He notes that in the UK and North America, about 20% of hysterectomies are vaginal (as opposed to abdominal), also a procedure that requires considerable skill. "Encouraging a group of surgeons to suddenly increase their rate from 20 to 60 percent would not be a meaningful way to evaluate the safety of the procedure," he writes. "Nor should all women have an abdominal hysterectomy because some are poor candidates for vaginal surgery and because some surgeons lack the skill or experience to support a safe, high vaginal hysterectomy rate. . . . Increasing the rate arbitrarily and randomising such a complex mix of patient and operator characteristics would compromise safety, yet this is what happened in the term breech trial."

Hannah brushes aside the criticisms. The study followed standard research protocols, she says, and excluding the questionable baby deaths after randomization would have "introduced bias." With a randomized trial, you assume that such surprise anomalies would be similarly distributed across the groups. On this, Kotaska is in agreement. As for his critique of the study overlooking "considerable skill," Hannah says Kotaska is "totally incorrect in his assumptions." Only certain practitioners at a center were signed off to participate in the study, and they had to be deemed "experienced" by their department chairs, she told me. Still, the centers with the most expertise did not participate, and Kotaska's point stands that those who participated had to meet a quota. Others have pointed out that in spite of the effort to mandate competence, nearly one-fifth of the women randomized to vaginal birth were attended by practitioners who had not been authorized.[17]

The critics were somewhat vindicated in 2004, when Hannah published follow-up results to the study.[18] It turned out that at 2 years following birth, there were no neurological differences between the babies born by cesarean and those born vaginally. In other words, the initial diagnosis of "serious neonatal morbidity" had not predicted damage. The only statistically significant outcome was "medical problems not otherwise specified," which was higher among the cesarean-born babies. The follow-up study concluded that "planned cesarean delivery is not associated with a reduction in risk of death or neurodevelopmental delay in children at 2 years of age." Kotaska transposes it: "A woman at term with a breech presentation has a 97% chance of having a normal 2-year-old regardless of which method of delivery she chooses."

Kotaska and others felt that the follow-up undermined the initial conclusion that cesareans are safer and should be routine breech policy. Marek Glezerman, MD, chairman of OB/GYN at one of the participating centers, in Tel Aviv, conducted his own analysis of the study and found that it was "based on serious methodological and clinical flaws that do not permit the results to be generalized." Glezerman called for a retraction. The researchers "should now accept responsibility and withdraw the conclusions," he wrote.[19] "The results of the study are the results," Hannah responds. "You don't withdraw them because somebody doesn't like them."

If nothing else, what the Hannah trial shows is that babies are "remarkably resilient," says Kotaska, considering the labor management typical of the centers that were included in the study. The protocol, after all, allowed for induction of labor and Pitocin augmentation; it allowed for epidurals and "controlled delivery" of the head with forceps. It is very likely that all of the women gave birth in the counterproductive lithotomy position, with practitioners shouting at them to push. The Hannah trial allowed for hands *on* the breech. "There's a feeling among OBs that the results would be different if a different protocol were followed," Hannah acknowledges, but "the protocol reflects current practice."

ACOG revised its opinion in July 2006,[20] citing Kotaska's paper, among others, and recognizing more recent studies that have supported the overall safety of breech birth when in judicious hands, such as a recent study of 641 breech births, 298 of which were vaginal with no deaths or serious injuries at the time of delivery.[21] Another study of 481 planned vaginal breech births found the same.[22] Still, the ACOG opinion concludes that cesareans "will be the preferred mode of delivery" because of "diminishing expertise" in vaginal breech birth.

Indeed, physicians with breech expertise are few and far between. I met one, a high-risk perinatologist in the Midwest (he also provides some stealth backup for an illegal midwife (Chapter 6) and therefore did not want to be named). He will deliver breech, twins, even triplets vaginally, depending on the patients' circumstances and interest level. His colleagues look down on it, but they can't stop him. "I'm a perinatologist. I'm as high as it goes in the obstetrical world," he says. Peter Bernstein in New York will support a woman who wants a vaginal breech delivery, but only if she asks. These practitioners are the exceptions to the rule, and even physicians amenable to breech or VBAC can't get around continuous fetal monitoring and other restrictive protocols, which generally means an unphysiological delivery.

The elimination of vaginal breech births has bred a generation of obstetricians who are not only inexperienced but also unprepared to handle an obstetric case that will surely face them in their career: the unexpected breech birth. There is a small movement (arising out of military hospitals) for simulation training with mannequins, but it is in its infancy. To Bernstein and others, this is not acceptable. Surprise breeches happen, and in the next 20 years or so, U.S. obstetricians will have only outmoded book knowledge of how to manage them. Furthermore, what of the woman who does not want a cesarean? Should she be forced to have one because of diminished expertise?

EVIDENCE-BASED

The premise of a randomized controlled trial (RCT) is simple and elegant: to determine whether a treatment is effective or not, compare a group receiving the treatment to a control group receiving a placebo. This works well with pharmaceuticals: compare drug A to drug B, or drug B to placebo. Patients can be randomized to one or the other group, and the study can be double-blind. That is, neither the patient nor the provider knows which pill they are giving or receiving, thereby eliminating bias. The RCT has been used to look at similarly binary questions in obstetrics: episiotomy or no? electronic fetal monitoring or no? induction at 41 weeks or no? "The RCT is best suited to study very specific, technical issues with specific, easily measured outcomes," writes Kenneth C. Johnson, a senior epidemiologist at the Public Health Agency of Canada.[23]

The Center for Evidence-Based Medicine, based in Oxford, ranks the randomized controlled trial among the highest-quality evidence, second only to a systematic review of several randomized controlled trials. But it has its limits in maternity care. "Important questions like the safety of home versus hospital birth and the short- and long-term benefits of breastfeeding versus formula feeding are not amenable to RCTs," Johnson writes. Even the straightforward questions are not so easily shoehorned into the RCT mold. For one, "blindness" is nearly impossible (both patient and provider certainly know whether a cesarean, an episiotomy, or a electronic fetal monitor is being used), ethical limitations abound (can you randomize a woman to major surgery? to a labor induction?), and criteria are often immeasurable (what one provider calls "failure to progress" another may call "needs more time").

Let's say a randomized controlled trial was designed to compare position during pushing, all-fours to recumbent. A trial could randomize two groups of women to assume either position and evaluate the pelvic floor following. But the results wouldn't be very meaningful. "The first problem is that you can't force a woman to deliver on all fours," says Johnson. Many of the study subjects would end up pushing in a position to which they hadn't been assigned. Each woman has a different history, a different pelvis, a different-sized baby. Her ability to be in either position might depend on the type of pain relief and monitoring she's hooked up to. Any number of other interventions might influence the outcome, such as directed pushing or episiotomy. Furthermore, observers of physiological birth find that women end up in various positions and frequently shift positions even while they are pushing. A randomized controlled trial simply can't answer what position is best, because there probably *is* no answer. What's best is different for every woman, for every labor, depending on several factors.

Hannah's breech trial was designed to answer a simple question— vaginal or cesarean?—but it could not produce a simple answer because there is no simple answer, argues Kotaska. (It depends on the woman's characteristics and the provider's expertise and practice style.) Yet because this was a randomized controlled trial, the gold standard, an immediate change in practice was felt to be "evidence-based." A policy change based on a single study, says Johnson, is not what Cochrane had in mind when he was crusading for more scientific rigor in medicine.

"The focus shouldn't be on individual studies," says Johnson, even large randomized controlled trials. "The real key is the weight of the evidence. That's what Cochrane was all about." Consider the hypothetical position study again. If instead of conducting an RCT we designed an observational study, we would gain a different understanding. We might find out what position women are *most likely* to labor in, we'd find out how many different positions women labor in, and if we studied enough subjects, we could measure mother and infant outcomes and compare those to a group of women confined to bed.

In 2005, Johnson and Betty-Anne Daviss, an Ottawa midwife for 30-plus years and researcher for 16, conducted an observational study of low-risk women planning midwife-attended home births in the United States and Canada.[24] Published in the *British Medical Journal*, their study of more than 5000 births is the largest prospective study of planned home birth internationally to date. Daviss and Johnson gathered their subjects through the North American Registry of Midwives, which credentials all certified professional midwives, who are trained to attend out-of-hospital births. Enrollment in the study was mandatory for all midwives with the credential in the year 2000, and the study cohort was prospective; that is, every client who began care with the midwife was entered into the study, a detailed history was taken, and she was followed from prenatal care to 6 weeks postpartum. "The midwives had to tell us what births they were going to do ahead of time, and then they had to account for each one of those births," says Daviss. Researchers conducted follow-up interviews with a sample of mothers to validate documentation.

The study included the outcomes of all subjects, including those who transferred to the hospital for any reason. A total of 12% transported to the hospital, and one-quarter of those were considered urgent. The study found that among all the participants, very few required medical intervention: less than 4% had cesareans, 2% had episiotomies, and less than 2% had forceps or vacuum. There were no maternal deaths. Among "low-risk" mothers—not twins or breech births—the number of babies who died during labor or within the first 30 days was 1.7 per 1000, which is comparable to low-risk hospital births. The study nearly replicated the findings of the 1989 study of birthing centers, which also found that women planning low-tech, physiological births had a 4% cesarean rate and an infant death rate no different than in the hospital.[25] "It's clear from our study that the vast majority of low-risk women—which are the vast majority of women—can safely deliver at home or in hospital with little intervention," says Johnson. "We really think that this study sets a gold standard for what is possible and what is normal—what's reasonable to expect in terms of necessary intervention rates."

Jonathan Kotch, MD, a professor of public health at the University of North Carolina, is familiar with Daviss and Johnson's study; as chair of the Maternal and Child Health section of the American Public Health Association, he used the data to argue for a resolution endorsing certified professional midwives. "Being a hardnosed scientific critic, it doesn't meet the standards of a randomized controlled trial," he says of the study. "But at the end of the day, 5000 women who had their deliveries at home by certified professional midwives did just as well or better than women who were delivered in hospitals," he says. "This isn't a proof. But it's the next best thing." And it's simply the best that can be done. "A randomized controlled trial for childbirth cannot be done. You can't ask women to take a chance based upon the flip of a coin," says Kotch.

The APHA resolution, passed in 2001 after years of deliberation, supports "efforts to increase access to out-of-hospital maternity care services and increase the range of quality maternity care choices available to consumers."[26] Daviss and Johnson's study was the third-most accessed *British Medical Journal* article in 2005 and has been translated into German, Spanish, and French. Yet because this study did not have the potency of a randomized controlled trial—or perhaps because its conclusions raise some uncomfortable questions—it has commanded little attention from the obstetric community.

DISTORTION OF RISK

During a uterine contraction, the muscle layer at the top of the uterus shortens, which in turn pulls on the lower segment of the uterus, which in turn pulls up on the cervix, causing it to open. The cesarean incision standard since the 1970s extends about 4 inches crosswise on the lower segment of the uterus, about an inch above the cervical opening. Vaginal birth after cesarean has its own dedicated risk factor due to this scar: uterine rupture, when the uterus separates, usually along the previous incision. The scar giving way has been a known risk of a post-cesarean delivery for decades. With the outmoded "classical" incision running vertically higher up on the uterus, where contractions originate, the risk of rupture was a little over 1%, and about one in three of those babies died;[27] with the low transverse scar standard in the United States today, the risk of rupture is about 1 in 200, and about one in ten of those babies are severely harmed or die.[28]

Up until the mid-1980s, "once a cesarean" was "always a cesarean." This was the dictum of Edwin B. Craigin, professor of obstetrics and gynecology at Columbia University, stated in 1916[29] and embraced in the United States for the next 60 years. But beginning in the late 1970s, women were agitating for VBAC, and studies were showing that it was safe—on balance, the risks of another major abdominal surgery outweighed the small risk of rupture.[30] A 1980 government task force on cesareans recommended that all women with low transverse scars be given a "trial of labor,"[31] and subsequent studies showed that about 75% of women who tried to give birth vaginally would succeed,[32] avoiding repeat surgery. In the next decade, the vogue was VBAC. In 1994, ACOG recommended that women be *encouraged* to deliver vaginally after a previous cesarean,[33] and the push was so strong in the 1990s that some insurance companies were refusing to cover repeat cesareans. The percentage of women with previous cesareans who had subsequent vaginal births rose from 3% in 1981[34] to 28.3% in 1996.[35]

Then suddenly VBAC wasn't in vogue. A 1996 *New England Journal of Medicine* study gave it some bad press, finding that women who tried labor but ended up with an unplanned repeat cesarean suffered twice the rate of surgical injury and blood loss as women who elected repeat cesareans; in other words, the risks of unplanned surgery in labor are higher than the risks of planned surgery before labor, which is true for women without uterine scars as well.[36] Overall, the article confirmed a very low incidence of uterine rupture, at 0.3%. In the following years, more articles raised hackles—including a case study of a woman who died following a VBAC[37]—and some highly publicized lawsuits. Influential opinion pieces ran in journals questioning the wisdom of promoting VBAC. ACOG began hedging. In 1998, it reversed its position.[38]

The revised VBAC policy didn't call for an outright moratorium the way the breech edict had, but it created a major obstacle: VBACs were to occur with a physician and operating room staff capable of performing a cesarean "immediately" rather than "readily," which was later specified to mean that an OB had to be on site from the patient's admission to delivery, along with an anesthesiologist, scrub tech, neonatologist, and pediatrician.[39] The recommendation led many hospitals to ban VBAC outright, convinced malpractice insurers to threaten withdrawal of coverage, and prompted obstetricians everywhere to add VBAC to their list of "indefensibles." The VBAC rate has since taken a nose dive. In 2004, it fell to 9.2%.[40]

What's interesting is that through all the yo-yoing, the rate of uterine rupture kept coming up the same in the literature: roughly 1 in 200, even in women with multiple cesarean scars, and the rate of neonatal brain damage or death among VBAC attempts was consistently about 1 in 2000.[41] Those are excellent odds—the risk of a U.S. baby not surviving labor in a *low-risk* pregnancy is about 1 in 1000.[42] But the emphasis in news reports, journal editorials, and ACOG opinions falls on the rare tragedies and on the necessity of a round-the-clock surgical team on hand to save the baby, even though a complication requiring immediate cesarean—cord prolapse, placental abruption—is just as likely to occur in a woman without a scar. Anne Drapkin Lyerly, MD, an obstetrician-gynecologist in Durham, North Carolina, and a member of ACOG's ethics committee, calls this perception a "distortion of risk." She is the lead author of a 2007 article on the phenomenon.[43] "It's a major issue," she told me. "Patients are prone to it, doctors are prone to it."

To minimize perceived risks, physicians are forfeiting their ability to attend VBACs. In Oklahoma, the malpractice insurer Physicians Liability Insurance Co. (PLICO) has a monopoly and no longer covers VBACs, essentially creating a statewide ban. The policy was initiated by the company's board, composed entirely of physicians, who decided, "the risk is just too great for the mother and the baby."[44] At St. Barnabas Medical Center in New Jersey, about 60 obstetricians who have a group plan with the malpractice insurer MDAdvantage made a verbal agreement with the company to cease attending VBACs, as well as vaginal twin births. "We're basically looking for ways to curb our liability," Donald Chervenak, MD, president of the group and liaison to the company, told me. "If you do a VBAC and you have a poor outcome, you will get sued and you probably will lose." Nothing is official; there is no directive in writing. "You can't tell someone how to practice," says Chervenak. Still, they have an understanding. The physicians in the group were informed of this by "word of mouth," he says.

"The decline in VBAC is primarily the result of a perceived increased risk of uterine rupture. And I underline perceived," says Mark Landon, MD, director of maternal-fetal medicine at Ohio State University College of Medicine and the principal investigator of a large 2006 study that again confirmed a less-than-1% risk of rupture.[45] At the same time, he says, "Malpractice insurers and hospital attorneys have concluded that offering VBAC is not a sound business decision."

If anything, says Landon, the earlier data overestimated the frequency, because there was no distinction made between rupture and a uterine dehiscence, or "window," which is an asymptomatic separation of the uterine muscle but not the outer layer (called the sercosa), such that the uterus remains intact. True ruptures are often called "catastrophic," but Landon says there's no such thing—only catastrophic outcomes. And these are infrequent and unpredictable. Ninety percent of ruptures end well, with a repaired uterus and a healthy mother and child, according to Landon's research. During a rupture, contractions stop and the baby's heart rate slows; the cord may become compressed—essentially, air pressure is lost in the uterus—and the placenta will, at some point, begin to detach. Landon says common sense dictates that a cesarean should be performed as quickly as possible, although there are data suggesting that the "immediate" policy doesn't prevent baby deaths.[46]

What is largely ignored in the VBAC debate is that the risk of uterine rupture increases with labor induction (the scarred uterus, it turns out, also demands patience), and dramatically so when the drug misoprostol is used. Misoprostol, which goes by the brand name Cytotec, is a prostaglandin. Originally approved as a peptic ulcer drug, obstetricians began using it "off-label" in the 1990s to induce labor, though adverse events reported to the FDA prompted the agency to issue a cautionary letter to physicians and require a "black box" warning on the drug's packaging. (Politics complicates providers' understanding of the drug's risks; the warning is against use in pregnant women, but Cytotec is also FDA-approved for use with the drug mifepristone in medical abortion—also known as RU-486.) One study found that misoprostol increased the risk of uterine rupture in VBACs by five times.[47] Other studies have found that artifical oxytocin and even epidural are associated with higher rates of rupture; a garden-variety labor induction doubles the risk.[48]

A 2006 study suggests that physiological VBACs are much safer. Researchers in Israel encouraged women who had previously given birth by cesarean to try giving birth vaginally. They waited for spontaneous labor, up to 42 weeks; if they had to induce, they avoided prostaglandins like Cytotec. Once labor began, they allowed it to progress normally and used artificial oxytocin sparingly. Out of 841 women who planned a vaginal birth, 80 percent had one, and just one uterine rupture occurred, hours after the baby was born.[49] The study suggests that the true rupture rate may be far less than 1 in 200 if active management is abandoned.

The risk–benefit analysis of VBAC versus repeat cesarean breaks down something like this: If you are a woman attempting a VBAC, you have around a 75% chance of delivering vaginally and avoiding another major surgery and at least a 99.5% chance of not suffering a uterine rupture. If you choose a repeat cesarean, you have a 99.8% chance of not suffering a uterine rupture (it can still happen)[50] and a 100% chance of having another major surgery, with all the risks and drawbacks that entails. These include longer hospital stay; longer and more painful recovery; higher risk of infection, organ damage, adhesions, hemorrhage, embolism, and hysterectomy; more blood loss; higher chance of rehospitalization; higher chance of a complication with the next pregnancy; less initial contact with the baby; less success breastfeeding; higher risk of respiratory problems for the baby; and twice the risk of the most catastrophic complication of all: maternal death.[51]

That information is not what I've seen on the terse consent forms that women planning a VBAC are required to sign at many hospitals. Nor is it what I hear from many physicians when I ask them about the risks of VBAC. The message, direct or implied, is that VBAC is categorically more dangerous than cesarean. I've been told that the rate of rupture is 2%, 3%, and even 9%, despite the fact that the data show it is half a percent. Physicians have implied to me that a uterine rupture means a baby death, when in fact the chance that a VBAC baby will suffer brain damage or death is less than one-tenth of a percent. And very rarely are the risks of cesarean section mentioned in the conversation. When I asked Gary Hankins, MD, chair of ACOG's obstetric practice committee, about the risks of surgery, he asserted that "a scheduled cesarean section has almost no risk."

Even physicians who offer VBAC often make it restrictive, both financially and medically. Some add out-of-pocket surcharges for the extra bedside time. Others impose arbitrary gestational size and age cutoffs. I've talked to physicians who will schedule a cesarean on the due date for a VBAC patient—only if she goes into labor early can she have a vaginal birth. (These restrictions are unsupported by ACOG clinical management guidelines.[52]) "You have to have a picture perfect labor," one obstetrician told me. "If you do that, then you have a 40% chance of having a VBAC."

Even if they will have a choice in how they will give birth, women may not be getting accurate information on which to base a decision. Landon says that physicians, if they have an agenda, wield enormous power in this regard. "I could talk most women into either option if that was what I truly wanted to do," he says.

In spite of the evidence, the opinion of influential obstetric leaders is broadcast throughout the news media. Hankins of ACOG told *USA Today*, "I think VBAC is dead."[53] Charles Lockwood, MD, chair of obstetrics at Yale and former president of ACOG, told the *Washington Post* in 2005 that "There's a lot of hard, irrefutable data on the increased risk."[54] And that risk is often presented as far too great for any respectable mother to take. W. Benson Harer, Jr., MD, who helped rewrite the ACOG guidelines, put it to me this way: "If airplanes crashed one percent of the time, how many people would take that risk?"

THE 'EXPLODING UTERUS' CARD

Linda Bennett is a retired midwife in Portland, Oregon, who spends her days monitoring online group lists where hundreds of women who've had cesareans lay their emotions bare. The Yahoo ICAN (International Cesarean Awareness Network) list has a robust 1500 members, and they post like mad. In just 24 hours after signing up, I had more than 100 new messages.

There's a sense among many of the women, says Bennett, that they were led down a road to a primary cesarean they didn't need. "Part of what upsets so many women is that they feel they were lied to," she says. This lack of agency is evident in the truncated birth histories with which many members sign off: "Failed induction 2003, forced repeat 2005" "Coerced cesarean for 'fetal macrosomia' 2005," "C-section after failed induction 2002; stupid reason repeat C-section 2004," "C-section for physician distress," "Primary cesarean for iatrogenic stupidity," "Cesarean 2001 for CPD [i.e. "the baby won't fit"]—14.5 inch head; HBAC [home birth after cesarean] 2005—14.5 inch head!!!! Take THAT @#@% OB!!!"

There's a deep distrust of medical opinion on the list. "They're told, 'You know, your baby's getting really big'—that's the 'big baby card,'" Bennett explains to me. "Or, 'Wow, your placenta is aging, we should get that baby out soon.' We call that the 'dying placenta card.' Or, 'You're so uncomfortable, let's just do an induction. You can get your mom flown in, give your notice at work, get someone to watch the kids.' We call that the 'convenience card.'" The women online are months, or even years, out from their cesareans, yet many are still coming to grips with them. And when they get pregnant again, they are often being told they must have another surgery; that their uterus could rupture and the baby could die. "We call that the 'exploding uterus card,'" says Bennett, which is usually followed by the "dead baby card." "Many, many people on the list can't find a VBAC provider."

In 2005, the American Academy of Family Physicians came out in support of VBAC, which it calls TOLAC—trial of labor after cesarean.[55] Based on a review of the literature conducted by the Agency for Health Research and Quality, a division of the National Institutes of Health, the organization recommends that all women with a low transverse incision be offered a "trial of labor," and, in direct opposition to ACOG, that VBAC "should not be restricted only to facilities with available surgical teams present throughout labor since there is no evidence that these additional resources result in improved outcomes." Such a policy, says the group, limits women's access to care and appears "to be based on malpractice concerns rather than on available statistical and scientific evidence." The Society of Obstetricians and Gynecologists of Canada also maintains that vaginal birth after cesarean is safe and should be available to women.[56]

One could argue that the "liability crisis" is to blame for the unique attitude in the United States, but it seems to me that suspended in the chasm between evidence and practice is a profound cultural denial that goes beyond malpractice anxiety or convenience. Somehow we are willing to accept repeated major abdominal surgery for women—mothers, who have to go home and take care of an infant, or twin infants, or an infant and toddlers, no less—when at the same time, in other surgical specialties, there's been concerted effort to *reduce* the frequency of exposing the abdominal cavity. Today, appendectomies, gall bladder removal, even gastric bypass surgery can be performed by less invasive, less traumatic laparoscopy.

There is also a striking double standard apparent in the denial of VBAC. Women must sign a dedicated consent form to have a VBAC, but there is no such a thing for a second, third, or subsequent cesarean, which carry risks of equal or greater magnitude. Nor is there a special consent form for labor induction, artificial rupture of the membranes, or episiotomy. The risk of miscarriage following amniocentesis, a common procedure, is 1 in 200[57]—the same as the risk of uterine rupture in an actively managed VBAC—yet there is certainly no campaign to ban amnio.

Meanwhile, obstetric leaders frame elective cesarean as a woman's "right to choose." "If women can make a choice to do things like breast augmentation or any other cosmetic surgery," says Hankins of ACOG, "then why would they not have the choice to have a cesarean delivery?" That is, women should have the freedom to choose the risks of surgery, but not the risks of vaginal birth. The rhetoric notwithstanding, women's choices just don't seem to factor into far-reaching policy decisions. I asked Hankins about the effective VBAC ban created by ACOG's policy: "I don't think we have an obligation to practice unsafe medicine," he responded.

Vaginal birth after cesarean and repeat cesarean both carry risks, and no birth is guaranteed a good outcome. What the ACOG guideline does is decide for women—and physicians—which risks they should take and which are unacceptable. Linda Bennett has come to this conclusion: "What you've got here are people who would rather have a controlled rupture of the uterus—what is a C-section but a controlled rupture of the uterus?"

With hospitals banning VBAC and physicians demurring, women who've read the research and want a vaginal birth are in many cases simply abandoning obstetric care. Stacey Escoffery, who lives on Long Island, New York, sought a VBAC at Winthrop Hospital. Her doctor told her he was a longtime supporter, but warned her that if she went into labor when he wasn't on call, he couldn't guarantee that the other obstetricians would honor her choice. He also asked her not to tell anyone that he was VBAC-friendly. "That sent up a red flag. I felt that if I got one of his partners, I'd be sectioned," she told me. Escoffery called several doctors to no avail, and finally, through a doula, found a nurse-midwifery practice farther out on the island, at Stonybrook Hospital, a 90-minute drive from her house. She knew they supported VBAC, but she still labored at home with the doula until she was 9 centimeters dilated. She arrived at the hospital practically crowning.

To Andrew Kotaska, this is the equivalent of abandoning care, a violation of the Hippocratic oath. "Instead of an OB saying I'm going to abandon you, which happens all over the States and Canada, women need to be saying, 'You have an ethical obligation to help me find someone to do it.' And I think empowering women to get those words out of their mouths is probably the biggest thing we can do. 'I understand your guidelines, but this is my body.' If they can request a cesarean and take all the risks, and nobody bats an eye, then they should be able to request a VBAC, or request a breech. And as a profession, I think we have a duty to help women fill those requests."

Some women will labor in the parking lot of a hospital known to be anti-VBAC, arriving on the L&D floor just in time to push the baby out. The "showing up pushing" strategy is discussed in full on the ICAN list. Fully aware that the hospital would have required them to plan a repeat cesarean, they try to time the birth so that when they get to L&D it's too late. This doesn't work for everyone, though. Susie Nalbach showed up at a Coral Springs, Florida, hospital ready to push in 2003. Instead, she was pushed into a wheel chair, separated from her husband, and taken into the operating room. There she remembers two nurses arguing with each other. "The younger one was telling me to push, and the older one was telling me not to push. I kept pushing because I couldn't help it," she recalls. "I remember being told to breathe into an oxygen mask. But it wasn't oxygen, it was general anesthesia. I did not consent to it. I never signed anything. I woke up later with a son." She says on her medical chart, the indication for the cesarean was "failure to progress." Legally, this is assault and battery.

As obstetrics becomes more didactic, women who are determined to avoid unnecessary surgery are shunning the hospital altogether and planning to give birth at home. "It's a matter of trust for most of these women," says Bennett. "The reason they're having HBACs is because they don't trust the hospital." Across the country, an untold number of midwives continue to care for the untouchables, in some places against regulations or illegally. In a number of states where midwives can obtain a license, practice regulations prohibit them from attending VBACs, breeches, and twins, which pushes these higher-risk births underground. In Arkansas, a woman who demanded anonymity chose a home VBAC with two licensed midwives who cared for her "under the radar." "As far as the state knows, I had an unassisted birth at home," she told me.

Although there is a solid body of evidence on the safety of midwife-attended out-of-hospital births for women with straightforward pregnancies,[58, 59, 60, 61] there are few data on home births that pose a higher risk—twins, breech, VBAC. One 1997 study of home births showed a higher infant mortality rate among such higher risk births.[62] In a 2004 study of roughly 1500 VBACs in birthing centers, there were 6 ruptures and 2 neonatal deaths connected to a rupture. But when researchers analyzed the data they found that the majority befell women who delivered after 42 weeks gestation and who had undergone two or more previous cesareans. For women without those risk factors, both the rupture rate and the rate of neonatal death was 2 per 1000.[63]

Certainly in the case of a uterine rupture, there would be a delay before a cesarean, putting the baby's survival in peril; the time to emergency care could also be life-threatening to the mother. In an ideal world, says Bennett, VBACs would occur with an OR close by. "But only if the hospital provides the kind of services and supportive care you can get at home—the ability to walk around, intermittent monitoring, the ability to change positions, not pushing anesthesia unless the mother is asking for it," she says. "Because most hospitals are not supportive, women and babies are probably safer at home." At the least one could argue that they are not receiving artificial oxytocin, epidurals, and other interventions that increase the risk of rupture. I asked the Midwestern perinatologist whether he thought it was safe for such women to stay at home. "Well my friend, let me tell you, if you want to have a vaginal breech, you better do it at home. You'll be cut in the hospital," he said. "That is also happening for VBAC. There are fewer and fewer physicians and hospitals who will allow a woman to VBAC."

touching his chest. "I felt his head descend quickly, got down on all fours, and let my uterus push him out into my hands," Goorchenko later wrote about the birth. "This was our first arrival, a little boy named Psalm Victor, who cried just enough to let us know he was okay, but otherwise settled into a deep calm. . . ." He weighed 7 lb, 10 oz.—average size for a singleton baby.

The video then fades briefly to black (husband Alex had put the camera down to help cut the cord and wrap the newborn in blankets), and next we see Goorchenko back on the toilet moaning and grunting, sipping water from a sports bottle, the phone ringing again in the background. Of the second birth, she writes:

> My friend Kari thankfully arrived at this point to help Alex, who was now watching our 2-year-old, holding Psalm, and filming the birth, all at the same time! I reached inside me once again to check on my progress, and felt momentarily confused as to what body part was presenting itself. It felt like a hand, possibly, tucked up near the head, but then I realized it was our daughter's foot. . . . I wasn't afraid, just surprised. My husband asked what he could do and I responded, "Nothing. Just film." A foot and leg quickly came out, followed by a second foot and leg (I could feel her literally pushing her knee out of me). Next came her body, hands, and arms, as I supported her with my hands reaching under me. Her head popped out and our daughter Zoya Olga was born, with spurts of blood coming with her and a train roaring by outside. . . . After 10 or 15 minutes, I clamped the cord with shoelaces, gave her to my husband, and birthed the placenta into a big glass bowl. Their two placentas had fused into one big butterfly with two cords emerging from it. (The girl was 8 lb, 11 oz.)

Goorchenko didn't set out to have an unassisted birth, at least not initially. She'd gone back to the midwifery practice that had attended her second pregnancy, but when her belly started measuring suspiciously large and an ultrasound confirmed twins, she was "risked out" of their practice in accordance with California licensing regulations. By law, the midwives had to refer her to an obstetrician.

"They gave me a couple names of OBs," says Goorchenko. "I remember looking at them and thinking, this isn't an option. Because in California, a twin pregnancy pretty much means you're going to have a cesarean section and a NICU stay for your babies even if they don't need it. That was really painful for us to imagine. And I had very little interest in surgery for no good reason." Indeed, there is no evidence to suggest that routine cesarean delivery of twins improves outcomes.[64]

Goorchenko was now in her third trimester, with twins, and had no care provider. She started calling midwives. Most said they couldn't take twins or didn't feel comfortable doing so. Finally one said yes, but with certain provisos. "She wanted a small team—a second midwife and an assistant and paramedics waiting. She had no breech birth experience. And I thought, what is she bringing to the table? Plus she was going to charge me the full fee even though it was about 8 weeks before my due date."

Goorchenko did meet with an OB with whom she was familiar and asked if she would support a normal vaginal delivery in the hospital. "She said, 'Sure, I will. But nobody else in my practice will,'" says Goorchenko. "She even said to me, which I'll never forget, because it sounded so strange coming out of a doctor, 'You know, it just sounds like you really want a home birth.'"

Goorchenko's first baby was born at the hospital. She was an unexpectedly pregnant 19-year-old and got "one heck of an episiotomy," she says. "I had a mirror set up so I could see the birth and all of a sudden I'm watching my vagina being cut with scissors." It took years to get over the psychological trauma. "And on top of that it just fucks up your vagina," says Goorchenko. "I had incontinence. I could barely feel sex for a year and a half." She intended to have a home birth with her second child but went into labor at 35 weeks, too early to give birth safely at home. The hospital birth was fine, but the NICU experience wasn't.

With this pregnancy, Goorchenko had a month to go, and still no provider. "We just decided there was no one willing to help us or qualified to help us," she recalls. "At that point, we just made the decision that we needed to be home alone. It was actually a very easy decision to make." Goorchenko had been a childbirth educator for years, and her husband was trained as an EMT. "I felt very confident in the birth process," she says. "I believe that women instinctively know how to take care of their babies. If you can be in that state of primal knowing—I hate to sound all cave-womanesque, but I think we have that wisdom still. But mostly what I wanted to do was protect the babies from intervention and interference with a physiological process."

There was one midwife, though, that someone had mentioned in passing, a woman who lived 3 hours away, had 25 years of experience, including twins and breech, and somehow ignored licensing regulations. Goorchenko and her husband met with the midwife and felt a connection—she was both qualified and willing. But everybody knew there was a good chance she wouldn't make it to the birth in time. "This is going to sound petty, but one of the major benefits I had was telling my family we had a midwife," says Goorchenko. "I didn't mention that she was 3 hours away and that my births tend to be really fast. But there was definitely that psychological peace of getting everybody off my back. I was worried that they were worried."

Goorchenko went a full 40 weeks. "I was the size of a small house," she says. (She gained 80 pounds during the pregnancy—and by the looks of her in the video, all belly.) Toward the end, she invited to the birth a close friend who also happened to be a labor and delivery nurse with experience in neonatal resuscitation. Goorchenko finally went into active labor at 7 a.m. on January 25, 2004. She called the midwife, called her friend, and gave birth to the first baby at 9 a.m., before either had arrived. She told me that even in labor she had a "strong awareness" of her decision and an overwhelming sense of relief that she had stayed home. "When I felt my daughter was a footling, I knew that minute that I would have been in surgery, knocked out on general. Even if we were having a vaginal breech birth, there would have been hands all over her, and that's when it gets really dangerous. Instead it was this wonderful experience." The midwife arrived 45 minutes after the babies were born. Goorchenko was soaking in the tub, taking turns bathing each baby.

DO IT YOURSELF BIRTH

There are no reliable data on planned unassisted births. Most births classified as unassisted are those attended by cops and cab drivers, and in states where midwives are illegal, many midwife-attended births end up being recorded as unassisted. The number of intentional solo-birthers is small, but many believe it is rising—some are calling it a movement—based on several very active bulletin boards and e-mail lists dedicated to "freebirth" or "U-birth." On motheringdotcommune, the bulletin board of *Mothering* magazine, which has a robust 75,000 active members, there are 1500 threads in the "Unassisted Birth" forum. The members are women like Goorchenko, who can't find a care provider willing to support a normal birth; women like Nalbach, who feel so traumatized by their previous birth that they don't trust any care provider; women who are religious and feel that birth should be a private affair to which only the husband is privy. Then there are women like Laura Shanley, who simply believe that any outside interference with birth is unnecessary and potentially harmful. Shanley is the author of *Unassisted Childbirth*, published in 1993, and founder of the high-traffic website of the same domain name. If you simply search "childbirth" on Google, her site comes up sixth.

Unassisted birth isn't new. In the 1960s and 1970s it was often the only alternative to a hospital birth—a strapped down, separated from husband, guaranteed episiotomy birth—and the women who did it also gave birth to organized midwifery. "That's what we were doing in the 1970s before there were any midwives," says Peggy O'Mara, editor of *Mothering*. "It was part of the whole back-to-the-land movement and commune movement." It was also a natural extension of the early feminist, grab-a-speculum-and-mirror-and-reclaim-your-body ethos, she says. "And I consider it a really legitimate response to certain environments. Where I lived in southern New Mexico, for instance, the choices were so poor that we just wanted to figure it out ourselves."

Laura Shanley gave birth to her first child, with her husband and friends present, in 1978. But she came to unassisted birth a bit differently. Shanley was heavily influenced by the New Age you-create-your-own-reality principle. You get where she is coming from in the first paragraph of her book:

> In 1976, my husband David and I became aware of the concept that we create our own reality according to our desires, beliefs, and intentions. Undesirable events are neither punishments handed out by an angry God, nor chance happenings

that originate from without the self for no apparent reason. They are instead the result of an untrained mind that has not yet become aware of its own abilities.[65]

For O'Mara, unassisted birth was the best women could do under the circumstances; today, midwives outnumber obstetricians in New Mexico and attend nearly one-third of all births.[66] "Now, unassisted birth here would seem extreme," she says. Shanley, on the other hand, says there's "no such thing as a casual observer." She doesn't see most midwives as much of an improvement over the hospital. "The midwives will say, 'Doctors are not gods, but we are goddesses. We have the knowledge, we will hold your hand and help you,'" says Shanley, mimicking a good-witch tone. "Well, what if I don't want to hold your hand? What if I think *I* have the knowledge? I think there are people with big egos who like laboring women dependent on them," she says.

You can hear echoes of Shanley's own ego on the Yahoo group list C-birth, in talk of midwives "spoiling" the birth energy or "feeding off" birth energy and "taking over" births. "If you understand how your mind affects your body, and if you understand that birth is inherently safe, then it can be as natural and easy as going to the bathroom or making love," says Shanley. "You don't need help with those things, so I don't believe you need help giving birth—provided you are healthy and in right frame of mind." Shanley talks of a birth intelligence that healthy women need only tap into, an intelligence she feels is basically retarded by the hospital and is often supplanted by a midwife, who brings her own intelligence into the room. "There is an intelligence within us that knows how to grow a sperm and egg into a human being, and that consciousness knows how to give birth," she says.

It is likely that there has always been a tiny minority of women who felt confident enough to birth without professional assistance. But now, the unassisted movement feeds off the increasingly restrictive obstetric environment. O'Mara says U-birthers appeared on her radar only in the past 5 years, around the time when VBACs started being denied. Restrictions on midwifery care have contributed as well: in several of the states that offer licenses, such as California and Washington, midwives are under the same pressures as their cooperating physicians. Instead of inducing with Pitocin and Cervidil, they are often doling out herbs and castor oil at 41 weeks to "get labor going." If a client hits 42 weeks, they will be forced to transfer her out of midwifery care.

Goorchenko has become somewhat of a poster girl for the unassisted community, a defiant hero who blew the cover off birth—see, look, it works just fine by itself, even twins! She speaks to childbirth education classes and sells her video via her website. "Looking back at the birth of our twins, it was extraordinary yet so perfectly normal at the same time," she writes. "I realized how much of a big deal birth is turned into, when in actuality, it is such a straightforward and ordinary event."

The Discovery Channel got hold of Goorchenko's video and included it in a show titled "Amazing Babies" (one of the babies was born on a small plane, another had robotic surgery). Goorchenko sent me copies of both—the original video and Discovery's makeover. Her footage is notably absent of fear; there are smiles and laughter during and between contractions. There's excitement; the contractions themselves elicit distinctly orgasmic sounds. At one point Goorchenko actually says, "This is so fucking awesome." The produced piece notably edits out these moments, depicting her as though in constant agony. There's the obligatory mood music—ominous high notes that bring to mind the strings from *Psycho*, particularly with the shower in the background. With editing and voiceover, the program somehow reframes the labor as if on the brink of disaster at every moment—"Plans for a home birth go terribly wrong," the baritone narrator begins. After baby A slides out "too fast," we hear, "the baby wasn't making any noise." With baby B, "her left leg was actually sticking out of the birth canal, but her head was trapped inside!" The image of the dangling foot is stretched over nearly two suspense-filled minutes, when in real time the baby emerged, toe-to-head, in 60 seconds flat. When disaster never comes, it's presented as a dodged bullet. "Even when faced with dire complications, they took it all in stride."

Just as there are no data on the frequency of unassisted birth, there are no data on its safety, only anecdotes. The issue is extremely divisive for midwives. "Frankly, it's a sticking point," says Angelita Nixon, a midwife in Charleston, West Virginia. "If pressed, I'd have to say that I have some reservations—I don't think that every woman who chooses it is necessarily as informed as I would want her to be. But on the other hand, in terms of women's rights, it is a decision that women should be able to make. And we have so much culturally prescribed fear around childbirth, I really admire a woman who's been able to actively resist that, who believes in her body's ability to give birth." Lisa Block-Wieser, a midwife in Tucson, Arizona, is less charitable. When I mentioned Goorchenko's video she shook her head and raised her voice. "You know, I'm happy that it went well for her, but it's really irresponsible of her to put that out there," she said. The story reminded her of an unassisted birth of twins in Tucson just before her arrival in 2001—one of the babies died. Even though there was no midwife present, "it cast a cloud over the whole midwifery community," she said. "They think of it as all the same."

"Look," she went on. "There are people who can do it with Zen and finesse, but they're setting other women up for failure. Most women need support. These people are forgetting what midwifery is about, which is supporting women."

In a sense, Shanley believes she is the über midwife, empowering women to be completely independent. The notable lack of support and not infrequent hostility from midwives initially came as a shock to her. "These are women who really encourage women to trust themselves, to listen to themselves—but only to a point," says Shanley. "I have more faith in women."

Women who feel wholly disempowered and demoralized by an interventive birth often find power in that sentiment, and yet I find a sad militancy, too, in holding up a woman alone in childbirth as the ideal. Giving birth is a natural bodily function, but even in the best of environments it is not always easy and not always harmless, and historically, across cultures, women have sought support.[67] It's part of what separates us from animals: our babies are helpless, *neonatal*. Easing out that evolved brain from a narrow bipedal pelvis is more of a challenge than it is for other mammals. We can recognize ourselves as animals and take some hints from animal behavior during labor—rarely do mammals lie down on their backs for the duration, and rarely do they stay put. But our brain size is what makes human birthing a bit more complicated, and it's what makes us smart enough to get the village in on it.

Shanley argues that the growth of unassisted birth is just one aspect of "the psychological revolution" taking place. O'Mara, on the other hand, sees it as a marker of regression. "I think it's a sign, just as it was in the 1970s, that the births available to mothers have become over-medicalized, that the hospital is being perceived as a dangerous place, and that women don't have options."

PHYSIOLOGICAL V. INDUSTRIAL

I wonder if there's something the breech babies are telling us—have been telling us for decades—about birth. Do their mothers really require such different care than most mothers, or does their heightened sensitivity to active management make them emissaries of normal birth? In other words, should we be treating all births with fewer hands and more brains? "That's a big question," says Kotaska. "An unmedicated birth in an environment where a woman feels comfortable, where she's adequately supported, where she has a degree of privacy that allows her brain and her uterus to do the dance that we understand very poorly called labor, is a physiological birth. And once you start messing with any one of those factors, put her in hospital with noise and light, take away her privacy, you go down a slippery slope toward industrial birth."

And I wonder if there's something that the freebirthers are telling us; I wonder if they and the "perineal sparing" crowd are really just two sides of the same coin: going unassisted and signing up for an elective cesarean are both coping mechanisms of a sort, the goal being to avoid a traumatic labor and delivery.

I asked Kotaska what was going through his mind while he was watching Goorchenko's video. He said knowing the ending colored the experience—the parents wouldn't be selling a video of a birth gone bad, after all. But in general, he told me, it was a reminder that birth works. "For caregivers, the best thing to realize is to sit on your hands if you don't need to intervene—to be vigilant, not hyper-vigilant," he says. "That's the art of obstetrics: learning to do nothing."

If vaginal breech birth is a lost art, then the art of obstetrics—as Kotaska sees it, anyway—is fast becoming so. During the breech conference, midwives and physicians shared technique and experience, and it was extraordinary in this regard. "A big revelation for the physicians was the all-fours technique," Kotaska told me. The breech baby, that ever-demanding creature, drew the two modalities together, and essentially reeducated medical attendants in a key aspect of normal, physiological birth: active, upright positions. On the whole, however, there is scant collaboration between midwives and doctors. Obstetricians are increasingly isolated from the mechanisms of physiological childbirth. The same forces pushing higher-risk women toward cesareans, or toward unassisted home births, are pushing away low-risk women with straightforward pregnancies who simply want a normal, vaginal birth.

That's all L, a professor in New Jersey, wanted (she also didn't want me to use her name because she's in trouble with her university for breast-feeding once during a class—more isolation from normal bodily processes). L didn't think she was asking for much: to be able to move around in labor, birth in a comfortable position, and keep her baby close immediately following delivery. With no birthing centers nearby and home birth prohibitive at $2000 out of pocket—even after partial coverage from her health insurance—she initially settled on giving birth at a hospital with a nurse–midwife. "She bent over backwards for me," says L. "She arranged with the head nurse that the baby would stay with me—hospital policy was that he would be taken away for a battery of tests."

But then she and the midwife came to an impasse: the fetal monitor. "I was really upset, I thought why is this so damn hard—to have a baby the way you want to have a baby?" L had done the research and knew monitoring would mean a bedridden labor and an increased chance of surgery. "To have to lie on your back during labor was anathema to me," she says. "I was like, 'This is my body and my birth, why am I agreeing to this if there's no demonstrated medical need?'"

L opted instead for the nearest birthing center, in Pennsylvania Dutch country, a 2-hour drive from her home.

She labored with the blinds shut. "There was no sound. I loved the silence, I loved the darkness," she told me.

When she felt the urge to push, she announced the baby was coming and dropped into a squat. "The final contractions right before she crowned were incredibly intense. You feel like you're splitting open. There was a burning sensation, but then suddenly her head came out and then her body came out all in one push. It was this amazing sense of relief. It's true that you forget all the pain. I just started shouting, 'Give me my baby!' It was the most amazing moment."

CHAPTER 4

Consequences

THE RISING CESAREAN RATE was a major story in the 1980s. "Too Many Caesareans?" asked *Newsweek* in 1980.[1] "Rise in Caesarean Births Stirs Dispute" was a 1981 *New York Times* headline.[2] "'Runaway' C-Section Rates Reflect 'Crisis,'" announced the *Los Angeles Times* in 1987.[3] In 1979, the National Institutes of Health, the research arm of the Department of Health and Human Services, appointed a 19-member task force on "Cesarean Childbirth" and in 1980 held the first U.S. conference on the issue. "The rising caesarean birth rate is a matter of concern," read the final consensus statement, part of a 537-page report. The trend "may be stopped and perhaps reversed, while continuing to make improvements in maternal and fetal outcomes, the goal of clinical obstetrics today."[4] The data available at that time showed the cesarean rate just clearing 15%.[5]

The 1980 conference attributed the rise in surgery to two main causes: a spike in diagnoses of "dystocia" during labor, also termed "failure to progress," and the policy of automatic repeat cesareans, which together accounted for nearly two-thirds of the C-sections performed in 1978. Similarly, it found that the rush to surgery wasn't saving any more babies or preventing brain damage. Among the panel's recommendations were investigation and peer review of the "dystocia" diagnoses, encouragement of vaginal birth after cesarean where appropriate, and further "research clarifying the factors which affect the progress of labor, including the effects of emotional support, ambulation, rest, sedation, and [synthetic] oxytocin administration." The conference noted a two- to fourfold greater risk of maternal death with a cesarean birth than with a vaginal birth.[6]

Leading obstetricians were not only amenable to these recommendations, they were behind the conference itself. Mortimer Rosen, MD, at the time a professor of reproductive biology at Case Western Reserve University and director of OB/GYN at Cleveland Metropolitan General Hospital, led the task force and conference panel. For the next 15 years he agitated for broader obstetric reform. In 1985, he was appointed professor at Columbia University and chair of OB/GYN at Columbia Presbyterian Medical Center in New York, where he led a New York State task force on the cesarean rate, which monitored hospitals with higher-than-average numbers. In 1989, he chaired the NIH panel on prenatal care that found many of the routine tests and procedures to be of dubious value,[7] and he also published the consumer-friendly book *The Cesarean Myth*. "Patients and doctors alike have come to believe that cesareans are as safe as vaginal birth, that they are necessary in a wide range of cases, and that they guarantee a good outcome." These beliefs, he wrote, "are myths."[8]

The feeling was that too many cesareans were happening for no good reason, and the medical community was being held accountable. Laws passed in Massachusetts and New York mandated that hospitals disclose and disseminate their rates. Hospital quality assurance committees held weekly sit-downs at which doctors would be called out on cesareans they'd performed and asked to defend them. "There were these bright yellow forms we had to fill out," recalls New Jersey obstetrician Richard Fain. "For years we were all reviewing every case," says Andrew Garber, also in New Jersey. "You had to explain to all kinds of people why a patient had a cesarean." Managed care got the fever as well, because fewer cesareans meant lower bills. There were even reports of insurers offering hospitals incentives to lower their cesarean rates and mandating trials of labor after cesarean regardless of the woman's wishes.[9] "I think they were pushing a little too hard for VBACs," Garber says in retrospect.

During his tenure at Columbia Presbyterian, Rosen instituted a protocol to tighten up admission to the OR. He set more stringent guidelines for cesarean sections, appointed a policing review board, and integrated nurse–midwives onto the labor ward. Columbia's rate dropped from 25% in 1985 to 19% in 1989. He told the *New York Times* in 1989 that he expected to lower it even further.[10] Other hospitals achieved even more dramatic results. The most famous was Mount Sinai Medical Center in Chicago, which required second opinions for all non-emergency cesareans, among other rules, and the rate dropped from 17.5% to 10.2% in 4 years. University Medical Center in Jacksonville, Florida, saw cesareans plummet from 28% to 11% in just 3 years. In Denver, St. Luke's Hospital reported that not even 6% of their clinic patients required cesareans under its initiative.[11]

"These were public health examples," argues Sidney Wolfe, MD, director of Public Citizen's Health Research Group, a consumer advocacy organization, which in 1989, 1992, and 1994 published reports titled "Unnecessary Cesarean Sections," calling for swift reform. The feeling was that if tertiary-care hospitals with high-tech neonatal intensive care units, accepting patients with all manner of risks and complications, can do it, "it can be done in many other places," Wolfe told me.

The American College of Obstetricians and Gynecologists maintained that there was no way to calculate what an appropriate cesarean rate might be,[12] but in 1990, the U.S. Centers for Disease Control and Prevention set 15% as a "Healthy People 2000" goal.[13] The number seems to be a conservative interpretation of a 1985 World Health Organization resolution that determined between 10% and 15% as the ideal rate.[14] Prior to that, in 1983, Edward Quilligan, MD, former dean of the School of Medicine at the University of California at Irvine and editor of the *American Journal of Obstetrics and Gynecology*, had come up with a similar number, calculating that individual hospitals could safely range from 7.8% to 17.5% and that the country at large should fall between 12% and 14%.[15] Based on Quilligan's calculation, Public Citizen estimated that about half of cesareans at the time were unwarranted.[16]

The buzz seemed to be having an effect. In the 1990s, the cesarean rate held at about one-quarter of all births, even dipping to 20.7% in 1996.[17] The VBAC rate was climbing. In its 2-inch-thick 1994 report, which listed the cesarean rates at thousands of hospitals across the states, Public Citizen wrote that "Cesarean section, while at times a life-saving intervention for both mother and child, can be a cause of significant harm to mothers and provides no additional benefits to infants when performed outside of certain well-defined medical situations. We are beginning the long road back from an epidemic of unnecessary surgery."[18]

Not exactly. The main vehicle for lowering the cesarean rate was pushing VBAC, which undeniably had a swift, dramatic impact. What few hospitals or practitioners did, however, was take a close look at that red flag, the rate of dystocia diagnosis, and the management practices that led to it, as the NIH panel had suggested they do. Although the VBAC rate kept climbing, peaking at 28% in 1996,[19] (see Appendix B) the number of women undergoing unplanned, in-labor, first-time cesarean surgery held and could not be attributed to any increase in maternal risk factors.[20]

When ACOG revised its policy on VBAC, the weekly accountability sessions at hospitals ceased, and the stigma of a high cesarean rate lifted. At the same time, the burgeoning subspecialty of urogynecology began to gain a foothold in the literature. Urogynecologists deal in disorders of the pelvic floor, the diaphragmatic muscle that is suspended in the lower abdomen like the net under a trapeze artist. They spend their days looking at organs that have fallen from their perch, treating conditions such as chronic incontinence and uterine prolapse, which occurs when the uterus protrudes into the vagina. And many blame vaginal birth per se. The research has not, so far, borne out any connection.[21] Nevertheless, urogynecologists, who generally don't attend births, have been some of the main proponents of elective cesarean, or "perineal sparing," as it has been termed. The idea is that surgery now could save you pelvic floor surgery later. That logic was further amplified by Benson Harer in his treatises on "prophylactic elective cesarean."[22] And in 2000, he was appointed president of ACOG.

What had been a medical problem in the 1980s was by the late 1990s a consumer trend. Malpractice premiums started to make headlines. Posh Spice, who elected surgical over vaginal births, made headlines. "Doctors report rise in elective caesareans," was a 1998 *New York Times* headline.[23] In 2000, the government backed off its original Healthy People Goal, lowering the bar to 15% for "low-risk," first-time mothers only,[24] strategically dodging the VBAC debate. Trude Bennett, PhD, a professor of maternal and child health at the University of North Carolina Chapel Hill was a member of the committee that set the Healthy People 2010 goals. "It had become too controversial to recommend VBACs," Bennett told me, and the CDC adopted ACOG's cautionary approach.[25] "There's a lot of debate about how much that's been driven by best scientific evidence, how much it's been driven by the bias of individual researchers, and of course how much all of this is driven by providers' fear of liability." In 2003, ACOG widened the justifications for surgical birth to include maternal request.[26] Now women could be directly responsible for unnecessary cesareans.

By 2006, the cesarean rate was double the number held up to the light in 1980. Yet there is little concern from obstetric leaders, government health institutions, and even public health organizations. When a labor enters that gray zone today, there are no second opinions required, and rarely a second thought. "Now if you don't do a C-section," says Andrew Garber, "everybody's wondering why."

THE MATERNAL MORTALITY RATE IS RISING IN FLORIDA

When the World Health Organization came up with 15% as an acceptable cesarean rate, the number was based on an informed calculation: the known conditions that called for surgery, how likely they are to occur, and the known complications of surgery. Logic held that unnecessary cesareans should be avoided, and that if they weren't, needless injury and death would result.

But many obstetricians didn't buy it. In 1999, four prominent Boston obstetricians made headlines with a *New England Journal of Medicine* editorial arguing that arbitrary target rates were threatening patient safety and patient choice, and charged that the 15% guideline had no scientific basis.[27] That sentiment stands today: Harer told me that WHO is "hung up on statistics that they developed in the 1970s." Frederic Frigoletto, MD, one of the authors of the editorial and chief of obstetrics at Massachusetts General Hospital in Boston, told me the number "was determined by people sitting around a table. There's no basis for that recommendation." The 2006 NIH conference on "Cesarean Delivery on Maternal Request" concluded, "artificial declarations of an ideal rate should be discouraged."[28]

José Villar, MD, who directs reproductive health research at the WHO, admits the 15% figure was consistently doubted and debated. "It was always challenged because there weren't any hard data behind it," he told me. "We now have solid data behind those numbers."

In 2005, Villar led a WHO study of 100,000 births at more than 100 hospitals in Latin America, looking at the connection between adverse outcome and cesarean birth. The study, the largest ever on the topic, was published in the *Lancet* in June 2006.[29] It found that after controlling for risk factors so that poor outcomes could be attributed to the delivery method alone, the rate of "severe maternal morbidity and mortality"—infection requiring rehospitalization, hemorrhage, blood transfusion, hysterectomy, admission to intensive care, and death—rose in proportion to the rate of cesarean section.

The risk held true for cesarean babies as well: preterm birth and infant death rose significantly when cesarean rates exceeded between 10% and 20%. This supports the 2006 study led by CDC statistician Marian MacDorman, which found that low-risk babies born by cesarean were nearly three times more likely to die within the first month of life than those born vaginally.[30] What these epidemiological data show, explains Villar, is that the medical logic of the 1980s actually hit the bull's-eye. "There is a point roughly below 15% at which the side effects start increasing," he says.

The rise in cesareans is perhaps attributable to another logic, an illogic, that assumes that what successfully treats an unhealthy individual will prevent disease in a healthy individual. "Our results show how a medical intervention or treatment that is effective when applied to sick individuals in emergency situations can do more harm than good when applied to healthy populations," Villar and his colleagues conclude. "High rates of cesarean delivery do not necessarily indicate good quality of care or services. Indeed, institutions that deliver a lot of babies by caesarean should initiate a detailed and rigorous assessment of the factors related to their obstetric care."

One argument made by proponents of elective cesarean is that delivering at 39 weeks eliminates the risk of a stillbirth at 40 or 41 weeks—at 41 weeks, that risk is 1 in 1000.[31] This may be true, but the data suggest a net loss. And there's some indication that women who deliver by cesarean are actually more likely to suffer a stillbirth in their next pregnancy.[32]

The term *morbidity* is derived from the Latin *morbus*, for "disease," although a maternal morbidity is not strictly such. In the context of labor and delivery, it is defined by the CDC as "an adverse impact on a woman's physical health during childbirth, beyond what would be expected in a normal delivery." The CDC considers cesarean section a morbidity in and of itself, even if surgery is successful. By that standard, they calculated that between 1993 and 1997, 43% of women giving birth in the United States suffered some morbidity. The CDC did not count episiotomy, which would have driven the number higher, and they based their calculation on a cesarean rate of 25%. Today, according to this formula, the proportion of women suffering morbidity is probably well over half.[33]

A cesarean section is a wound that impedes normal digestive function, function that must resume following surgery. Breast milk is delayed. Seven layers of tissue and muscle are severed. There is also significant blood loss. In a vaginal birth, 300 to 500 milliliters—fittingly, about eight or nine menstrual periods' worth—is normal; anything over 500 is considered a hemorrhage. The average blood loss during a cesarean is 1000 milliliters.

Most women recover well from cesareans, although the recovery is much longer and generally more painful than recovery from a vaginal birth. The *Listening to Mothers* survey found that among women who had cesareans, 80% said incision pain was a problem, 31% had "bowel problems," and, surprisingly, 17% reported incontinence issues.[34] A 2006 study followed 800 low-risk women from pregnancy through 5 weeks postpartum. The authors concluded that women who gave birth surgically were in "significantly worse physical health" than those who gave birth vaginally.[35] And though a "bikini" scar sounds aesthetically benign, women often complain of a permanent disfigurement colloquially termed either the "pooch," "apron," or "overhang"—a flap of skin or fat that bulges over the cesarean scar, which is sometimes so bothersome that it prompts later cosmetic surgery.

Serious complications afflict a minority of cesarean patients, as with any surgery, but not an insignificant minority. The most common is infection. Estimates of just how many women get infections vary widely, from 10% to 50%[36]; 19% of respondents to the *Listening to Mothers* survey who had cesareans reported infection. The infection rate in women who give birth vaginally is 1% to 3%,[37] though all hospital patients are susceptible to increasingly antibiotic-resistant strains of bacteria.[38] Women who have scheduled cesareans experience fewer infections than women who have unplanned cesareans, but still more infections than women who give birth vaginally. Scars can heal improperly and sometimes reopen, requiring more sutures and, often, rehospitalization. In 1994, Public Citizen estimated that 25,000 serious infections a year result from unnecessary cesareans.[39]

Much of the risk of cesarean emerges in the next pregnancy, 91% of which today will be delivered by repeat surgery.[40] Surgeons refer to the layers beneath the skin as "planes," and those planes become harder to distinguish after just one surgery, sticking together in places like melted cheese. These adhesions, as they are called, develop in the majority of abdominal surgery patients. Adhesions themselves can cause problems—pelvic pain, infertility, abnormal bowel function. They also complicate the next surgery. Navigating and separating those adhesions means more time on the operating table, which means more blood loss and the possibility of organ damage. The surgeon could accidentally nick the surface of the intestine, for instance. If that nick goes unnoticed, it could form scar tissue and lead to what is called a bowel obstruction, which thwarts blood flow to the intestine. This life-threatening complication might not manifest for months.

The uterine scar can of course rupture in a future pregnancy. The scar can also interfere with the placenta. Miscarriage and ectopic pregnancy, implantation of an embryo outside the uterus, are more common in women with scarred uteri. An abruption, detachment of the placenta before birth, is twice as likely after just one cesarean section and is a major cause of infant death.[41] Placenta previa, which occurs when the placenta grows over the cervix, is 50% more common after surgery and can cause complications for both mother and baby.[42]

The scar poses a further risk. Accreta, increta, and percreta are grisly, catastrophic placental complications, listed here in order of increasing severity. A placenta accreta implants along the scar from a previous cesarean, an increta is more deeply embedded, and a percreta extends through the scar and often into the bladder. The problem comes after the delivery of the infant: in lay terms, the placenta basically rips open the uterus and possibly the bladder with it as it detaches. This results in a severe hemorrhage, often requiring several blood transfusions and hysterectomy. If the bladder is involved, further reparative surgeries are often required.

Data suggest that such complications have risen 30-fold in the last 30 years. Whereas approximately 1 accreta in 19,000 births occurred in 1970,[43] the proportion narrowed to 1 in 2500 by 1980[44] and was recently reported as high as 1 in 533 births in 2005, according to an analysis by University of Chicago researchers.[45] "[P]lacenta accreta is rapidly becoming the most dreaded complication facing the obstetrician and, in the vast majority of cases, is the result of a previous cesarean delivery," writes Robert Resnik, MD, in a 2006 editorial titled "Can a 29% Cesarean Rate Possibly Be Justified?"

Accreta babies are much more likely to be born premature and underweight. Most mothers lose their uterus; as many as 1 in 15 die.[46] The rise in such disasters is related to the number of cesareans performed, but there is also some controversy over cesarean stitching methods: the classical method is a "double layer" suture of the uterus, but increasingly common is a single layer, which has been associated with more implantation problems and with a fourfold increase in the risk of uterine rupture.[47]

Regardless of the closure technique, the risk of the complication increases with each successive surgery, so a woman having her fourth cesarean has a 1 in 50 chance of an accreta, compared to a chance of 1 in 400 for the first repeat surgery.[48]

There are rarer and even more devastating complications. Necrotizing fasciitis, the flesh-eating bacteria, afflicts 1.8 per 1000 surgical patients[49] and is profoundly disfiguring or fatal. There's the less vicious but still virulent MRSA, an antibiotic-resistant staph infection that is becoming more and more common in all hospital patients. There's pulmonary embolism: a blood clot forms in the legs or pelvis as a consequence of immobilization, travels to lungs, and causes death if not caught in time. There's amniotic fluid embolism, or AFE: amniotic fluid and debris somehow enter the mother's bloodstream and clog the arteries leading to the lungs, although the precise pathology is still poorly understood. This complication is also associated with labor induction and the use of forceps and vacuum. AFE is difficult to diagnose and often fatal. Disseminated intravascular coagulation, DIC, is another rare and often fatal occurrence that can be triggered by AFE or placental abruption; blood begins to clot throughout the body, which pulls platelets from circulation, threatening a hemorrhage.

For each of these complications, there is profound human tragedy, of course. Tanyka Brydson, 25, gave birth to twins via a planned cesarean section in 2001. She was due to go home from the hospital when she began running a fever. "That was the last time I spoke with her," her father, Rodney Brydson, told me. She had contracted necrotizing fasciitis and spent several more weeks in the hospital, heavily sedated, undergoing multiple surgeries to remove the infected tissue. "I lost count of the number of surgeries," says Brydson. "By the time she passed, she had about 55 percent of her body flesh remaining." One of the twins died following her death. In 2004, a Texas woman had a cesarean section after a failed induction and died of an amniotic fluid embolism 30 minutes following surgery. In 2003, a 32-year-old woman in Philadelphia suffered massive blood loss following the cesarean delivery of her fourth child. She survived but was left in a vegetative state.

The midwife and author Ina May Gaskin began collecting such stories in 2000, after learning of a nurse in California who died of a bowel obstruction 9 months—plus two additional surgeries and a colostomy bag—after having a cesarean. Gaskin has sewn these stories into a protest quilt that she has unfurled around the world at conferences and colleges, as well as at the CDC and NIH. She calls the campaign the Safe Motherhood Quilt Project. She'll stitch on a square for anyone who's lost someone to a maternal death since 1982 and can document it. This is the last year the official U.S. maternal death rate declined significantly; it hasn't budged since.[50] At the end of 2006, the quilt had 125 squares.

A woman giving birth by cesarean is more likely to die than a woman giving birth vaginally—four times more likely.[51] There is a heightened risk independent of any medical condition that might have been cause for the surgery itself (i.e., preeclampsia or diabetes). The most recent study looked at 65 deaths in mothers with no risk factors and found that mortality was 3.6 times as likely for those who had cesareans, even those who had surgery before labor.[52] Even planned repeat cesarean carries twice as great a risk of death as vaginal birth.[53]

According to a WHO study, the main cause of maternal deaths in industrialized countries is complications from anesthesia and cesarean section,[54] which suggests that one way to reduce the number of deaths is to reduce the number of cesareans.

In 2006, the U.S. maternal death rate officially rose for the first time in decades. Jeffrey C. King, MD, is medical director of maternal-fetal medicine at Riverside Methodist Hospital in Columbus, Ohio, and heads ACOG's maternal mortality special-interest group. "Our maternal mortality ratio is higher than it is in a variety of developed countries," says King, and he gives several reasons for this: general health status (high rates of obesity, diabetes, and hypertension), lack of access to care, more multiple-gestation pregnancies created by reproductive technology, and the medical malpractice climate, all of which result in more cesareans. "We know that cesarean section, by its very nature, has higher mortality associated with it," he says. With more primary cesareans being done, either legitimately or defensively, and with VBAC waning, more repeats will be done. "More cesareans lead to more repeat cesareans, and repeat cesareans are associated with higher risk of hemorrhagic complications, including placenta accreta leading to hysterectomy," says King. "It's almost like a runaway train. In the long run, this will lead to more maternal deaths."

Still, maternal deaths are rare, so rare that in industrialized countries they are measured per 100,000 births. In the United States, the most recent reported rate is 13.1 per 100,000,[55] a value difficult to bring down to scale. Even a large hospital that delivers 5000 babies annually might just see one maternal death a year or every other year. A doctor or midwife could practice an entire lifetime and never lose a mother.

The truth is, however, that we don't know what our true maternal mortality rate is. The U.S. Centers for Disease Control and Prevention acknowledges that pregnancy-related deaths are underreported by as much as three times.[56] "Most of us believe the maternal mortality rate is probably upwards of mid-twenties to 30 per 100,000," says King, which he projects out to about 1200 maternal deaths a year. Compared to the

Healthy People goal of 3.3 per 100,000, thought to be the irreducible minimum, that is 1000 too many.

In the UK, each and every death occurring in a woman who gave birth in the 12 months prior to her death is investigated; a detailed report, called "Why Mothers Die," is published every 3 years. José Villar says the U.S. needs equivalent surveillance, or at least a large-scale, nationwide study similar to what he led in Latin America. "That is what your neighbors to the north, in Canada, are doing," he told me. The Canadian report is due to be published in 2008.

With the liability climate in the United States, there is a disincentive to investigate deaths—courts have tried to subpoena case information from mortality reviews in malpractice cases. Further, more accurate nationwide surveillance is nearly impossible because we have no consistent terminology or tracking across state health departments. For example, a woman who dies of a bowel obstruction 9 months following her cesarean would be counted as a maternal death in Massachusetts, which includes pregnancy-related deaths up to a year postpartum, but not in Virginia, which counts them through only 42 days postpartum.

In some cities and states that have conducted their own detailed reviews the number of pregnancy-related deaths is two to three times the national reported rate and shows a staggering racial disparity. In North Carolina between 1995 and 1999, the rate was 42 per 100,000 for black women and 12 per 100,000 for white women.[57] In New York City there were 22.9 deaths per 100,000 births between 2003 and 2005, with a similar racial disparity.[58] In Florida between 1999 and 2002, the rate was 12.2 per 100,000 for white and Hispanic women and 38.1 per 100,000 for black women.[59] Even in places where there are no in-depth reviews, the reported numbers are high: in Jackson, Mississippi, the total reported maternal death rate is 25 per 100,000. For women of color, it is 36 per 100,000; for white women it is 17 per 100,000.[60]

Across the board, black women are four times more likely to die in childbirth than white women, according to the CDC.[61] And this is not because they experience more disease. A 2006 study found that conditions such as eclampsia and preeclampsia were equally prevalent in white and black women but that black women were two to three times more likely to die of either condition.[62] "There's no biological reason for this to happen," Cynthia Berg, MD, a CDC epidemiologist who focuses on maternal mortality, told me. "It suggests that we need to be looking at things like access to care, quality of care, and broader social issues." Berg, however, declined to comment on how the cesarean rate relates to maternal mortality.

Isaac Delke, MD, who is chief of maternal-fetal medicine at the University of Florida Medical Center, is also a member of Florida's Pregnancy-Associated Mortality Review committee. He says the connection between the rising cesarean rate and maternal mortality is an "evolving" issue, and what's becoming clear is that while the risks of VBAC are trumpeted, the risks of repeat cesareans are an "untold story," a story that's emerging from Florida's data. Seventy-two mothers died during or following childbirth between 2003 and 2004, roughly one-third from embolism or hemorrhage, both complications related to surgery. "None of them died from VBAC," says Delke. "On the other hand, there are patients who died during a cesarean for placenta accreta, where they couldn't control the hemorrhage." King says we should be looking to Florida as a bellwether. "The maternal mortality rate is rising in Florida," he says.

Still, prominent physicians continue to present cesarean delivery as nearly risk-free. In spite of the evidence to the contrary, Gary Hankins, MD, chair of ACOG's obstetric practice committee, told me that "a scheduled cesarean section absent labor, in a controlled environment, actually has a lower mortality for mom than an anticipated vaginal birth." Benjamin Sachs, MD, professor of obstetrics and gynecology at Harvard Medical School and chair of OB/GYN at Beth Israel Deaconess medical center in Boston, was a coauthor of the 1999 editorial (cited earlier in this chapter) condemning efforts to lower the cesarean rate[63] and continues to insist that such efforts are misguided, even in light of the data that have emerged. "I'm underwhelmed," he says of the WHO and CDC studies suggesting that excess cesareans cause more injury and death in both mother and baby. "We know in Massachusetts that it hasn't caused a rise in mortality or severe morbidity, as far as we can tell."

Sachs was referring to his analysis of data from Massachusetts, which he presented at the 2006 NIH conference. Though he did not publish this analysis.[64] Still, when asked at the conference what he would tell a woman who asked what chance she had of dying from an elective cesarean, Sachs answered, "Based on last year, zero."

"CESAREAN DELIVERY ON MATERNAL REQUEST"

L&D lingo for the cesarean is simply *section*, used as both verb and noun. Hence "We're going to section her" or "She needs a section." No other operation uses this term. No malignancy is being removed (ectomy), nothing is being repaired, corrected, or rerouted (plasty, fusion, bypass), and nothing is being inserted (transplant, replacement). *Section* is another word for cut or incision.

Historically, the decision to proceed with cesarean section, as with any surgical intervention, always entailed a careful weighing of the risks versus the benefits of the procedure. Early on, the risk was absolute. There was no condition riskier than the cesarean itself, and a baby was delivered abdominally only if the mother was dead or dying. Gradually, as medicine gained the ability to anesthetize the patient and prevent infection, other reasons for performing a cesarean accumulated: deformed pelvis, preeclampsia, obstructed labor. The qualifying threat was generally to the mother, not the fetus.

The concept of an elective cesarean, performed as a preventive measure, isn't new. As early as 1906, a Boston physician advocated it for "an exceedingly small class of overcivilized women in whom the natural powers of withstanding pain and muscular fatigue are abnormally deficient."[65] But the idea of preemptive surgery remained controversial for decades, and until the 1970s, the vast majority of cesareans were strictly emergency procedures. Before that time, a cesarean performed without a compelling indication was derided as the mark of a lazy, lackluster physician. "Anybody who can use his hands and has a few tools can do a cesarean section," said J. Whitridge Williams, who exerted great influence over obstetrics through the first third of the century (and who lives on through his textbook *Williams Obstetrics*, which is considered the bible of obstetrics). In his own practice, Williams achieved what today seems an implausibly low cesarean rate, less than 1%, and obstetricians' surgical restraint through the 1960s can be partly attributed to his philosophy.[66]

Surgery was not only unfashionable but still quite risky, with a much higher mortality rate than vaginal birth, even after antibiotics and blood-banking became available. The risks of not doing surgery still had to outweigh the risks of doing it, and the operation usually lost out in that calculation. But in the late 1970s, with surgery in general becoming safer, the scales began to shift. The risk–benefit analysis was thought to favor surgery for more cases—first came the breech babies, then the twins, and later the diabetics, the women of "advanced maternal age," and the "suspected macrosomias."

What was so profound about the 2006 NIH conference on "Cesarean Delivery on Maternal Request" is that it expanded the risk–benefit analysis to be all-inclusive. It asked whether the benefits of a planned cesarean might now favor *all* expectant women, not just those with tricky breeches or chronic disease. And the answer they came up with was "It might."

The cesarean is a landmark achievement of modern medicine, a life- and health-saving procedure. Still, it is major surgery. The CDC considers all abdominal surgery a trauma to the body, a morbidity. A deep wound is created, the uterus is entered, and the mother loses blood. Her body takes a beating. One woman who had a planned repeat cesarean told me, "It was like I was in a car accident and had a baby at the same time."

Given the risks inherent in cesareans as well as the latent risks to future pregnancies, how did the NIH panel arrive at the conclusion that there was "insufficient evidence to fully evaluate the benefits and risks of maternal request cesarean delivery"? Because there are no studies that compare *requested* cesarean to vaginal birth, even though there is a solid body of evidence on the dangers of the cesarean itself. In other words, it was only because the topic was "cesarean delivery on maternal request" that the panel could have reached this conclusion.

"If they had structured it around 'low-risk, non-indicated cesarean,' that would have been a different question, and a more important one," says Eugene Declercq, the professor of maternal and child health at Boston University. "Instead, they could say, 'Well, we don't know, we have to do more research.'"

Declercq coauthored, with two CDC epidemiologists, one of the first expert presentations, commissioned by the NIH, over the 3-day conference. The work severely undermined the premise of the gathering. CDC data collected over the past 15 years show a rise in cesareans without a medical indication—1 in 9 first-time mothers in 2003 had a cesarean for no apparent reason.[67] But researchers warned the panel several times that it is unclear "whether these cesareans were the result of maternal request or because of physician recommendation" and that there's "very little evidence" to suggest that women's choices are affecting the rising cesarean rate. The presentation also cited, as the only indicator of women's opinions on the matter, the 2005 *Listening to Mothers* survey. It found that just one woman out of 1500 requested a primary cesarean— less than one-tenth of 1%,[68] compared to the 2.5% claimed by HealthGrades.[69] Given these uncertainties, the conference seemed misguided from the start.

An NIH conference is organized when the proposed topic is deemed to have enough "importance," says Barnett Kramer, MD, director of the Office of Medical Applications of Research at the NIH. His office makes that decision, at which point a planning committee is formed, a date is set, and the ball gets rolling. But given the data limitations on patient choice, and the legions of women who cannot request a vaginal birth after cesarean, why would the NIH devote precious research dollars to what is probably a sliver of a much larger phenomenon? And further, when CDC epidemiologists are telling us that the cesarean rate is attributable to changes in provider behavior, why make it about a woman's choice?

The focus on maternal request originates with the National Institute of Child Health and Human Development, a division of the NIH. In July 2003, Catherine Spong, MD, chief of the pregnancy and perinatology branch of the NICHD, formally proposed the conference with two others in a memo titled "Proposal for State of the Science Conference on Elective Cesarean Delivery." The final wording of the conference title was hammered out in planning committee meetings for which she served as chair, but the focus was laid down from the outset.

I spoke twice with Spong. Weeks prior to the conference, she told me, "A lot of women are asking for this," although she didn't cite any specific data or studies. When I spoke with her a few months after the conference and asked her directly what data prompted the NICHD to propose a conference on the subject of "maternal request" cesarean, again she did not identify a single study by name. "I think there are some reports and some studies out there to show that some women are asking for this. There's been media attention," she said, mentioning Britney

Spears. I pressed for specifics, and she finally admitted that "The data on the incidence of cesarean delivery on maternal request are very poor."

The HealthGrades study was never cited by name in any of the conference literature, and when I mentioned it to Spong she seemed only vaguely aware of it. However, it does appear in the initial conference memo. "The numbers were right out of HealthGrades," says Declercq. "Which is doubly ironic, because these are theoretically the people who are most interested in scientific research, not a non-peer-reviewed publication generated by a company that's trying to build up its business." The NIH's use of the HealthGrades study but not the *Listening to Mothers* survey revealed an inconsistency, if not a bias. When I asked Kramer about these contradictions and data gaps, he told me, "We stand behind the process, not the product."

Howard Minkoff, MD, chair of obstetrics and gynecology at Maimonides Medical Center in Brooklyn, New York State's largest maternity ward, was asked to serve on the NIH conference planning committee. An obstetrician for 25 years, he is also a member of the ACOG ethics committee that wrote the 2003 opinion condoning patient-choice cesarean. I asked him, as a conference insider, why he thought it was focused on "choice," in the midst of such a high cesarean rate. "That's a straw man," he said flatly. "No one has come up to me and said, 'I have absolutely no indication, but I'm like Britney Spears and I'm too posh to push.' Maybe that happens where women do lunch, so to speak. But that's never happened to me. What is happening is that the threshold for doing a cesarean has dropped."

Sanctioning patient-choice cesareans removes that threshold entirely, effectively sanctioning physician-choice cesareans as well, he says. "Doctors are sort of saying, *sotto voce*, 'Well, since we're allowing elective sections, then why should I worry about sectioning somebody in labor for mediocre reasons?' Now we don't need any reason," says Minkoff. "I don't think anybody is saying that out loud—I don't even think they're conscious of it."

Minkoff says the cesarean rate should be high up on the public health agenda. One of his mentors served on the 1980 conference panel, and the first article Minkoff ever published, that same year, was titled "The Rising Cesarean Rate: Can It Safely Be Reversed?"[70] "There are now a million women a year giving birth with a scar in their bellies—you can do the math and count how many women are going to have accreta, how many are going to have placenta previa, how many babies will be stillborn," he says. "Rather than focusing on the less than one percent of this that may be attributable to cesarean by choice, it's time to reopen the question that hasn't been looked at in 25 years, when the section rate was roughly half of what it is now."

I asked Catherine Spong why the NIH didn't convene a conference on the rising cesarean rate in general. "Having a conference on the rising cesarean rate really isn't a question for a state of the science or a consensus conference," she said. Yet that's exactly what the NIH did in 1980, and today there is a far larger and more rigorous body of research evidence on cesareans. I asked Spong why they didn't call the conference "medically unnecessary cesarean delivery" or something to that effect—a more neutral, more scientific description that doesn't project a zeitgeist of patient choice. She said the point of the conference was "to provide women with information on the risks and benefits so that they can make informed decisions."

Carol Sakala, PhD, formerly a scientist with the U.S. Agency for Healthcare Research and Quality, which oversees the systematic evidence reviews conducted in preparation for a conference, now serves as director of programs of Childbirth Connection. Childbirth Connection is the nonprofit research and advocacy group that sponsored the *Listening to Mothers* surveys. Two years prior to the NIH conference, Sakala conducted a systematic review of the benefits and risks of cesarean section versus vaginal birth. Months of research and the resulting hundreds of pages were condensed and neatly packaged in a 30-page consumer-friendly booklet called "What Every Pregnant Woman Needs to Know About Cesarean Section."

Sakala's review evaluated hundreds of studies, and it concludes as follows:

> Without a clear, compelling and well-supported justification for cesarean section or assisted vaginal birth, a spontaneous vaginal birth that minimizes use of interventions that may be injurious to mothers and babies is the safest way for women to give birth and babies to be born.[71]

A systematic evidence review examines the available literature on a particular topic for its overall thrust. The NIH commissioned a review for the conference, but it bore little resemblance to Sakala's and arrived at a far different conclusion. For one thing, says Sakala, the NIH review considered only the short- and long-term outcomes of the initial cesarean, not the risks associated with future repeat cesareans. "Placenta accreta was not mentioned in the report, placental abruption was not mentioned in the report. The only place where adhesion appears in the document is in the 'need for more research,' section," she says. "There's a high rate of scar tissue with any surgery—any surgeon knows this. Yet this was completely swept under the table."

Michael Klein, MD, professor emeritus at the University of British Columbia, was among a number of experts asked by the NIH to review the systematic evidence review prior to the conference.[72] "It was fundamentally flawed," says Klein. "It was so fundamentally flawed in my view that it couldn't be fixed." Klein took issue with a number of things, foremost among them the exclusion of future pregnancy outcomes. "The data is absolutely unambiguous," he says. "The enhanced risks for placenta previa, accreta, percreta, ectopic pregnancy, and infertility go up after the first cesarean section. There's a huge amount of morbidity associated with subsequent births. And they chose simply not to look at it."

Klein also took issue with the methodology. Because there are no randomized controlled trials comparing primary elective cesarean to planned vaginal birth—and probably never will be—the researchers had to improvise and use what are called proxy groups. One they used repeatedly was Mary Hannah's breech trial, because it was a randomized controlled trial. In Sakala's review, the breech trial did not pass muster because "all babies were breech, and results may not apply to other populations." Women considering an elective cesarean are by definition low-risk, and therefore the proxy groups were supposed to represent women with no risk factors—that is, women with uncomplicated, singleton, vertex (head-first) births. Klein has harsh words about this. "Sorry folks, these are not vertex births!" he says. "This is just preposterous! But then it gets even worse. Having done that, they chose not to look at two-year follow-up, which showed no difference in mother–baby outcomes, including pelvic floor problems."

The only way to definitively settle the debate would be a randomized controlled trial comparing healthy women who schedule a cesarean to healthy women who plan to give birth vaginally. And during the conference, it was revealed by a physician in the audience that the NIH had already funded a study on the feasibility of such a trial. This study was being led by Anthony Visco, MD, the same researcher who conducted the systematic evidence review for the conference. The feasibility study gathered focus groups of childbearing-age women, pregnant and not, and asked them whether they would be willing to participate in a randomized controlled trial, risking randomization to surgery. They overwhelmingly said no.

It is here that the question driving the conference hits a brick wall. If a randomized controlled trial is the only research evidence that will convince, and if such a trial is neither feasible nor ethical, then data on the risks of cesarean section in low-risk women must suffice. And the amount of existing data is vast. Since her initial review, Sakala says she's amassed a pile of articles 20 inches thick. In early 2007, for instance, a large Canadian study found that otherwise healthy women who had cesareans were three times more likely to suffer complications than women who gave birth vaginally.[73] "The damning evidence is mind-boggling," says Sakala.

Klein submitted a thorough and detailed critique of Visco's systematic review to the NIH, as requested. "They thanked me very much and told me that they'd acknowledge me in the published review, to which I replied, 'No, you won't. I don't want to be associated with this in any way. Please take my name off it.'"

Pelvic floor problems were exhaustively researched by the NIH systematic review—Visco is a urogynecologist. But at this influential conference, no research was presented on the many known labor management practices associated with pelvic floor injury, such as episiotomy, manual pressure on the uterus, pushing in a recumbent position, and "directed," hold-your-breath-and-count-to-10 pushing. This was the point that the audience kept raising. If women are seeking cesarean section because they fear incontinence or sexual dysfunction, shouldn't they be informed of common labor management practices that contribute? Shouldn't clinicians be informed of those practices and avoid them? And if the comparison is between the outcomes of cesarean delivery and those of vaginal birth, shouldn't we be comparing cesarean to normal, physiological birth?

Instead, the conference implied something unprecedented about normal birth: if the trauma of cesarean section—cutting a birth canal in the abdomen—might be equal to or less than the trauma of a modern vaginal birth, then vaginal birth, as practiced in most U.S. hospitals, is so harmful that it rivals the injury of major abdominal surgery.

One of the arguments for "prophylactic" elective cesarean is that it will preempt problems like third- and fourth-degree perineal tears and long, exhausting labors that ultimately result in unplanned cesareans, which are more risky than cesareans that are planned. But rather than offering surgical birth as an alternative, critics like Sakala and Klein argue that labor management should be reformed. The fact is that few women who plan a spontaneous, physiological birth in a hospital setting actually have one. Elective cesarean, it follows, is prophylactic against actively managed birth, a "surgical solution to a non-surgical problem," says Klein. Says Sakala, "We should not ask mothers to choose between vaginal birth with avoidable harms and cesarean section."

If the goal of the conference was, as Spong says, to provide women with information so they can make an informed decision, the validity of that information has been called into question. The final statement, written by the panel, published as a consumer-friendly pamphlet, suggests that a primary cesarean section is equivalent in risk to vaginal birth. It does warn that "Given that the risks of placenta previa and accreta rise with each cesarean delivery, cesarean delivery on maternal request is not recommended for women desiring *several* children" (emphasis mine). "Several" is left up to interpretation, but the risks begin accumulating after the first cesarean. "The word should have been 'next' or 'subsequent,'" says Klein. The statement says that medically unnecessary cesarean may be a "reasonable" choice for women, but there is no mention that there will be a *lack* of choice to give birth vaginally the next time.[74]

What all this adds up to for Klein is a clear pretext to "normalize the cesarean section." He says this is evident in the very architecture of the conference, which flipped the traditional scientific burden of proof. Klein says, "If you have a conventional procedure, let's call it vaginal childbirth, and you're proposing a major deviation from that norm, cesarean section, then the burden of proof is on the people who want change." The NIH's conclusion, he says, is "a radical departure from medical norms."

Instead of cautioning physicians and women against the gamble of unnecessary surgery, the panel reaffirmed ACOG's position, that fulfilling a patient request is ethically sound so long as the patient is informed of the known risks. Klein says this is backwards and that elective cesarean should be discouraged until the science suggests that it is safe. That is the conclusion to which FIGO, the Geneva-based International Federation Gynecology and Obstetrics, came: "At present, because hard evidence of net benefit does not exist, performing Caesarean section for non-medical reasons is ethically not justified."[75]

At a press briefing in May 2006, Mary D'Alton, MD, chair of OB/GYN at Columbia University Medical Center in New York and chair of the NIH conference panel, told reporters that placenta problems are a growing concern (she sees an accreta once a month now at her hospital). "There's definitive information that the incidence of placenta accreta and perceta is rising due to the increasing incidence of cesarean section," she said. Seated next to her, Frederic Frigoletto (who coauthored the 1999 editorial condemning efforts to reduce the cesarean rate) talked about a recent case of placenta percreta at Massachusetts General Hospital in Boston—the woman required 25 units of blood. "We were very fortunate to save her life," he said.

Robert Lorenz, MD, director of maternal-fetal medicine and vice chair of obstetrics at William Beaumont Hospital in Royal Oak, Michigan, is, like Minkoff, a member of the ACOG ethics committee responsible for writing the 2003 opinion on patient choice. When we talked, he also voluntarily brought up the nightmare of an accreta. "You can't imagine," he said. "When a woman comes in for a scheduled cesarean, and her mother is flying in, and three hours later she's in intensive care, intubated, receiving her 20th unit of blood. . . . This is a disease that didn't exist before we were doing cesareans."

"The more times a lady has a cesarean section, the greater the risk—that is clear," says Gary Hankins of ACOG. "But if a woman is anticipating having only one or two children, there's no question that cesarean section is safer for both the mom and baby."

There is a disconnect here: bald recognition of the risks of repeat cesareans, yet at the same time a tacit—or, in Hankins's case, explicit—encouragement toward primary, patient-chosen cesareans and a revived mandate for "once a cesarean, always a cesarean." The fact that primary cesareans lead to repeat cesareans, and the fact that many women planning to have one or two children may later decide to have more, are left out of the equation.

"The number one problem right now is the absence of an appropriately aggressive leadership in the OB/GYN community," says Sidney Wolfe of Public Citizen—a new guard of obstetric leaders who are unwilling to buck the system. "It's interesting," says Eugene Declercq, "because this comes about at a time when there are more female obstetricians than there ever have been, and there was a lot of hope that that would change things, and it really hasn't." Female obstetricians are, in fact, more enthusiastic about cesareans than their male peers. When asked in surveys whether they would choose an elective cesarean for themselves or their spouses, the women said yes in higher numbers.[76]

Following this trend, Mary D'Alton is Mortimer Rosen's successor both as chair of an NIH conference on cesarean section and as the Willard C. Rappleye professor and chair of obstetrics and gynecology at Columbia University Medical Center. In both forums, however, she is leaving a markedly different legacy. Weeks before he died, Rosen told a reporter, "Cesareans are costly, dangerous and painful. This is not a neat, simple procedure. It is big-time, major surgery. The floor of the operating room is covered with blood and fluids. A woman loses two units of blood, undergoes anesthesia. She is scarred internally and externally."[77] D'Alton, on the other hand, told United Press International that she hopes to see a randomized controlled trial on planned primary cesarean section.[78] At Columbia, one of her first executive decisions was to effectively shut down the midwife-run birthing center housed within the hospital, the Allen Pavilion, which developed under Rosen's influence. She has also presided over a swift rise in the cesarean rate that Rosen had worked so diligently to bring down. In 2004, Columbia claimed one of the highest rates of surgical birth in New York City, at 37.1%.[79]

OPTIMAL V. NORMAL

On paper, Kristin Branske-Lotane, a corporate meeting planner in Chicago, was successfully induced into labor a week past her due date and gave birth to a healthy baby girl vaginally. Neither she nor her baby suffered any morbidity as it is defined by the CDC. But the birth was traumatic nonetheless. Planning to have an unmedicated delivery, Branske-Lotane had read up on pain. And one of the first things she read was that the pain of an induction is not normal pain. She knew that the Pitocin would be rough, "but what I was unprepared for was labor from 4:00 p.m. until the following morning at 3:00 a.m. without the option of an epidural" because she hadn't dilated enough, she told me. The pain was agony, the dilation agonizingly slow. A few hours in, a resident came and tried to break her water. She remembers him down between her legs, poking repeatedly with a metal instrument. Finally he looked up and said, "Did I do it?" She withstood 12 hours of increasing levels of Pitocin, managed only by moving around the small room, wheeling her IV bag in tow. "I vividly remember that the only thing that made it better was standing up and bending over the bed," she says, although the nurses kept telling her not to—it threw off the fetal monitor strip. "I was like, you're kidding, right?" If she had been confined to bed, she says, "It would have been a nightmare."

Finally, at 4 a.m., she got the epidural she'd been asking for. It provided some relief and allowed for a catnap, but by daybreak she was awake again and in pain. She was also exhausted and starving—food and drink were off limits. She begged to start pushing. "Pushing felt better," she says. "It feels better to be doing something." She pushed for 4 hours lying flat on her back. The shift changed while she was pushing, and a nurse–midwife she had never met ended up catching the baby. Branske-Lotane tore on her perineum as the baby emerged. "The baby and I both had a fever by the end and she needed to have a tube put down her throat to breathe," she says. The baby also had numerous cuts and scratches on her head, which Branske-Lotane attributes to the amateur attempts at breaking her water, though they could have also been markings from an internal fetal monitor. "We were both fine, but I attribute my initial breastfeeding failure to being so exhausted from the whole experience."

The crudest measure of a successful birth is survival: live mother, live baby. Next to that is "healthy mother" and "healthy baby." The baby is neatly assessed on a scale of 1 to 10 called the Apgar score after Virginia Apgar, a New York anesthesiologist who created the system as a way to hold physicians more accountable for infant mortality. The Apgar is a measure of a baby's vital signs. From zero to 2 points each are assigned for color, breathing, movement, heart rate, and response to stimuli, assessed at 1 minute following birth and again at 5 minutes. Thus a pale, motionless neonate who isn't breathing on his own after a minute has an initial Apgar of zero, and a kicking, crying, rosy-fleshed baby gets a perfect 10. The Apgar is a research tool—in the Breech Trial, for example, babies with an Apgar score less than 4 at 5 minutes were considered to have suffered "serious neonatal morbidity."

As useful as it is, the Apgar is merely a couple of snapshots, not the complete record. Branske-Lotane remembers her daughter having high Apgars. By the numbers alone, you'd never know the baby had been intubated, feverish, and lacerated on her scalp.

We have an even less comprehensive record for mothers. A "healthy" mother is generally defined by the *absence* of serious complications rather than by the presence of wellness. In research studies, if a mother required no blood transfusions and had no severe (third- or fourth-degree) perineal tearing, no infection that required rehospitalization, and no admission to the intensive care unit, then the outcome is considered good. This is how health is measured in general, although that view has been challenged in recent years. The World Health Organization defines health as "a state of complete physical, mental and social well-being and not merely the absence of disease or infirmity."[80] And in terms of the goal of maternity care, it amends "healthy mother and child" to include the "least possible level of intervention."[81]

In 2006 the American College of Nurse–Midwives developed a research tool to evaluate maternity care. Like the Apgar, the Optimality Index is a score. But rather than measuring an individual outcome, the index is intended to measure the quality of care across an institution or population. The index defines optimal care as the World Health Organization does: essentially, "no interference." Points are deducted for induction or augmentation, early vaginal exams, epidural, continuous electronic fetal monitoring, directed pushing, flat-on-back pushing, episiotomy, and separation of mother and baby.

Judith Fullerton, PhD, a certified nurse–midwife for 35 years, is one of the index's creators. She says the index values evidence-based care, and the goal is to measure the gap between evidence and practice, between normal and optimal. "Between 5 and 6 o'clock at night the traffic is normal at 5 miles per hour, but that is hardly optimal," she says. "Normal is customary and usual, but it may not be necessarily what the evidence shows to be best."

The Optimality Index is a promising tool, but so far it has been used only in pilot studies. Currently, there are gaps in what we know, gaps in what we measure, and assumptions that we make. The assumption promulgated by the early anti-cesarean crusaders was that if we could just prevent unnecessary surgery, we'd save women a great deal of trauma. Then the urogynecologists came along and said wait, there's trauma in vaginal birth as well. But what has been largely ignored is the trauma itself, regardless of the ultimate route of delivery, and its impact on women and babies.

Michel Odent has termed this area of inquiry "primal health"; essentially, it is the study of how the way we are born affects who we become. Odent founded the Primal Health Research Centre in 1990. He's interested in looking far beyond the 5-minute Apgar score to what we might call the 5-year, 25-year, and 50-year Apgar. He's put a database online, where one can search studies that have connected narcotics at birth with addiction in adulthood; induction of labor with autism; and cesarean section with immune disorders. The research is far from conclusive, but it points to the large, unknown territory of the impact of medicalized childbirth.

Odent places value on the process of physiological childbirth itself, of which we still have only limited understanding. How can we fully appreciate the risks of intervention, he asks, if we don't fully understand what is normal? The mother's body has spent 9 months growing and sustaining fetal life, and millennia of evolution have depended on spontaneous labor and its timed release of several hormones to transition the fetus from the womb to the outside world. Odent has compiled scientific evidence that each one of these hormones serves an important function in guiding the progress of labor and supporting the fetus—and that these hormones are interdependent. "What we're understanding today is that what happens at birth seems to be important," says Odent.

BAD-ASS CONTRACTIONS

Oxytocin, produced in the hypothalamus and secreted by the posterior pituitary gland, is the force that powers normal childbirth; labor would never progress to its ultimate conclusion without it. Oxytocin is an ancient hormone, present in all mammals. In addition to its star role of contracting the uterus during labor and birth, oxytocin is the hormone secreted, in both men and women, during the ecstasy of orgasm, the feeling of emotional connection with a friend, the rush of being in love, and the literal rush of milk to a suckling infant. We even get a jolt during a shared meal. For this, oxytocin has been dubbed the love hormone. In the words of Ina May Gaskin, "What gets the baby in, gets the baby out." And gets the baby fed, too.

Oxytocin opens the floodgates. It facilitates the male ejaculation reflex, the milk letdown reflex, and the "fetal ejection reflex," as Michel Odent describes the powerful finale of contractions that expel the baby from the birth canal. Oxytocin also works on our emotions, opening our hearts, cementing intimacy and community, and, in the case of childbirth, bonding mother to child. Oxytocin makes space for something, someone new.

It is often presumed that the oxytocin stored in a glass vial is no different from the oxytocin stored in the brain and that to be "Pitted," or induced, inflicts no extra discomfort or pain. "To a woman nine-months pregnant, an intravenous drip of synthetic oxytocin is a powerful elixir" is how *Chemical and Engineering News* magazine described the drug in its 2005 issue devoted to "The Top Pharmaceuticals That Changed the World." External oxytocin works powerfully on the uterus, but it does not cross the blood–brain barrier, so it doesn't provoke the emotional release that the body's own oxytocin does. Not only that, but it signals the body to shut down its own production of oxytocin. It is no elixir. There is no love in the synthetic love hormone.

For all the tons of synthetic oxytocin being given to women each year around the world, there has been scant research on how it feels. One randomized study of women who labored on their own or with synthetic oxytocin found that 80% in the latter group felt it had increased their pain.[82] A British midwife told a researcher that the sounds women make when they're on artificial oxytocin are hauntingly different: "It's a panic, it's a scream and it's different from the noise they make when they're working with their bodies. . . . It sounds like someone's being murdered."[83] Some point to the Dublin trials, in which 40% of women were receiving artificial oxytocin, as evidence of increased pain, because epidurals increased 12-fold under the active management protocol.[84] At the same time, women who are being induced, like Branske-Lotane, often spend varying lengths of time on the drug without the option of pain relief.

"It's very painful, and it's invasive," Judith Halek, a practicing doula for 20 years in New York City, told me. "It's one contraction after another, like bulldozers and gangbusters driving through her body. And I've got to tell you, I wouldn't expect any woman to go through an induction of Pitocin without an epidural. It's torturous." There is little disagreement among clinicians who've seen both Pitocin labor and normal labor. The latter starts off slow and builds. A Pitocin induction, it has been said, takes a woman from zero to 60 all at once. "These are not your natural, slow-building contractions that have a crescendo and decrescendo," says Jacques Moritz, MD, in New York. "These are bad-ass contractions. I personally think it's cruel and unusual punishment to give somebody Pitocin without an epidural."

Erin Morrison of Lanham, Maryland, experienced both. Her water broke at home and her doctor told her to come to the hospital right away. She was left to labor naturally for 12 hours and then given Pitocin. Before the Pitocin, she told me, she was able to breathe through each contraction—there was enough time between them to regroup. "You tell yourself, 'I can get through a minute.' But with the Pitocin, the contractions follow one right behind another. You almost have no chance to breathe." Branske-Lotane experienced natural contractions with her second baby, and she puts it in terms of music. Her body's contractions were a familiar refrain. The Pitocin contractions were "some crazy weird jazz." A normal contraction was "still really bad, but you understood it, you knew where it was coming from, and you felt like it was going somewhere."

In studies of labor stimulators, the measure of success is often the time from dose to delivery—speeding up labor is certainly one way to cut down on "dystocia" diagnoses. And the rise in the use of these agents may be partly attributed to efforts to lower the cesarean rate. Whereas Rosen's program at Columbia Presbyterian Hospital encouraged labor support, St. Lukes Hospital in Denver administered high-dose Pitocin when labor fell off the Friedman curve.[85] In other words, labors that would have ended in cesarean for "failure to progress" ended promptly in a vaginal birth, but at what cost to the mother? And at what cost to the baby? What if everybody had just waited?

A contraction is stressful on both mother and baby. Labor is essentially sprint training; that is, a contraction is followed by a resting period, during which the fetus replenishes oxygen and the laboring woman gets a literal breather. As labor progresses, the contractions become stronger and more frequent, culminating in the "ejection reflex" documented by Odent. Pitocin has no such intelligence. And with an epidural deadening the body's natural pain threshold, staff can keep upping the dose, which can lead to contractions that fire like a machine gun or that last for minutes, during which time the fetus is oxygen-deprived. This is called hyperstimulation. It is not uncommon and would be considered a trauma—beyond what is normal. In half of the cases of hyperstimulation, the fetal heart rate drops below normal (this is called a "non-reassuring" heart-tone). If it stays there, it's fetal distress.[86]

Kathleen Rice Simpson, the perinatal safety expert who has studied the nurse–physician conflicts over synthetic oxytocin, says that hyperstimulation has been somewhat trivialized and is often ignored until the baby's heartbeat dips, which is the wrong response. The drug should be turned down or off immediately. Cytotec also causes contractions, and because it is a pill administered vaginally and absorbed quickly, an adverse reaction can't be reversed.

At its worst, hyperstimulation can escalate to a uterine rupture or premature detachment of the placenta. And the interventions that often accompany the Pitocin—amniotomy, insertion of an intrauterine pressure catheter, placement of a fetal scalp electrode—are to blame for nearly half of umbilical cord prolapses.[87] A recent ACOG survey found that in 43% of malpractice suits involving neurologically impaired babies, Pitocin was to blame.[88]

"Mismanagement of oxytocin is a significant liability risk," says Simpson, "even though most of the time it doesn't harm the baby." Clinicians and women have the impression that it's harmless. "Most babies are so healthy, they're so resilient, they can take just about anything. You can't predict which baby is going to turn out with an adverse outcome and which will not."

Marsden Wagner, the neonatologist formerly with the WHO, argues that the extent of the damage caused by hyperstimulation is unknown. He specifically implicates the drug misoprostol, or Cytotec. Wagner has testified in 16 malpractice suits involving the drug and involving hyperstimulation; in four of these cases the mother died, and in four the baby died.

But Pitocin is also a concern. A 1997 study at one hospital found that it doubled the odds of oxygen deprivation during labor.[89] "The situation is somewhat analogous to holding an infant under the surface of the water, allowing the infant to come to the surface to gasp for air, but not to breathe," the childbirth activist Doris Haire, founder of the American Foundation for Maternal and Child Health, told UNICEF's 1997 Birth Without Borders Conference. Even *Williams Obstetrics* offers a sobering history: "Oxytocin is a powerful drug, and it has killed or maimed mothers through rupture of the uterus and even more babies through hypoxia from markedly hypertonic uterine contractions."[90]

Writing in the *British Medical Journal* in 1994, Richard Lilford, a research director in the UK's National Health Service, commented that "if oxytocin had been discovered in the 1990s we would not sanction its widespread routine use and would conduct further clinical trials."[91] Lilford banned use of the drug at his own hospital, Leeds General Infirmary.[92] Wagner draws an analogy with skydiving: "With all the risks associated with oxytocin, using it . . . to speed up labor is like designing a streamlined parachute—you may get there quicker but you may pay a big price."[93]

Odent argues that the price may be higher than we can measure. "We have to ask questions in terms of civilization," he cautions. Before the advent of artificial oxytocin, women had to rely on their bodies to go into labor and give birth. Now, many women are relying on manmade hormones or surgery. He calls this "a turning point in the history of childbirth."

There are several other unknowns. "We do not know the psychological effects of giving birth without the peak levels of oxytocin that nature prescribes for all mammalian species," writes Sarah J. Buckley, MD, an obstetrician and family practitioner in Australia who has documented the hormonal physiology of normal birth.[94] Normal oxytocin function is essential to the behavior that makes us human. It is crucial not only to reproduction but also to social interaction, communication, and our participation in culture. Malfunction of the oxytocin system factors significantly in autistic spectrum disorders, for instance. A 2004 study out of Australia found that autistic children were twice as likely to have been born without natural labor, either by elective cesarean or induction.[95]

There's a tendency to look upon a labor intervention, such as induction, in isolation, when it should be regarded as more of a package deal. With Pitocin comes amniotomy, internal fetal monitoring, immobilization, epidural, and urine catheter; oftentimes a blood sample will be taken from the fetus's scalp to confirm a heart tracing, and an intrauterine pressure catheter will be inserted to measure the contractions' strength within the womb. Intervention leads to intervention—chaos that the body may not be capable of resolving on its own. The term *cascade of interventions* is often employed, and it calls up a powerful image. Even the most benign and isolated of routine practices, such as intravenous fluids, introduces a foreign element into the delicate ecosystem of childbirth. IV fluids, for instance, dilute the body's own oxytocin levels and can throw off a person's electrolyte balance. The prominent Dutch obstetrician G. J. Kloosterman puts it this way:

> Spontaneous labour in a normal woman is an event marked by a number of processes so complicated and so perfectly attuned to each other that any interference with them will only detract from their optimal character. . . . The danger will arise that the physiological part of obstetrics will be threatened by doctors who all too often will change true physiological aspects of reproduction into pathology."[96]

TO BE BORN IS TO BREATHE

Although modern medicine can chemically mimic dilation and contractions with manmade prostaglandin and oxytocin, it has not been able to fully explain or successfully replicate the onset of labor. The moment when spontaneous labor begins is a moment that remains mysterious, a private hormonal conversation between mother and fetus that scientists have yet to fully decode. And research suggests that this moment is extremely important.

"What we understand now is that the baby participates in the initiation of labor," says Odent. "In particular, the baby gives a signal when its lungs are mature. For a baby to be born it implies that the lungs are ready, because to be born is to breathe. When you induce labor, or when you do an elective cesarean section with no labor, the baby has not given the signal. The baby has not said, 'I am ready, I am mature.'" In other words, induced labor is premature labor.

In the womb, the lungs are filled with fluid, and the fetus receives oxygen through the umbilical cord. The remarkable process by which the fetus adapts in seconds from water to air is still unclear, but the current understanding is that it begins purging its lungs of fluid in the days prior to birth. "Somehow, the fetus comes to know that it is about to be born," is how Lucky Jain, MD, professor of pediatrics at Emory University, puts it.[97] Jain has studied this transition from one respiratory medium to another and has found that the process continues during spontaneous labor and birth. Hormones are released that prime the lungs for air, and the squeezing effect of the birth canal helps purge the lungs of excess fluid.

Cesarean babies often must be heavily suctioned or intubated to facilitate breathing; Jain says that a significant number of those admitted to NICUs are in fact term or near-term respiratory cases, and cesarean birth has been linked with childhood asthma in a number of studies. One 2006 study found that babies born by planned cesarean were significantly more likely to spend their first few days of life in the NICU, and those delivered before 39 weeks were twice as likely to develop a lung disorder as were babies whose mothers went into labor.[98] ACOG discourages cesareans prior to 39 weeks gestation—this was reaffirmed by the NIH conference—but there remains a margin of error in determining gestational age. Jain estimates that for every 1 million cesareans, there will be 25,000 cases of respiratory distress and 5000 cases of outright failure.[99] He reports that in Brazil, where private hospitals deliver some three-quarters of babies by scheduled cesarean, the NICUs are overflowing.

Labor induction and scheduled cesareans together are implicated in a veritable epidemic of fetal immaturity in the United States. A 2006 study by the March of Dimes noted that the most common length of pregnancy in the United States has now slipped from 40 weeks to 39 weeks,[100] prompting a public education campaign titled "I Want My 9 Months." Jane Haley, the nurse manager at Winthrop Hospital on Long Island, has observed this firsthand. "I see a lot of babies being delivered at

35, 36, 37 weeks," she told me. "We're thinking they're term babies, but they're not." The number of scheduled cesareans and the number of labor inductions add up to roughly half of U.S. babies being delivered before they've "given the signal."

Preterm babies have a harder time with a number of functions. It goes without saying that if breathing is a problem, so is breastfeeding. And here, too, our efforts to replicate nature pale in comparison: breast milk is inimitable. A recent Save the Children "State of the World's Mothers" report states that "Immediate breastfeeding is one of the most effective interventions for newborn survival."[101] (This is one of the reasons why the Baby Friendly Hospital Initiative, a joint effort of WHO and UNICEF, requires hospitals that wish to achieve "Baby Friendly" status to refuse to dispense free formula samples.)

Babies born vaginally with minimal obstetric interventions are more likely to breastfeed immediately, and babies who breastfeed immediately are more likely to continue breastfeeding. The CDC calls breastfeeding an "extremely time-sensitive relationship." The World Health Organization recommends that newborns be put to the breast within the half hour after birth; a "Baby Friendly" hospital in the United States must recommend and facilitate breastfeeding initiation within the hour, prioritizing immediate skin-to-skin contact over routine weighing, measuring, and testing in order to allow for bonding and nursing first.

The most common reason why babies are not put to the breast within the first hour is the cesarean section, and cesarean babies are more likely to be given milk substitutes in the nursery while the mother is recovering. A 2002 study found skin-to-skin contact to be "almost nonexistent" among post-operative mothers and their babies.[102] Babies born to mothers who were medicated during labor are also at a disadvantage. "Medications and procedures administered to the mother during labor affect the infant's behavior at the time of birth, which in turn affects the infant's ability to suckle," says a 2005 CDC report.[103] Procedures such as aggressive suctioning or intubation of the baby also affect breastfeeding. The tube irritates the baby's mouth and throat, making feeding unpalatable. Branske-Lotane's daughter would not latch on for weeks; she remembers the strained sound of her baby's cries in the hospital: "She sounded hoarse."

Maureen Corry of Childbirth Connection argues that even if there are no marquee consequences, such as were absent in Branske-Lotane's case, the way most U.S. women are giving birth—vaginal or cesarean—is not healthy. "The typical childbirth experience has been transformed into a morass of wires, tubes, machines and medications that leave healthy women immobilized, vulnerable to high levels of surgery, and burdened with physical and emotional health concerns while caring for their newborns."

Yet the value of spontaneous vaginal birth—the conditioning of the fetal lungs, the priming of the breastfeeding relationship, the infusion of the "love hormone," the physical proximity of mother and baby—is a radical notion among some obstetric leaders. I asked Gary Hankins whether, in promoting the cesarean as safer than vaginal birth, he's factoring in the benefits of the normal labor process. "Well, tell me what they are," he responded.

SCARRED MOTHERS

On paper, Birgit Amadori had two successful cesarean sections. Picture-perfect physical recoveries, she says. No problems breastfeeding either time. The first was in 1999 in Germany, Amadori's home country She was under the care of midwives, as is customary for normal pregnancies there, but during labor the baby's heart rate kept dipping abnormally. She was transferred to the hospital for an obstetric consult and had a cesarean that afternoon. The umbilical cord was wrapped tightly around the baby's neck.

The cesarean was a disappointment—painful, traumatic, unexpected. But she recovered, and with time it faded from memory. Five years later, in Torrance, California, Amadori became pregnant again. She assumed she would give birth vaginally. It wasn't until her 20-week appointment that her obstetrician told her no VBAC; it was "policy." Amadori had never heard of such a thing. She argued, she pleaded. Her insurance would cover delivery only at Torrance Memorial Hospital, and she called every obstetrician with privileges there. Just one told her she would allow a vaginal birth, but she added that Amadori was too far along to transfer care. Amadori then called the birthing center; they wouldn't do

VBACs either. She called a hotline for midwives; they told her it was outside their regulations.

Amadori didn't know what to do. She was just beginning to comprehend the U.S. health care system and was mystified by the politics of childbirth. She wrote to the ICAN e-mail list and they suggested that she either show up at the hospital pushing or stay home and go solo. "I have a lot of respect for women who do unassisted home birth," she says. "But I was too scared personally, without a midwife, without my family here. And my husband was not into it at all." Amadori argued with her physician at every prenatal appointment, often breaking down in tears.

"I ended up scheduling the cesarean," she says, "just like a sheep, just giving in to fate." She couldn't find another way out. "I scheduled it and didn't want to go. It was this big dilemma. I knew it was going to be bad. Not for my baby but for myself."

Amadori is an artist. I knew her birth story in images before she described it to me in words. The artwork is accessible online, with a dedication to "all the scarred mothers."[104] The series of computer illustrations, 28 in all, amount to a graphic novel of sorts, haunting allegorical renderings that document a bloody scene from all angles. The victim is lying prostrate beneath us, bound several times with blood spilling from the belly down over her face; she is upright, tied to a tree as though a witch about to be burned; she is floating above us, blood gushing from the gaping abdomen; she is sitting with a swaddled infant, dressed in full black as if in mourning.

A recurring motif is the red, swollen crescent of the sutured incision, which appears on the abdomen as well as on the face, in place of a mouth. "Smile, you have a healthy baby" is the caption beneath one image. In another, we see only disembodied, groundless legs and blood between them; "Earn your baby," reads the caption. "You go to your room and see your baby as soon as you can move your legs." Amadori didn't "earn" her baby for 5 hours and 33 minutes, she notes.

She sobbed through the operation. She remembers her doctor saying she'd never seen anything like it. "She said, 'You have a look on your face like you're going to be executed,'" recalls Amadori. "She said, 'I'm sorry, I'm just a surgeon, I'm just doing what I think is best.'"

Amadori's doctor appears once in her artwork. She and a team in blue scrubs and masks are standing atop the patient as though they have just completed an expedition. The lead doctor, with a yellow martial arts belt round her waist, has one foot up on the round belly, and she is raising the still-attached, screaming infant like a trophy. There is blood on the doctor's hands.

I'm not familiar with any other cesarean-inspired art, but the emotional thrust and the themes Amadori handles are ones that I've heard many times in the stories of women who've had or watched unwanted cesareans. Michelle McSweeney, the woman who was reluctantly induced in New York, later said that retelling her birth story was like reliving a war. She expressed the same feelings of being manipulated, of being overpowered, of being disabled. The loss of dignity notwithstanding, McSweeney's chief regret was the initial inability to bond with or care for her daughter.

"The saddest thing of all was that when the baby came out and they held her up for me, I didn't cry or feel that joy that you're supposed to feel. And I'm an emotional person. I didn't have that moment of ecstasy. I was so out of it," she told me. It took hours for the drugs to wear off. "I couldn't breastfeed right away. My arms barely worked. I couldn't pick the baby up if she was crying. I just had no abdomen, no muscles. I was pretty much an invalid for the first few days."

Many women experience difficulty connecting. Ashley Dees, an elementary school teacher in Houston, Texas, told me that it took 3 weeks before she felt anything for her first baby, who was born by cesarean after a failed induction in September 2005. "Probably the biggest thing I remember was the difference in bonding," she says. "I remember thinking, 'Who is this kid? Is he mine?'" She remembers a nurse holding him up to her on the operating table. "They were nice about it and everything, but when you're lying there gutted like a fish, you can't really relate. You're in a drugged state. Your hands are strapped down. You can't touch him."

When she arrived home, the haze wouldn't lift. "I felt like I was going through the motions," she told me. She was having a hard time nursing, the post-op antibiotics left her with a systemic yeast infection, her scar popped back open two days later ("They said don't lift anything but sent me home with a 9-pound baby"), and she was on Vicodin, which her obstetrician prescribed for 3 weeks. "I was on drugs," is how Dees explains it, now that she has another birth to compare it to. The Vicodin took away the excruciating pain but dulled her heart and kept her distant. "I handed the baby off to every person who came in my house. 'Here, take it for a while,'" she remembers telling visitors. Now, she believes that the narcotic, passed on via breast milk, left the baby unable to bond as well: "He was sleeping all the time," she recalls.

Cheryl Beck, a professor of nursing at the University of Connecticut, has spent 20 years researching the psychological fallout of childbirth. She began with postpartum depression and developed the screening tool used to diagnose the condition. But in 2002, while she was on a trip to New Zealand, Beck's research took a new turn, toward what has been termed "birth trauma." And what she learned is that somewhere between 1.5% and 6% of mothers are suffering from post-traumatic stress disorder (PTSD) as a result of their birth experience—with all the flash-backs, avoidance, and paranoia that plague survivors of rape and war.[105]

Beck began to study what PTSD following childbirth looked like, and she found that common among women suffering from it was a high level of medical intervention at birth. What leads to PTSD, however, isn't necessarily what happened during delivery, but *how* it happened. "The common element is that these women are systematically stripped of their protective layers," says Beck. "They do not feel cared for, they're not communicated with, they're powerless. They talk about being stripped of their dignity." Having interviewed nearly 100 women suffering from birth trauma, she says many characterized it as a rape. One woman titled her birth story "And He Scored a Perfect 10," referring to her baby's Apgar, which was announced by the obstetrician to cheering from the onlookers. Meanwhile, the mother's vagina had just been torn with forceps after only an hour of pushing. "She told me, 'Everyone was rejoicing, meanwhile I'm lying on the table thinking I'm being raped. Raped on the delivery table, with everybody watching,'" says Beck.

The horror-film quality of Amadori's work is consistent with the notion of birth trauma, according to Beck's research. Some women have reported that the anesthesia did not work properly, many remember seeing their own vivisection reflected in the overhead lights. McSweeney was numb, her line of sight blocked, but she says she "had the sense that all my organs were spread out across my stomach." Amadori also takes aim at the often casual rapport in an operating room, whereas in every other major abdominal surgery, patients are deep under general anesthesia. Not so for women undergoing cesareans. Amadori remembers which songs played on the radio and recalls conversation about the party the doctors had attended the previous weekend. "We're awake," she says, "It's not like we're sleeping."

Many of the women who post to the ICAN Yahoo group list are experiencing symptoms consistent with PTSD. Some women call their experiences "birthrapes." Carrie Mason, at the time living in New Jersey, writes that her cesarean was "damaging," "assaulting."

> I felt raped. Lying naked on a cold table, strangers sticking tubes up my body, pulling my innermost organs out to fondle. I could not even pull myself out of bed for the first 3 weeks. My life was hell for months. I could not bond to my child. I had a feeling that they pulled her out from under the table. I now live with adhesion pain; numbness from hip to hip and up to my belly button; pain during intercourse. I am not healthy! This is not birth. I went in pregnant, and I came out a bleeding, empty woman.

Many, including Mason, forgo celebrating their baby's first birthday. For them it is like the anniversary of an attack; this phenomenon is Beck's latest area of inquiry. There is certainly a feminist critique of obstetric practice as sexual violence, but the connection has also been made by public health figures. Sidney Wolfe has called the high rate of unnecessary cesareans "doctor-caused violence against women."[106] Judith Lothian, PhD, a board member of Lamaze International and professor of nursing at Seton Hall University, says it plainly: "Women are being abused."

Beck says postpartum depression is underdiagnosed. The 2005 *Listening to Mothers* survey incorporated some of her screening tool into its questions, and the results suggest that nearly two-thirds of respondents had depressive symptoms.[107] Post-traumatic stress disorder is even less accurately diagnosed. It is something most clinicians would never suspect, says Beck, because childbirth is as ideologically removed from war-grade trauma as one can get. PTSD arises from an event considered beyond the range of usual human experience, so the disorder following childbirth is paradoxical, a perversion of the quintessentially human as the inhumane.

Like Amadori, many women who are refused a VBAC contend not only with symptoms of depression but also with persistent anger. "Anger filled my every thought for months," one mother wrote to me. Another wrote that her VBAC was "sabotaged" and 17 months later is still suffering from nightmares, flashbacks, and panic attacks from the repeat surgery. "I'll never, ever place my children or myself under the risks of walking into a hospital without reason again," she wrote. Amadori says, "Not a day went by when I didn't think about it." She mediated her own anger late at night, with her baby and husband asleep, through art.

Amadori posted the series online in the spring of 2005, and e-mails from other mothers began trickling, then pouring, in. Since then she has received more than 1000 —long, revelatory e-mails validating her anger.

"Nobody talks about the emotional side effects from unwanted cesareans," she told me. "So I would hope that this would be taken into consideration as a serious side effect. And what happens when you don't let women choose how they want to give birth—the outcome is people like me who have a really, really hard time getting over it."

There's no research to date on secondary psychological effects to birth attendants who witness traumatic births—partners, doulas, nurses. But many report similar symptoms, nagging feelings of grief and loss and anger following a traumatic birth. Ina May Gaskin calls these individuals the "walking wounded."

For Sharon Breidt, a labor and delivery nurse for 15 years in Keene, New Hampshire, the emotional toll of routine cesareans and inductions came to be too much. "I loved it to death," she says of the maternity ward. But by around 2000, things started changing. It started with the hospital banning VBAC. "I had women who literally hung out laboring in the parking lot so they could come in and deliver before anyone could get a C-section ready," she remembers. She silently applauded these efforts. But when a woman came in early labor expecting a VBAC, Breidt's ethics were put to the test. "Now I'm screwed. I have to protect my license, and yet she wants to do something that I know is perfectly safe," she says. "As caregivers, it is our responsibility to give full information and support patient choice."

Breidt started seeing medically unnecessary cesareans as a matter of course. "I started seeing women being sectioned because they thought the baby was too big," she recalls. Or they would label a woman with a suspected big baby "high risk" and give her a "trial of labor" with continuous electronic fetal monitoring (Atypically, Breidt and her staff offered intermittent Doppler monitoring so that patients could remain ambulatory). "That's not really a trial of labor," she says. "That kid doesn't have a chance to get out, because she's flat on her back." She also saw more sick babies—babies born too early, needing resuscitation, and then not able to breastfeed. "The attitude was 'It's OK, it's not a problem, we'll call the pediatrician, give him some oxygen,'" she says. "To me it was like, No, that *is* a problem. This kid shouldn't come into the world not being able to breathe or nurse. That's not right."

The inductions were equally disturbing, often leading to "long, horrible, miserable labors." Recounting her last year in L&D, Breidt sounds as though she herself had been suffering through them: "I wasn't sleeping anymore, I was dreading going to work. My husband noticed I was angry all the time, and that's not me. I couldn't do it anymore—something that I love more than anything else in this world. Because in my heart I knew that there was a much better way." In 2003, she quit L&D and moved to the emergency room. "I went to the ER to relax."

CHAPTER 5

Mothers' Helpers

IN DECEMBER 2004, VICKI HEDLEY attended a birth in New Jersey as a doula. This word, borrowed somewhat awkwardly from Greek in the 1980s—it translates as slave or female servant—is now the popular term for a woman who helps prepare a woman for childbirth and stays by her side for nonmedical support through the event as well as postpartum. Hedley remembers this particular birth well. Her client was deathly afraid of childbirth, a "very nervous woman." So nervous, in fact, that she had initially requested a cesarean, which her obstetrician had agreed to do. But toward the end of the pregnancy, she changed her mind and called Hedley. "She came to me and said, 'I decided that I really want to do this.'" It was an 11th-hour change of heart, 2 weeks before she would give birth.

At the time, Hedley had attended more than 200 births over 10 years and had trained dozens of other women to be certified with DONA International (formerly Doulas of North America), the largest such organization, which at last count had 5500 members, up from 750 in 1995. She had also been teaching childbirth education classes for years, trained by Lamaze, Bradley, and Birth Works, all independent organizations with slightly different philosophies, and by this time she had melded them into her own. As a doula, Hedley's full fee is $1100—in the Northeast, the going rate is between $1000 and $2000 out of pocket. But when I spoke with Hedley she told me she was on hiatus. "Burnt out isn't the right word," she said. "It hurts me to see these women being treated the way they're being treated."

That's when Hedley told me about this particular birth. Soon after she got the call, she invited her new client over for tea. She talked to her about the normal labor process, trying to allay some of her fears. The day before she was scheduled to be induced, Hedley's client went into labor on her own, and Hedley left for the Valley Hospital in Ridgewood, New Jersey, to be with her. When she got there, her client was dilated 4 centimeters, with contractions 4 minutes apart. Hedley did her usual; she tried to keep the lights low, to keep her client as comfortable and relaxed as possible. Had her client not already been given Stadol, a narcotic painkiller, and been hooked up to the electronic fetal monitor, she would have tried to get her up and moving, but "she never once got up from the bed from the time she was admitted to the hospital," says Hedley. At 1:30 a.m., she got an epidural.

Pretty quickly, says Hedley, things started going downhill. "Her doctor was so unsupportive," Hedley recalls. "She pretty much abused the woman, verbally and physically. She broke her water without telling her. She put in an internal fetal monitor without telling her. She was hurting her while she was breaking her water." Hedley says her client was screaming for her doctor to leave her alone, but that the doctor responded with a scolding, "Stop it! This doesn't hurt!" Hedley remembers her client being "extremely upset." After 10 hours on an epidural, she ended up with a cesarean—the cesarean rate at Valley in 2004 was 41.8%;[1] Hedley knew it would be an uphill battle. "Her blood pressure tanked, labor slowed down. They had to give her another drug to get her blood pressure back up. It was really, really horrible," she says.

Hedley was able to stay with her client during the surgery and postpartum. She arrived at the hospital at 11 in the evening and didn't leave until 3 p.m. the next day. Then she returned 3 hours later to help the mother initiate breastfeeding. "The baby was in the nursery for 8 hours!"

Hedley tells me, looking over her notes from the birth. "That baby didn't get to breastfeed for the first 8 hours."

I asked Hedley whether her client would talk to me, and the next day I got a call from a woman whom I'll call Maria. "I was so scared and so anxious," she told me. She read everything she could get her hands on, but "the more I read, the more panicked I became." She took a Lamaze class and even that scared her—one day the instructor spread out on a table several delivery implements, including the Kiwi vacuum and forceps, which "stirred it up in me," said Maria. "So I went and scheduled it. I was going to have a planned C-section. And then my husband and I had a long discussion. He felt like the baby should be brought into the world on his own time. That's when I decided to try for a vaginal birth, and I found Vicki."

After eight and a half months of worry and even a session with a psychotherapist recommended by her obstetrician, "Vicki was very welcoming and gentle, she educated me in a lot of different ways about the emotional stages of the birth process," said Maria. "If I had known her earlier on, if I had been able to take one of her classes, I would have felt more accepting of it." But when she went into labor, the fear still lingered. "I think I worked myself into an unnatural fear—and I do think that it interfered with my birthing process. I do think my state of mind increased the pain."

I asked her to describe that birthing process, expecting to hear some of the taut indignation in Hedley's voice. But I heard none. "The contractions were extremely strong," she said. "I had an epidural, then an additional 10 hours of labor, and they said, 'Look, the baby's not progressing, I think it's about time we do a C-section.' And I was fine with it, because I just figured I don't want the baby to have any complications. I was just so worried about the baby."

She said her recovery was "very painful, and it took a good 6 weeks. I had to have family members come and help take care of the baby. It felt like my insides were falling out."

I began to wonder whether this was the same woman Hedley had told me about. Surely their emotional recall would match up more closely. I asked Maria if she was glad to have had a doula with her at the birth. "Vicki was wonderful," she said. "She held my hand through everything, she stayed with me through the C-section. My husband was in there too, but I feel that the support of having someone who's had her own children and knows the birth process, and who has experience with other people giving birth—it's important."

I asked a different question: Was she happy with her obstetrician, and would she go back to the practice for her next baby? "I would definitely go to the same practice. The practice was very good. I think they were very professional, very sympathetic to my fears," she said. "But I do feel like if they'd given me someone like Vicki or another doula, or if I'd met Vicki sooner, if I'd gone to her classes sooner and had more time to process, I think I might have gone with the idea of natural birth."

This was her only criticism, and it seemed almost tacked on, more self-criticism than anything else. I wrote to Hedley asking if Maria was indeed the woman whom she felt had been "abused." Yes, she said, this was the woman. "I am *constantly* amazed at the way women are able to compartmentalize or simply ignore treatment of this type," she wrote back. "This is truly amazing to me, as almost a year later I am still processing and working through her birth and the treatment she received, not to mention the trauma on her baby and all the [breastfeeding] problems that ensued as a result of that. At the time of her birth she was devastated by this treatment."

Hedley added that in spite of all the births she'd seen, something about the behavior of this doctor stunned her into silence. "I felt muted. And I'd been a doula for a long time."

One could argue that Hedley overreacted—that the staff were perhaps a little brusque, but the medical care was appropriate and necessary. Or maybe Hedley, not being a medical professional, didn't understand the rationale or urgency and unfairly maligned the physician. But having attended scores of births in the area, and having taught childbirth education and doula training for years, I think both of those explanations are unlikely. Hedley was accustomed to waters artificially broken and monitors inserted, time limits and epidurals; it wasn't the first time she had seen a woman's blood pressure drop (a common side effect of epidurals) or a resulting cesarean. Hedley's theory is that it was part birth amnesia and part psychological coping—that Maria blocked out the treatment so it wouldn't manifest as depression or worse. Hedley, on the other hand, was disturbed, partly by what she saw as a violation, and partly because she was unable to stop it.

R$_X$ FOR A NORMAL BIRTH

In surveys, women tend to report positive associations with maternity care. Eighty-three percent of the mothers surveyed by Childbirth Connection in 2005 called it "good" or "excellent," regardless of how they gave birth.[2] Yet if every maternity ward in the country were assessed on the Optimality Index (see page 133)—with demerits for near ubiquitous immobilization, high rates of induced and augmented labor, still frequent episiotomy, increasingly frequent cesarean section, and separation of mother and baby—we'd see failing grades across the board. We already have such an assessment from the CDC: at least 43% of mothers suffer morbidity.[3] According to UNICEF and WHO, only 55 U.S. hospitals could call themselves "Baby Friendly" in 2006, compared to 19,000 centers around the world. Even fewer institutions are considered "Mother Friendly," according to the U.S.-based Coalition to Improve Maternity Services. As of January 2007, just one U.S. hospital, Three Rivers Hospital in Grants Pass, Oregon, had met all of this body's mother-friendly requirements.

Optimal maternity care, according to the systematic evidence reviews conducted by the Cochrane Collaboration, can be distilled into six characteristics:[4]

1.   Labor begins spontaneously.
2.   Women have freedom of movement during labor.
3.   Interventions are medically justified rather than routine.
4.   Women have continuous emotional and physical support.
5.   Pushing occurs in any position but flat-on-back.
6.   Mother and baby are not separated.

Among the women surveyed in 2005 by Childbirth Connection, just 2% had an optimal experience.

The survey suggests another disparity. Although 80% of women agreed that they should be informed of every possible side effect before consenting to a procedure, less than half could correctly identify the risks of induction, and less than one-third were familiar with the risks of cesarean section. This suggested that they were not fully informed, and the responses to another question suggested that they were not solicited for consent: only 17% of women who got an episiotomy reported having a choice in the matter. And race was a strong determinant. A mere 4% of black women had a say in whether they were cut.[5]

The gap between reality and perception leaves a ringing dissonance. As Christiane Northrup, MD, author of *Women's Bodies, Women's Wisdom*, remarked in 2006, "Why are women willing to put up with so little?"[6]

Enter the doula. Her increasing prevalence in hospital delivery rooms suggests that women may be striving for something more. In 2005, doulas attended between 120,000 and 200,000 births, and demand for doula training has grown each year for the past decade. Doulas are currently the most highly rated form of labor support in the hospital setting, above doctors, nurses, partners, and even nurse–midwives.[7] Most doulas are hired privately by women with means, but hospitals and community groups have begun volunteer doula programs as well. A group in Chicago specifically works with teenage women, a group in Minnesota with Somali and Latina women, and a group in Washington State with incarcerated women. The term *doula*, if not exactly a household word, is at least something most expectant women have heard of.

The doula is a vestige of the female labor support that existed gratis for much of history. Midwives attended birth and were generally the only ones to examine the woman in labor, but other women from the community, as well as relatives from far away, would arrive to cook and launder, take care of other children, keep the house warm, fetch supplies for the midwife, and help physically support the woman during childbirth itself—often propping her up in a seated position to give birth. Unlike the midwife, these women were not paid, but service was expected in kind when they gave birth. In North America, social birth disappeared in the twentieth century: women no longer needed labor support because they were unconscious. When women woke up, the doula was roused from a long slumber as well.

"Doulas sort of slipped in the back door," says sociologist Christine Morton, PhD, who studies doulas and childbirth educators and who practiced as a doula herself for 6 years. With delivery rooms beginning to open to fathers in the 1970s, women started bringing along their Lamaze teachers and friends. The doula acquired her title and tolerance thanks to the patients' rights movement of the 1970s and 1980s and from a series of compelling studies conducted by the pediatricians Marshall Klaus, MD, and John Kennel, MD, which gave scientific credence to the notion that labor support is clinically beneficial.

Klaus and Kennel actually stumbled on the findings. Their primary interest was mother–infant attachment—what is now known as bonding. Their discovery came while they were studying whether support through labor and postpartum would facilitate bonding. What they found was that the support not only enhanced bonding but also seemed to ease the labor itself, resulting in fewer complications. They subsequently conducted several randomized controlled trials, published their research, and adopted the term *doula*. Although many in the field preferred the less loaded *childbirth assistant* or *labor support professional*, for better or worse, *doula* stuck.

Klaus and Kennell's work suggests that "high-touch" birth, as opposed to high-tech birth, is healthier for both mother and child. They discovered that the mere presence of another woman, even when she was assigned to "observe" rather than support, seemed to lessen the duration of labor and the need for intervention. (Either the observers ended up supporting anyway, because it's human to hold a hand in need, or the medical staff were on their best behavior because someone was watching them.) The researchers replicated their findings several times in the United States and elsewhere. One 1988 study of clinic patients in Houston found that among women who had doula support, there were half as many cesareans, one-third as many uses of forceps, and minimal requests for epidural anesthesia—11% compared to 60% among the unsupported group.[8]

Kennell saw the irony coming: "If I told you today about a new medication or a new electronic device that would reduce problems of fetal asphyxia and the progress of labor by two-thirds, cut labor length by one-half, and enhance mother–infant interaction after delivery, I expect that there would be a stampede," he wrote.[9] But the doula is not a commodity. She has a demedicalizing, decommodifying effect on birth. Perhaps that's why medicine hasn't embraced her.

At the same time, however, the doula is a product of medicalized birth, a response to it. She is a distinctly American creation, arising out of a social deficit in maternity care and a consumer demand to fill it. Even while women say they're satisfied with the care they receive, the doula movement is "an implicit critique of the medicalized system," argues Christine Morton. With central fetal monitoring and two or three labors per nurse, with endless forms to fill out, and with more and more non-clinical duties to complete during shifts, nursing staff have no time for handholding. "Now, nurses are caring for machines," says Morton. A doula restores hands-on care.

That is the doula's official purview, anyway. DONA International defines the doula as "mothering the mother"—as providing her with emotional and physical support and "assistance in acquiring the knowledge necessary to make informed decisions about her care." But as Barbara Stratton, a Maryland VBAC activist and former doula, points out, there's little physical support possible in many hospitals. Walking the halls is out of the question; showers and baths are rarely available or allowed; even changing positions or standing is often forbidden because it disrupts the fetal monitor strip. Stratton offers a descriptive scenario: "Here I was trying to help this one client—you know, you want skin-to-skin contact to stroke and comfort," she tells me. But there was little skin available. On the woman's left arm was an IV, on her right arm was a blood pressure cuff. "You can't rub her back because she's got two monitors, the contraction monitor and the baby's monitor. And then this particular hospital puts leg cuffs on anyone confined to bed, so her legs are covered from the top of the thigh to the ankle. So I spend the whole time rubbing her shoulders—that was all I could get to."

Today, doulas say they end up serving a far different, far more demanding role than simply that of handholder or cheerleader; they also serve as advocate and witness. Brenda Lane, a board member of DONA and practicing doula in Baltimore, Maryland, says most women hire her as "security." "I'd say the majority do not like the level of intervention in the hospital. They want access to it, they want to know it's there if they need it, but they don't want to feel like they're on an assembly line." A doula on Long Island told me that women are hiring her as "a sort of insurance policy against unnecessary medical intervention that they feel will be foisted upon them." The doula tries to normalize birth, get more pillows or a steeper angle on the bed, and slow down the hospital's time clock. She is often the go-between, the negotiator. Judith Halek, a doula who has been practicing in New York City for 20 years, calls what she does "holding the space," and describes maintaining a protective bubble around her clients so that physiological labor can progress unheeded and unhurried.

Priming that space happens before birth as well. Doulas might suggest that clients ask their doctors questions clarifying their policies, or they might subtly nudge clients away from providers or facilities they know to be unsupportive of normal birth. The doulas hired privately by women, unlike those who are affiliated with a hospital program, are in a unique position to give such advice. They "work" at each of a community's hospitals. When they are present in L&D wards, the walls have ears—and eyes as well. They get to know how a variety of obstetricians and nursing staffs perform. They are the "secret shoppers" of maternity care.

Knowing so much puts doulas in a difficult position, however. Should the doula tell her client that continuous electronic fetal monitoring isn't evidence-based but will be required by the hospital she's chosen? Should she tell her client that her doctor is quick to cut an episiotomy? DONA instructs its doulas to support the woman's choices and not to give medical advice. "It's a really tough issue," says Brenda Lane of DONA. "If a woman asks me point blank, 'Have you worked with my doctor and has this happened?' I won't lie. But I don't offer. That's not my place. I want to empower her to ask questions. I want to empower her to get a second opinion."

"The doula role as it was being constructed was carefully crafted so as not to impinge on the roles of the nurse and the physician," explains Christine Morton. This was a political calculation, because doulas have no absolute right to be in the delivery room. "They cannot afford to piss off the people in power." And yet doulas find it difficult not to push those boundaries, because they care about birth and about their clients' well-being. "Doulas are struggling," says Morton. "They get it through the training that childbirth is a natural, healthy process, but most doulas are working in hospitals where that view is not supported."

During labor, doulas are often put in the position of watchdog, even bodyguard, although many object to that terminology. "I think what we're here to do is advocate, so that nothing is done to them without their knowledge or permission," says Judith Halek. "That's different from body guarding." Many doulas report witnessing procedures that are not consented to, and intervening if they can. This frequently comes up with episiotomy. "I had a client who told me that she absolutely did not want an episiotomy," says Elan McAllister, also a doula in New York. "My client was fully dilated and pushing, and the baby's head was crowning. The midwife had a tray of instruments next to her, and every time the baby's head showed through, she'd reach for the scissors and then pull her hand back." McAllister was keeping one eye on the midwife while trying to help her client concentrate on pushing. "After a few minutes she picked up the scissors and said, 'I'm just going to make a tiny cut—to help this along a little.' My client nodded. I looked her in the eye and said, 'She's about to cut an episiotomy. Is that OK with you?' And at that my client sat straight up and screamed, 'Noooooo!'"

Today's doula is compensating not only for a social deficit in maternity care, but for a power deficit as well. So often, she becomes a shield, a buffer between the competing interests of the woman and of the hospital. In her research, Morton interviewed some 50 doulas practicing in the Seattle area, and she heard numerous stories like McAllister's, where the doula sees something going on that she knows the woman doesn't want and has to quickly disarm the provider without overstepping her bounds and getting kicked out of the delivery room entirely. Doulas and their clients often work out code words and signals in advance. Somehow, the doula has to bring what's going on to the woman's attention "in such a way that she can then act on it," says Morton. "Because the doula can't. That's how her role is defined." And that, says Morton, is asking a lot. Shifting the power dynamic "takes an immense presence of mind, an immense attention to the nuance of the interaction. And they're not trained to do that. They get a 4-day workshop."

Doulas have to navigate their own involvement philosophy carefully, and some come to be more proactive than they are taught to be. Vicki Hedley in New Jersey confessed that even while she was teaching her DONA trainees not to come between patient and doctor, to support women's choices at all costs, she began to feel an obligation to tell her clients when she knew their provider was a bad match. "I used to say things like 'So, how do you feel about Dr. M____?' I don't do that anymore. I tell them, 'It depends what you're looking for, but she's very medically interventive.' I don't beat around the bush," she says. "If you're not with the right group, you're in trouble." A doula in New York told me, "One of the most rewarding parts of this job is directing women away from doctors who won't give them the kind of birth they want."

Doulas are not the only agents in word-of-mouth channels. One maternity fitness instructor told me, "I have all the poop on the doctors." She has her students fill out birth questionnaires during their postpartum tummy workouts, including their provider's name and the facility they birthed in, and keeps a sort of blacklist of doctors whom she notes as cutting a lot of episiotomies and C-sections. She doesn't distribute the list, but if a prenatal client comes to her asking what she thinks of her doctor, she'll look that doctor up, and maybe help her find someone new.

A disempowering delivery is often the catalyst for becoming a doula. Candice Hilton, the woman who had an induction followed by an unwanted episiotomy in Mississippi, says she was so demoralized that she left the hospital "not wanting any more children." Two years later she got her doula certification and has since assisted 19 births, 18 of which were vaginal, all but one without an episiotomy. She also had two home births of her own. Hilton is unabashedly an activist—she doesn't want women to go through what she did. "I will speak up for my clients," she told me. "I've taken women off the monitor." She has also thwarted episiotomies. "I had a doctor standing at the woman's vagina with lidocaine in one hand and scissors in the other, and I said, 'She doesn't want an episiotomy.' And the doctor said, 'Well, sorry.' And I said very loudly to the woman, 'You have to speak up now. You have to be the one to say it.' I had to be loud and forceful."

Doulas often help women labor at home and advise them on when to go to the hospital; some advise them to go as late as possible. Some even advise them to lie about when labor started (to minimize the chances that it will be labeled "prolonged"). Some help their clients try herbal methods of labor induction in order to avoid Pitocin; others sneak food and drink into the delivery room or help their clients to the bathroom, where they can lock the door. (Some nurses have told me of performing similar acts of subversion: "losing" Cytotec pills, "forgetting" to up the Pitocin, encouraging their patients to keep going to the bathroom so they don't have to be "nailed to the bed.")

Jackie Levine, a doula on Long Island, urges her clients to ask their physicians to agree to certain banner stipulations—such as intermittent monitoring, no IV, food and drink allowed—on a prescription pad. She calls this the "Rx for a Normal Birth." She warns her clients that their doctor won't be with them for most of the birth, even if he's the one on-call, so the script will neutralize any resistance from nurses or residents. "The worst club held over the heads of women who come into the hospital to deliver is 'hospital policy,'" says Levine.

Many doulas are emotionally devastated by the treatment they're privy to. "If you care about birth, doing hospital births is very hard on your psyche," says Barbara Stratton. "It's hard to watch what they do to women." And yet part of the doula's mandate is to make the woman regard her experience as a positive one. The doula ultimately can't throw herself in front of a scalpel, but she can figuratively throw herself in front of the woman's psyche. "What doulas do is reframe what happens," says Morton. "They focus in on the things that are positive. They look at the woman and say, 'You were so brave,' 'You were so tired, you labored for so long.' They praise her over and over again."

And this, perhaps, best explains the chilling disparity between Hedley's and her clients' birth stories. Hedley didn't tell Maria what she thought of her doctor; she didn't yell, "Stop it!" when staff broke her client's water without getting informed consent. Instead, Hedley kept holding Maria's hand, wiping her brow, and telling her what a great job she was doing. And that is what Maria remembers. As doulas "reframe" the birth experience for their clients, they are also shielding the hospital and its care providers from criticism and complaint. Hedley did her job so well that even though she felt her client was "abused," her client will go right back to the same obstetrician and hospital for her next pregnancy.

"The unanswered, fundamental question is whether [doulas] are making birth better for women, or just making women feel better about their births," write sociologists Bari Meltzer Norman and Barbara Katz Rothman.[10] They raise a fair critique of the doula as an enabler. By supplementing the handholding and informed consent conversations that nurses and doctors should be doing, and by buffering the level of intervention, they are perpetuating the very system that they are in the business of changing.

Vicki Hedley was worried about the very same thing; that's why she stopped taking clients. Briefly. Within a couple of months she was back attending births. "I feel sorry for people," she told me. "They need help. So I tell them I'll attend their births. And then I feel sorry for them when I leave." On some level, says Hedley, women must know this as well. After all, hiring a doula is in a sense a vote of no confidence in the prevailing system. It is a woman's admission that the baseline maternity care she's purchased is at best inadequate, at worst dangerous, yet it is not something she's willing to reject. Norman and Rothman take doulas to task for working within the system, but that's where their clients are.

"Doulas are caregivers," says Morton in defense. "They're not social change agents." At the same time, however, doulas may have more of a humanitarian responsibility to testify than they've so far acknowledged. "What doulas see at birth needs to be explored more," says Morton, "because they are the only critical, objective witnesses." As a group, doulas haven't yet found a voice to communicate to the public; many haven't yet found a voice to communicate honestly with their clients. "It took me a lot of years to come around to that," says Hedley of her willingness to dish about a provider's style or reputation. "We're taught that you're supposed to be supportive." Morton doesn't blame individual doulas. The majority of them, she says, are working for little to no pay, have children of their own, and are giving precious time and energy to virtual strangers. Instead, she sees the lack of political engagement as a failure on the part of the certifying organizations, not only for the health of women but also for doulas themselves. "This is the hidden story of what goes on in birth. We've got folks talking about it as medical rape. Doulas are witnessing these things, and it's eating them up inside."

A LITTLE GAME

For $23.95, a childbirth educator can purchase something called the "Go with the Flow" Birth Plan Game. The game—quasi-maternity Tarot—consists of a set of ten laminated cards with various outcomes on either side, such as "Episiotomy/Tear" "Long Labor/Short Labor" and "Forceps or Vacuum/Spontaneous Delivery," each with a stock clip art graphic to match (for the vacuum, the upright Hoover; for a long labor, the clock).

To play, you, the parent-to-be, arrange the cards in accordance with the kind of birth you want. Then the educator tells you to flip one card over—now you have an unsavory element to ponder. How are you going to feel if you end up with Pitocin? Flip another card over. What if the anesthesiologist is called to the ER and you can't get the epidural you wanted 15 minutes ago? Another card: Long labor. "By the end of the game, you end up with your worst case scenario," says Sue Cooter, executive director of Prepared Childbirth Educators, Inc., the creator of the game. The goal, she says, is to prevent postpartum anguish over an unrealized "fantasy birth." "If they kind of learn that they have to go with the flow, then the outcome is much better," she says.

Cooter's birth plan game is her answer to the birth plan itself, an idea that was introduced in the 1980s by natural childbirth educators whose intention was to empower women to refuse the ritualistic enemas, pubic hair shaving, stirrups, and episiotomies—and they suggested you put it in writing. As the number of tubes, drugs, and sensors multiplied, so did the pages of birth plans. But where its original purpose was to help patients avoid unnecessary medical interventions, now it can help make a case for using them.

The birth plan is usually a list of statements that begin with the conditional "I would like . . . " or "I would prefer . . . " or "We wish to have . . . " The plan may be pages long—several websites have interactive templates that allow the user to set dozens upon dozens of preferences and generate a custom wish list. There's the etiquette section: "I would like people to respect my privacy by knocking before entering the room." The atmosphere section: "I would like the environment to be kept as quiet as possible." The scissors section: "I would prefer to avoid an episiotomy." And often a molecularly precise pain-relief section: "I would like the following pain relief medication to be administered as soon as possible: Stadol, Nubain, Demerol, Low-dose Epidural, Epidural Block." Or, "If induction is necessary, I prefer the following methods: Pitocin, Prostaglandin Gel, Amniotomy, Cytotec."

In the nonjudgmental mold of the doula, many sites put best practices and harmful practices side by side and ask women to choose: "I would like an episiotomy" some offer as an option. Babycenter.com, however, offers only the choice of optimal care—you can't choose an induction, episiotomy, or Demerol here. And just filling out the form would educate the user in active birth positions (flat-on-back is notably missing), non-pharmacological pain-relief options, and the concept of a doula.

No matter which website, the emotional reward of creating a plan is a sense of power and control, even if it is a little like online shopping. The expectant woman is making choices, doing her homework, exercising her right as a consumer. It's your body and your birth, the act seems to imply. At Childbirth.org, the interactive plan prompts, "You may choose intermittent *or* continuous monitoring" and asks the user to select the fetoscope, the Doppler, the external electronic monitor, or the internal electronic monitor. Babycenter.com asks whether you'd like to "be allowed to progress free of stringent time limits" and to "walk and move around as I choose." Would you also like to bring music, to dim the lights? Will you be bringing a birthing stool, a beanbag chair, and/or a birthing tub? Click, click, and click, submit, and print out your receipt.

The only problem is that the hospital may not be amenable to any of your choices. In today's malpractice climate, I've never heard of anyone bringing their own tub to a hospital, let alone actually birthing in one. Oftentimes hospital staff snickers at birth plans. A labor and delivery nurse in Minnesota told me, "We have a running joke, it's like 'uh oh, they have a birth plan, prep the OR.'" Many hospitals won't allow intermittent monitoring, for instance—they don't have the nursing staff. That nixes walking or "moving around" much. Many hospitals have epidural rates of 85% or more, which might indicate a near ubiquitous demand for drugs, or an institutional expectation that women labor stationary and silent. Creating the lounge atmosphere (dim lights, music) is nearly impossible and is an utterly comical notion in any large teaching hospital. "Couples think they have decisions in areas where they really don't have decisions," says Cooter, who was a nurse for 30 years.

Studies show that a woman is more likely to have a positive birth experience when she feels she is in control.[11] Interestingly, whether or not she experiences pain has little impact.[12] And the doulas, the check-box birth plans, the Bradley, Lamaze, and Hypnobirthing classes—these all give women a sense of control. They also suggest that women are seeking control. The question is, if women have so much control, why are only 2% having optimal birth experiences? Why are 43% suffering morbidity in childbirth?

One possibility is that women aren't being warned. "They are going into hospitals expecting to have perfectly normal births, maybe with an epidural, but they're coming out traumatized," says Judith Lothian, professor of nursing at Seton Hall University and board member of Lamaze International, which was founded in 1960 to promote "natural childbirth." After Christine Morton plumbed the doula scene for answers, she moved to childbirth education classes. What she found was that, like doulas, childbirth educators often bite their tongues even when they have information that is crucial to a woman's decision making. "There's this naïve belief that's really becoming clear in my research, where these folks think, 'If I can just give them unbiased information—if there is such a thing—they'll make the choice that's best for them. That's their mantra," says Morton. "It's very individualistic, and in that sense it's very American. This notion of choice, that people have individual choice, that somehow they're getting all the information they need. But guess what? The childbirth educators aren't telling their students that this hospital has a 90% epidural rate, an X-percent cesarean rate."

Sue Cooter of Prepared Childbirth says that's not a childbirth educator's place. Women need to do their homework, she told me. "If they're going to a hospital with a 99% epidural rate and they want a natural birth, or if they want to walk around and hospital policy is to put in an IV, then they're at the wrong place," she says. "But that's not for us to tell them." Her company trains nurses who teach primarily in-hospital "prenatal classes." If anyone knows a hospital's culture, it's the nurses. Still, says Cooter, all childbirth educators can do is encourage their students to "be consumers," to call the hospital, call their doctor, ask questions, and make sure their goals are realistic. "Sometimes it does dawn on them that they're at the wrong place," she says.

I asked her what the childbirth educator's responsibility is if she has a student who believes she will have an option—say, intermittent monitoring or the ability to walk around—that the educator knows will not be tolerated at the hospital. "The responsibility is to refer them to the healthcare provider. You don't really answer. You don't make them upset," says Cooter. "You have to know your place as a nurse. That's why you have to be really careful in what you say and what you don't say in these classes."

Morton calls this "imposed self-censorship," similar to what many doulas end up doing, deferring to the woman's choice, even if they know it's not in her best interest. "What women need during this time is a reliable source of information they can trust," says Morton. Yet their doulas and childbirth educators are telling them to "check with your provider" rather than telling them, "You know, the hospital you've chosen is very restrictive—are you going to be OK with that?"

The motto for the International Childbirth Education Association is "Freedom of choice based on knowledge of alternatives in family-centered maternity and newborn care." But freedom of choice does not exist without full information. Judith Lothian says that the "support the woman's choices" mantra is based on a false premise. "I think we have dangerously bought into the fact that women are making truly informed choices. And they're not," she says.

I asked Cooter if "go with the flow" is just another way of saying to a woman, "you will have no control." "No," she said. The point is that "some things happen that you don't have control over. She might have said, 'I don't want any Pitocin,' but if her labor slows down, the choice might be between Pitocin and a cesarean." Women are disappointed, she says, when they don't accept that they can't write their own medical charts. "These woman couldn't go with the flow. Really we do this to ourselves," says Cooter. "What was her goal? Was her goal to have a healthy baby or not?"

Childbirth is, by definition, a loss of control over the body—contractions and expulsion, and the bleeding and fluids and pain, are as involuntary as orgasm and sneezing. The British childbirth educator and researcher Sheila Kitzinger puts a lyrical spin on it, writing that in physiological birth a woman needs to "joyfully surrender her body to the creative experience."[13] But in the hospital, the surrender is usually of the body to the provider. Women often lose control over what's *done to* the body, rather than over what the body *does*.

Cooter's birth plan game prepares women for the former kind of surrender. Lamaze was criticized for the same thing in the 1980s. "Rather than being alerted to which hospital procedures are arbitrary or might be unnecessary in her case, the woman is taught instead how to ignore— 'breathe through'—enemas, perineal shaves, repeated examinations, transfer from bed to stretcher and so on," wrote Barbara Katz Rothman in 1982.[14] In her qualitative study of childbirth education classes today, Morton found that with the exception of the Bradley method, which encourages women to "be an advocate for yourself and what you want," most are focused on a similar acceptance of medical routines.

But being an advocate for yourself is difficult, says Judith Lothian, who wrote *The Official Lamaze Guide: Giving Birth with Confidence*. She told me that when she entered birth advocacy in the 1970s, "if you could avoid twilight sleep and have your husband with you, you were good to go in a hospital." Today, she offers a dismal analysis of the notion of control once a woman enters a hospital. "It's an illusion," she says. "No matter what anybody tells you in prenatal classes, or what your friends say, or what you read in books, the bottom line is, you will follow the rules of the hospital, and you will do what your doctor wants you to do. No matter what you think going into it. Sometimes I say your choices are very limited, but in point of fact, I don't think women *have* any choices."

These are radical words coming from a registered nurse who is chair of Lamaze's International Certification Council, an organization that was built around medicalized childbirth. For years, Lamaze offered certification only to registered nurses. Its first training manual stated that a woman "should be encouraged to respect her own doctor's word as final . . . [and that] she is responsible for controlling herself and her behavior."[15] Lothian says all the birth planning and so-called education is just a facade. "You know, we're just playing a little game here," she says, "And it does women a disservice because they really do think that they have choice, and then they don't."

STAYING PUT

In 1823, the metal eyelet was invented. The eyelet was no zipper or Velcro, but when threaded with laces, the small reinforced hole—you now see it on boots, sneakers, and draw strings—was a highly effective fastener. It allowed for new fashion possibilities, including one women's-wear trend that would hold tight for the next three generations: the corset. Although today this word simply describes a top or undergarment that hugs the torso, the Victorian corset was designed to actively constrict and permanently reshape. The laces were drawn ever tighter over the course of time, molding the pelvis and ribs into the vaunted hourglass shape, forcing organs above and below the tiny rounded waist—hence the term *tight lacing*. The saying went that a woman's waist shouldn't measure more in inches than her age of marriage in years—and most women married by age 21.

Historians have debated the prevalence of tight lacing, or "waist-training," but as the sociologist Leigh Summers argues, the profusion of advertisements, fashion plates, and lively debate among feminist "dress reformers" over 20-inch waists suggest that most women across the class divide in the latter half of the 1800s wore "stays," as the corsets were aptly called—wore them tight and wore them young. Young girls grew up with softer training corsets, which acquired whalebone or metal panels and were cinched around the waist by early puberty, just as the uterus was developing. Women even tight-laced during pregnancy, using stronger, reinforced "maternity corsets" manufactured to push back and conceal their swelling abdomen.[16]

Today, a "dazzling constellation," as Summers puts it, of Victorian ailments is attributed to the corset, from constipation, nausea, and vomiting to headaches and backaches, leg pains, and menstrual disorders. The corset exerted up to 80 pounds of pressure per cubic inch, cramping circulation, often causing swelling in the legs and a visible pulse at the temples. Pelvic floors deteriorated, uteri prolapsed, and miscarriages (some deliberate) ensued. The corset even created its own syndrome, chlorosis, a term that referred to the triad of menstrual cessation, shortness of breath, and fainting spells—a severe form of anemia. This condition, originally attributed to the fragile female constitution, mysteriously disappeared with the arrival of the drop-waist flapper dress.[17]

What effect did the corset have on childbirth? "The rigours and dangers of labour experienced by American and English women were considered by many authorities as the consequence of generations of corset-wearing," writes Summers. Oscar Wilde, as editor of *Woman's World*, wrote that the corset had "by slow degrees deformed the figure." The female body had "lost its elasticity and had ceased to develop according to the laws of nature."[18] In Joseph DeLee's 1913 textbook *The Principles and Practice of Obstetrics*, five chapters are devoted to the "contracted pelvis," including 83 pictures and diagrams. (In 1000 pages, the corset is only mentioned once.)[19] An 1882 book devoted 68 pages to misshapen pelvises; a 1921 textbook devoted 75.[20] Many of the deformities were caused by rickets, but how many by the corset?

Alice B. Stockham, one of the first female doctors in the U.S., saw a connection between the corset and reproductive complications. "The corset, more than any other one thing, is responsible for women's being the victim of disease and doctors," she wrote in her book *Tokology* in 1883—the Victorian *Our Bodies, Ourselves*. "The corset should not be worn for two hundred years before pregnancy takes place." Stockham believed that childbirth itself should be relatively painless, and that the corset was in large part to blame for difficulties. She also looked to tight lacing as "the chief cause of infantile mortality."[21]

But Stockham was in the minority. The general ill-health of women was written off as "female complaints." Being a woman meant being sick most of the time. Most physicians cast no blame on the corset, and even those who did made no specific mention of its widespread use during pregnancy. According to Summers's research, not one medical article between 1876 and 1900 addressed the corset's effect on childbearing; the surgeon general William A. Hammond even endorsed a specific corset brand. Newly organized medicine was largely silent on the entire subject of corsetry. The physician Charles Graham Cannaday wrote, in an 1894 paper called "The Relation of Tight Lacing to Uterine Development and Abdominal and Pelvic Disease," that the medical community "lived in the presence of such an injurious custom" yet failed to offer "a united protest" against it.[22] In a cruel irony, corsetry came to be known as therapeutic for the very debilities it caused, a necessity to maintain the integrity of the frail female form, in particular when it was with child. Patents and advertisements even claimed it prevented miscarriage.

Corsets were painful—hours of wear left scar-like purple indentations on the skin or chafed it to bleeding. They crushed ribs, which sometimes punctured lungs; the cloth sometimes gave way, and loose, sharp whalebone and metal stays sprung into the flesh. Yet it was out of this pain-ridden existence that women began demanding a pain-free childbirth.

Even as the corset fell out of fashion and the chlorosis epidemic waned, the demand for obstetric anesthesia grew stronger. The cause was taken up by suffragists who advocated twilight sleep in the same language in which they called for voting rights—physical as well as political liberation. At one of several rallies organized by the National Twilight Sleep Association in 1914, one woman held up her baby and called the audience to action: "If you women want it you will have to fight for it, for the mass of doctors are opposed to it."[23] Access to twilight sleep was, in part, what drove childbearing women from home to hospital in the first half of the twentieth century. Between 1900 and 1955, that proportion soared from 5% to 95%, with a majority undergoing episiotomy and forceps deliveries while they were sedated.[24]

In the 1940s, women were presented with an alternative. The pain isn't necessary, said Grantly Dick-Read, an English obstetrician; it is in fact unnatural. "Healthy childbirth was never intended by the natural law to be painful," he wrote.[25] Pain was simply the manifestation of fear and tension—the blood pulled away from the uterus in a fight/flight response. If women could simply overcome fear, then the uterine muscle would work efficiently and effortlessly, tension would dissipate, and pain would be abolished. Dick-Read laid out this theory in *Childbirth Without Fear*, which was written in 1933 but not published in the United States until 1944.

Soon after Dick-Read in 1951, the French physician Fernand Lamaze offered his own variation on the theme. He'd witnessed women in Russia who had prepared for childbirth with "psychoprophylaxis," learning in advance how to sublimate pain with relaxation techniques. His vision was to combine psychoprophylaxis with labor support. That is, the same nurse who instructed the woman in the relaxation technique would be with her during birth. What came to be emblematic of the Lamaze technique in the United States is now a worn-out cliché: the rhythmic panting, which Lamaze no longer even teaches. And in 1965, Denver obstetrician Robert A. Bradley wrote *Husband-Coached Childbirth*, promoting natural childbirth through spousal support.

All three physicians were moved by personal observations: Dick-Read by a woman who "kindly but firmly" declined chloroform and later asked whether childbirth was "supposed to" hurt; Lamaze by the deeply relaxed women in Russia; and Bradley by difficult labors made easy once the husband came into the labor room. It was based on these men's theories that natural childbirth activists argued for women to reject the drugs and instead be "awake and aware."

At the time, the choice was between being "awake and aware" and being unconscious and out-of-control, with no memory of giving birth and no contact with the baby for hours. Faced with this dichotomy, the natural childbirth movement blossomed. And after a series of letters to the editor were published in 1958 in *Ladies' Home Journal* detailing the brutality witnessed in maternity wards while women were under twilight sleep, women began to fear what would be done to their bodies more than they feared the pain.

In the 1970s, the culture of childbirth was changed by another material invention: plastics. Prior to the commercial availability, in the 1970s, of the flexible nylon catheter, a woman's access to regional anesthesia was a "one shot" deal. Anesthetic would be injected into the spinal fluid, blocking all sensation from the waist down for a good 2 hours or more. Called the "spinal," this technique has a numbing effect so strong that it is still suitable for cesarean section. The catheter, on the other hand, allows the anesthesiologists continuous access to the epidural space surrounding the spinal cord. Here, instead of acting on the spinal fluid, anesthetic and opiate "bathe" the spinal nerves, as William Camann, MD, director of obstetric anesthesiology at Brigham and Women's Hospital in Boston explains. "Today we use very low doses of medicine in the epidurals. The woman usually still retains the ability to move her legs, to feel contractions. She might feel a slight ache or pressure, but it's not really painful." The walking epidural—an even lower dose of anesthetic and narcotic—allows for even more sensation, though not usually walking.

What happened to the natural childbirth movement? "The epidural," says Judith Lothian. Prior to it, the only way to stay awake and aware was to mentally overcome the pain. With the refinement of the epidural, women were told they could have it all: awake, aware, and pain-free. In the late 1980s and 1990s, women voted with their lower backs. Use of epidural anesthesia in childbirth at large hospitals increased from 22% in 1981 to 66% in 1997 [26] and is estimated to be 80% today.[27]

"We didn't do a good job," Lothian tells me, referring to how the natural childbirth movement handled the concept of maternal pain. "Basically what we said is that pain is an unnecessary side effect, and you come to childbirth education classes to learn ways to deal with it other than having nitrous oxide and scopolamine." This, she says, engendered the notion that pain was unimportant, a psychosomatic response that had no physiological role. It also implied that in the absence of drugs, women needed to prepare themselves using some "method." As Suzanne Arms wrote in 1975, Lamaze had "the unfortunate side effect of greatly altering a woman's natural experience of birth from one of deep involvement inside her body to a controlled distraction."[28] Lothian argues that the pain is important. It is not a side effect, rather it is a central component of normal birth—*not* something from which mothers should be distracted.

Pain communicates, and sometimes it tells us important information—that we should take our hand off the hot stove, for instance. The pain of Victorian corseted life should have told women to burn their corsets and let their organs breathe. By the time they did, however, perhaps they could no longer distinguish between "good" pain and "bad" pain. All pain had become associated with oppression, sexism, and disenfranchisement. Women rejected the pain, and with it, normal birth.

In 1999, the Joint Commission for Accreditation of Health Care Organizations developed new guidelines on pain management. The goal was to ensure that pain would be recognized as the "fifth vital sign"—pain relief as every patient's right, not a privilege. And these guidelines were designed no differently for maternity wards than for the ER. "Adequate pain control is the humanitarian thing to do," says Camann, "whether it's a trauma patient, someone who's had surgery, or someone who has cancer. Childbirth is the same way. To ignore pain in childbirth is not proper."

That doesn't mean you push epidurals on every woman, adds Camann. There are alternatives that don't involve drugs. "Laboring in water is extraordinarily effective at relieving pain," he says. But under the Joint Commission's standards, nurses are obliged to offer relief of some kind repeatedly, and very few can offer bathtubs or massage.

I asked Camann about the many grievances often cited against the epidural: that it lengthens labor, necessitates artificial oxytocin, increases the likelihood of a vaginal tear or episiotomy, ups the chance of a cesarean section, and disrupts breastfeeding. All have been associated with the epidural, he acknowledges, but the studies aren't proving cause and effect. Sometimes it's indirect. An epidural, he says, "makes it more convenient to do an episiotomy," because the area is already numb. Pitocin and the epidural have a "very strong association," but which comes first hasn't been isolated in the literature. Was it an induction that led to more pain and an epidural request, or was it an epidural that slowed down labor and warranted Pitocin augmentation? The same is true for cesarean section, he says. There's no way to separate out the effects of the epidural from what he calls "the whole package."

A drop in blood pressure is a common side effect of epidural anesthesia—Camann says it occurs in 20% to 30% of women and is treated with ephedrine. About 15% to 20% of patients develop a fever. Whether or not it signals an infection, it usually means that mother and baby will be separated immediately after birth so the baby can be tested and possibly treated with prophylactic antibiotics. (Camann scrupulously points out that with all the other pathways to infection—the internal monitors and vaginal exams—it's again unfair to blame the epidural as the sole cause of a fever.)

Lothian and other childbirth activists point to risks to the baby. Camann says that systemic drugs like Demerol, Nubain, and Stadol, which are administered via IV, do pass through the placenta and to the baby and that it may take several days after birth for a newborn to metabolize them. "With an epidural, the doses are much less than they used to be, so very little medication is getting to the baby," he says.

As safe and effective as the epidural is in relieving pain, what's emerging from research is that the pain is chemically linked to the progress of labor.[29] Rather than grouping childbirth pain with the agony of a broken bone or a gallstone, there's a compelling scientific argument that the pain of childbirth promotes a healthy birth.

Oxytocin is but one hormone in the bath of birth. Endorphins, natural opiates that are also secreted during sex, reach peak levels during birth and are responsible for the altered state of consciousness that women often describe toward the end of labor—a reproductive version of the "runner's high." The endorphins stimulate release of prolactin, which is central to breastfeeding. Adrenaline and nonadrenaline, the fight-or-flight hormones, are released in both mother and baby. In the baby, these prime the lungs and protect the brain against the stress of birth.[30]

Epidural anesthesia blocks adrenaline as well as the endorphins, which can be advantageous in the first stage of labor because it melts fear and anxiety, which keeps oxytocin's pathway clear. Toward the end, however, it is counterproductive because it thwarts that final energy burst. "A woman giving birth with an epidural will thus miss out on the fetal ejection reflex, with its strong final contractions designed to birth her baby quickly and easily," writes Sarah Buckley.[31] Studies have also shown that epidural anesthesia causes a drop in prostaglandin, yet another hormone involved in the birth process, which keeps the uterus supple enough to contract and bounce back. This can result in a less responsive uterus, a malpositioned fetus, longer labor, and a higher risk of hemorrhage.[32]

"The pain of labor is part of the physiological process," argues Michel Odent. Take away the pain, and the endorphins don't get released; without endorphins, prolactin lies dormant. The endorphin–prolactin connection may explain recent data suggesting that epidurals hamper breastfeeding.[33] Odent argues that the interplay of hormones is part of a complex biofeedback mechanism that scientists are just beginning to understand, and that that mechanism also keeps oxytocin flowing, which is what powers labor, culminating in birth. Take away the pain, and you take away progress, necessitating artificial oxytocin. "You cannot extract the pain and keep the rest. It's a chain of events," says Odent. "So the objective should be that women are in such an environment that they can make the birth as easy as possible."

Lothian now tells women that the pain of childbirth is protective. The revamped Lamaze motto might be "awake and aware of the pain."

"What do we do when we experience pain in general? We respond to it," says Lothian, offering the analogy of the toe blister—you protect the wound with movement. You shift your gait, lift your heel, or even kick off your shoe. You move. And that, she says, is precisely what a woman needs to do in labor. "She's got to move to get this baby to get through the pelvis more easily." The baby's position is key, and if a woman's water is broken and she's immobilized, the baby will have a harder time angling itself into the pelvis and working its way down and out. "If the woman can feel labor," says Lothian, "she's moving, she's tightening, she's releasing, she's moving her hips."

Lothian interrupts herself to make it clear that she's not anti-epidural: "It's wonderful when it's truly needed." But when women are routinely not able to feel the pain and respond to it—to move their bodies—they are more vulnerable to injury, she argues. "When we've got a baby that rams through because this mother doesn't feel anything, we're increasing the risk of damage to her pelvis, to her vagina, and to her pelvic floor. And we don't know whether we're increasing risk to this baby. We've taken a hugely protective part of physiology and gotten rid of it."

GETTING CONTROL

A labor and delivery nurse in New Jersey shared an observation: "You know, all the methods for childbirth, whether it's Bradley or Lamaze, they've all been developed by men," she said. "I don't want to sound like a feminist, but it kind of bothers me because there's no real childbirth process or plan or whatever you want to call it that's been developed by a woman." What she's missed, or perhaps what she's never been exposed to, is the body's own method. This is the conclusion Lothian has come to after years of advocating Lamaze. Physiological childbirth, pain and all, is the original, time-tested, made-by-women-for-women method.

And if women want to use that method, says Lothian, they have to have the "freedom to do whatever they need to do to cope with the pain." The climbing epidural rate doesn't surprise her. "If we put women in hospitals with restrictive policies—they're hooked up to everything, they're expected to be in bed—of course they're going to go for the epidural, because they're unable to work through their pain," she says.

Tricia Anderson, a midwife in England, calls this a "torturous and fiendish environment." She writes:

> Let us bring them into harsh rooms with bright lights. Let us make them lie on their backs on hard narrow beds. Let us tether them to machines so they cannot move. Let us make them stay silent and make no noise with their pains. Let us expose their most private parts and threaten them with cold steel. Let us make them push their babies upwards, against the pull of the earth . . . In these conditions, labour swiftly becomes unbearable and pain relief becomes a woman's only hope. . . . This is not the natural cry of a woman in labour bringing a child to birth, although if you have only ever witnessed childbirth in a medicalized setting you might be

forgiven for thinking so. This is the screaming plea of a tethered animal in pain.[34]

Lothian believes that most women are unaware of the restrictions that await them in the hospital. "I go wild with nurses and childbirth educators who say, 'Women don't want to experience the pain, and they don't want to work hard in labor. They just want to come in and have their epidural.' I say, 'And even if they *don't* want to come in and have their epidural, they come to *your* hospital, and they have no choice. They have no choice. This is not an intellectual decision at that point. They can't manage their pain because *you won't let them.*'"

"Women are not stupid," she adds. "Deep down they know it's the only option they have. And I also don't buy the fact that today's women are not willing to work hard. They work extremely hard at a lot of things." They also seem, as many doctors have observed, to be trying to exert some control over the process. The birth plan, that wish for control in black and white, is an anomaly in medicine; no other medical event has inspired the patient to bring with her a list of Dos and Don'ts.

Like the birth plan, however, the epidural confers dubious control. It has been framed as a feminist right to choose, just as twilight sleep was at the turn of the century. But then as now, a woman under anesthesia actually surrenders motor control, control over her bladder, and control over her perineum. Christine Morton points out that because women are numb, their bodies are vulnerable to the exigencies of teaching hospitals. "She can get more vaginal exams than she needs, and rougher exams," she says. With an epidural, it's more likely that an episiotomy will be cut, and it's more likely that she'll tear because she will rely on coached pushing. She may have avoided pain in labor, but women describe the pain of recovering from sutures in their vagina as "excruciating." Several told me that it was the worst part of giving birth.

The question deserves raising again: why do women put up with so little? Lothian has another answer: "Americans trust doctors and they trust hospitals, and they equate the two with health. And people want what's best for their babies. They assume that you decrease your risk by going to a hospital and having a top-flight doctor. What they don't understand is that obstetricians are surgeons, and they know pathology, but they really suck at wellness." They are trained to sew up a tear, but not to prevent one.

The larger question is whether the needs of a woman in physiological labor can coexist with the needs of an institution. Lothian understands a woman's impulse to want the technology there in case it's needed—she gave birth to all four of her children in a hospital with an obstetrician. But for women seeking normal birth, she now advises against it. "I really think birth needs to move back out of the hospital. I think the whole model has to change," she tells me. "Hospitals never should have been where healthy women went to have babies; doctors never should have gotten involved."

Like Lothian, Lamaze has become somewhat radicalized over the years. In 1993, the board passed a resolution acknowledging the benefits of out-of-hospital birth—and lost a sizable chunk of its membership. "I wouldn't have said this 10 or 15 years ago," says Lothian. "Then I thought we could fix it. I felt, if we just had less restrictive hospital policies. But it's never going to happen."

Several nurses and childbirth educators I spoke with said the same. "Don't deliver in the hospital unless you have a risk," Sharon Breidt in Keene, New Hampshire, told me. "I'm a strong home-birth advocate. That's the only place where I see providers truly respecting the process." Jill Jernigan, the director of childbirth education at Florida Hospital, says that if a woman wants a physiological birth, she suggests a birthing center an hour's drive away. "I tell them you gotta go somewhere else. Because there's no hospital where they're going to get that kind of birth." Even Sue Cooter—although she would never say this to a client—told me, "I think if you really want a non-medicated birth, then you really need to go to a birthing center."

CHAPTER 6

Underground

IF A WOMAN WANTS to give birth outside the hospital with a midwife in Taos, New Mexico, she's encouraged to do so by the local obstetrician, by her friends, and even by the state Medicaid office, which will pay for it. In 1997, obstetricians Heidi Rinehart, MD, and Rudy Fedrizzi, MD, husband and wife, moved to Taos and joined local midwives to form the Northern New Mexico Women's Health and Birth Center, possibly the only freestanding birth center in the United States in which physicians worked alongside independent midwives in a nonprofit institution. The birth center provided the full range of maternity care, from a home water birth to an elective repeat cesarean. For the past decade, about one-third of the predominantly Latina and indigenous childbearing community has received care through the center. And they probably comprise the highest percentage of out-of-hospital birth in the country.

"I tell women they're better off going with the midwives," Rinehart told me, seated in her office, the purple Taos mountains in the distance behind her. "It is very clear that doctors and hospitals look for pathology in healthy women when none exists." When I visited in 2002, the center's cesarean rate was 15%, which Rinehart lamented as "still too high."

Rinehart and Fedrizzi have since moved on—the nonprofit business structure didn't quite hold up for the doctors. The center, now called the Northern New Mexico Midwifery Center, is now run solely by midwives, so their clients are women with normal, uncomplicated pregnancies, a "low-risk" population for whom a high percentage of normal, uncomplicated deliveries should be expected. Like the Daviss and Johnson home-birth study,[1] the center's statistics suggest that in such a population, necessary intervention is minimal and complications are few. Among nearly 350 women giving birth, more than half for the first time, close to 90% had spontaneous, vaginal births. Only 2.4% required forceps or vacuum, 2.7% had an episiotomy, and 8% had a cesarean section. Among the same mothers, 14% gave birth in the water, 11% gave birth at home, and 86.5% were still breastfeeding at 6 weeks, compared to 61% in the general population.[2] There was one stillbirth, and there were no neonatal or maternal deaths.

Rinehart and Fedrizzi moved to Taos to test their philosophy that midwives should care for normal birth, obstetricians for complications, which is the norm in most industrialized countries. "We are trying to change the culture around birth," Rinehart told me, but she also said that at times she felt like she and Fedrizzi were "hiding" in the small mountain town, isolated and insulated from the gestalt of twenty-first-century obstetrics. "There's no framework in most physicians' belief systems to incorporate the science that says that midwifery care is superior and out-of-hospital birth is safe. It doesn't fit, so they reject it," Rinehart said. "A lot of the things I do are outside of what the herd is doing. If I lived in a medium or large-sized city, I might be attacked or ostracized or black-balled, medically or professionally."

The two doctors met and married during medical school at Vanderbilt University in the 1980s. Rinehart, who was chief resident, stands about 5 feet tall, with short-cropped brown hair and a gymnast's build; Fedrizzi stands a head above her, a slim runner with a long nose and a shiny bald head.

During their residency in Nashville, both were struck by the high cesarean rate and disturbed by several maternal deaths on the operating table. "What we were doing didn't quite seem right," Fedrizzi told me. "I knew there was something better." Rinehart had seen Ina May Gaskin speak and wrote to her, "Can I come to The Farm?" She spent two weeks there, learning from the midwives. "I came back from that experience having been to three births in which there was an absence of fear," says Rinehart. "And I don't want you to think that meant the midwives weren't alert. We had two very hard births—one postpartum hemorrhage and one baby that was in a difficult position. The midwives were alert and attentive and ready to use their skills, but they weren't afraid."

When Rinehart became pregnant with their first child a few years later, the couple chose to get prenatal care and give birth with the midwives at The Farm, 80 miles away, rather than on their own maternity ward. "We were grateful for a birth that was not a delivery of a package but a transformation of a family," Rinehart told me. She gave birth to their second child at home.

New Mexico remains the most midwife-friendly state in the nation. In 2004, midwives outnumbered obstetricians. Nearly one-third of births were attended by midwives there,[3] compared to 8% nationally.[4] In other states, women have fewer options. There are just 175 independent birthing centers nationwide; 25 of them are in Texas; Massachusetts has two; there is just one in the entire state of Georgia. In 12 states, there are no birthing centers. Meanwhile, hospitals have dissolved nurse-midwifery practices in Austin, Chicago, Cleveland, Des Moines, Manhattan, Nashville, Richmond, and most recently in Syracuse, New York.

In the United States, midwives generally fall into two categories, those who are registered nurses and those who are not. Certified nurse–midwives, or CNMs, are licensed in all 50 states and recognized by the American College of Obstetricians and Gynecologists as legitimate maternity care providers. *Your Pregnancy and Birth*, ACOG's guide to childbirth, tells women that "Four types of practitioners offer medical care for pregnancy and birth: obstetrician-gynecologists (ob-gyns), maternal-fetal medicine specialists (high-risk ob), family physicians, and certified nurse–midwives." But there is another trained, credentialed provider whom ACOG does not recognize, and that is the certified professional midwife, or CPM.

New Mexico and 21 other states license CPMs; this is the credential held by the midwives at the Taos center. Any recognized provider is entitled to Medicaid reimbursement by law, although many states do not comply. Certified professional midwives work autonomously and are trained to attend out-of hospital births. Nurse–midwives are trained in hospital protocol, and most are subordinate to obstetricians. There are some other differences: CNMs are licensed to start IVs, suture perineal tears, and write prescriptions; CPMs must refer out for such services. Both credentials require training in neonatal resuscitation.

Ten states and the District of Columbia not only disregard the CPM but have case law or legislation *prohibiting* these midwives from attending births. In Alabama, Illinois, Indiana, Iowa, Kentucky, Maryland, Missouri, North Carolina, South Dakota, Wyoming, and the District of Columbia, a CPM who attends a home birth is subject to a misdemeanor or even a felony prosecution. The Midwest is a particularly hostile region. Several states there have actively investigated and prosecuted midwives in recent years, and all except Wisconsin have quashed licensing efforts. Illinois is in a class all its own, as the only state in the nation that prohibits freestanding birth centers. There, the Taos midwifery center would be legally tantamount to a brothel.

The landscape is a patchwork of conflicting and often vague labels and laws, where what's covered by Medicaid in one state is criminal in another. Consumers are confused by the various brands of midwives— "certified," "licensed," "lay," "direct-entry," "nurse," "traditional." The labels don't always reflect a midwife's skill set or experience level. Karen Brock, for instance, had been attending births for 20 years in Alabama when she was charged with practicing nurse–midwifery without a license. She pled guilty in 2003, received a 30-day suspended jail sentence, 18 months of unsupervised probation, and $1000 in fines, and at the same time applied for and received midwife licensure from the state of Tennessee. In one state she is an illegal "lay" midwife; in another, she is a licensed healthcare provider. Brock still lives in Alabama but attends births in a private house that she rents just over the border, or sometimes in hotel rooms. She says 95% of her clients are from Alabama or other "illegal" states. Some have traveled as many as 5 hours to give birth with her. "Because of distance, about half of the women who contact me do not birth with me," she tells me. "They are worried about the drive. Many choose under-the-radar midwives or unassisted home births."

Even in states that offer licensing, some midwives remain underground because they object to increasing restrictions on their practice. Washington State, for example, was one of the first to recognize independent midwives[5] and has a colorful history in obstetric reform. It was in Seattle that a man handcuffed himself to his wife's maternity bed so he could stay with her during the delivery, garnering national attention. But in recent years the state health department has launched investigations against some 30 midwives, and several have been charged for attending VBACs, breeches, and twins, even though nothing in their regulations had prohibited it.

"Washington State looks really good on paper for midwives, but we're being driven out of practice," says Shaheeda Pierce, a midwife who has practiced for 30 years and now lives in Puget Sound. In 2005, Pierce spent $32,000 in legal fees fighting charges that she overstepped her bounds by attending a breech birth. Also a paralegal, Pierce refused to hand over her clients' records when investigators showed up at her door. She calls the case a partial win. Pierce preserved her license (after a year's suspension) and Washington midwives' legal sanction to attend frank and complete breeches. But a similar case against a midwife who attended a VBAC did not end so well, and the midwives' malpractice insurer no longer covers VBAC.

Licensing has backfired in Washington, say Pierce and others, and a number of midwives have given up their papers entirely and gone back to being outlaws. "I give licensed midwifery three more years," Pierce told me, although she is unsure if she would practice without the protection. As of early 2007, about 40 midwives had lost or retired their licenses.

Midwives have faced administrative and criminal challenges in many states, even in those where they are licensed or where their practice isn't prohibited. Their homes have been raided. They have been subjected to sting operations—a couple pose as expectant clients, then return later bearing badges and handcuffs. They have spent their savings on legal fees; some have lost their homes.

In 2002, the Associated Press reported that 300 independent midwives had been criminally charged, sued, or disciplined in the previous decade, mostly for practicing medicine without a license. At least 50 had been sentenced to prison.[6] Since then, a midwife in Wisconsin has been sentenced to 6 months in prison; a midwife in South Dakota spent 30 days in jail for practicing nurse–midwifery without a license; a midwife in Indiana who had attended more than 2000 births was charged; and at the start of 2007, a Pennsylvania midwife who serves the Amish was facing $30,000 in fines for practicing without a license. Her first hearing attracted 300 plainclothes supporters to the courthouse in protest.[7]

Yet in spite of the costs, hundreds of midwives continue to practice illegally nationwide.

MIDWIFE ON WHEELS

Before I met Linda in the flesh, she would often return my calls from the road. Her voice would come in broken, and then her cell would cut out, and she'd call back a few minutes later to say it was the snow or the hills interrupting the signal. This was my first clue to her peripatetic life. Linda lives in the rural flatlands of the Midwest; any hills are about an hour away from her home, an old farmhouse a few miles off the highway surrounded by rusted evidence of her husband's opposite tendency to nest.

Linda defies several midwife stereotypes; for instance, she prefers black leather to anything billowy. If it weren't for all the birth gear, I could easily see her zipping off-road on a motorcycle, peeling into the gravel driveway of one of the many Amish or Mennonite families who call on her, materializing as though from the future next to horse and buggy.

One night while I'm driving with her on a dark divided highway, Linda tells me that back in the '50s her town was offered the interstate. She shakes her head, tsking. "And they said, 'No thanks, we don't need it. We've got the railroad.'" She chortles. "And I just think that's a shame." At first I'm not sure why she'd prefer the interstate and its attending cloverleaf of exhaust and fast food. Instead, a downtown still exists, the nearest Applebee's is 10 miles away, and a sign at the edge of town boasts the "winningest" high school athletic team.

But it becomes clear that Linda simply wants to reach all her clients faster. One primary demand of the home-birth midwife is mobility. There are midwives in Alaska who double as bush pilots, and in Puget Sound, Shaheeda Pierce keeps horses handy in case of an earthquake. Linda drives. She drives a truck into the ground every 18 months and clocks 50,000 miles a year.

The maze of country roads requires not only more driving time, but precious brain time. With a caseload of about 30 women, most of whom don't come to her, Linda has a lot of directions to remember. She has to recall the subtle landmarks and turns, for the call may come at 3 a.m. from an Amish man who's walked half a mile to the community phone to say his wife is dilated 7 centimeters, with contractions 5 minutes apart, and the only available landmark will be a kerchief he ties to the fence post.

Linda allowed me into her world for two weeks, provided that I did not reveal her real name or location. All names have been changed. Much of our time was spent in her pickup truck, driving from one client to another. Linda trained with midwives in another part of the state and moved to her current residence a few years back. Between clients inherited from a midwife who was retiring, word of mouth, and a few oblique flyers posted on bulletin boards ("Interested in home birth?"), Linda's practice grew rapidly. By 2006, she had attended around 400 births and had reached a saturation point. Not that she'd saturated the market, by any means; rather, the market had swamped her, and she had more clients than she knew what to do with. If she were a legitimate business, she'd be fulfilling the American dream—ready to expand, recruit employees, and open a satellite office.

The state considers Linda to be "practicing medicine without a license," a felony offense. She wouldn't be recognized even in a state that offers licensing, because she currently doesn't hold a CPM credential. Because it affords her no protection from the state, obtaining it hasn't been a priority. Shortly after she began taking clients, Linda was served a Cease and Desist order by the state. Several other midwives in the state were investigated as well, and of those, Linda is the only one still practicing.

In such an environment, providing care requires discretion. After receiving the letter, Linda stopped posting flyers and began screening her calls. Now, it is only by asking the right questions of the right people that women find her. For example, Rachael, a 20-something client who is bouncing a wide-eyed 4-month-old on her hip when we meet, moved to the area from Alaska when she was well into her second trimester. "I had called a birthing center in Alaska," she tells me. The center didn't know of anyone in the new area, but she remembers the woman on the other end of the phone reassuring her, "Oh, there will be a midwife there. She may not be visible, but there'll be one somewhere. You just need to start asking people." Rachael began her search with a list of doulas she got off the Web. "When I got here I just kept calling and asking," she says. She did this for 6 weeks. "I was about to cave when I found Linda." Like many home-birth clients in states where midwifery is illegal, Rachael didn't find a provider until her maternity clothes were well worn, at 7 months.

Similarly, I found Linda via a circuitous route of recommendations. A home-birth dad in Connecticut put me in touch with an activist in Pennsylvania, who put me in touch with a lobbyist in Virginia, who gave me the name of a midwifery student who knew Linda and suggested I speak with her.

Linda's is not a fly-by-night operation, but at times it has the air of such: her office is a trailer, which she hitches up to her truck when she's heading to a faraway client who is in early labor. She also rents an RV hookup one day a month in the nearest city and holds back-to-back prenatal appointments for her growing population of clients there. They heave their bellies up the shoebox-width stairs and into the stuffy cabin, sometimes with partners and kids in tow, and the whole RV rocks suggestively as everyone gets situated. Before she had the trailer, Linda asked clients with big living rooms to take turns hosting prenatal days. Before that she held court in a corner of the public library.

Linda feels she'd be too much of a target holding regular appointments at her home, so she moves about. Prenatals are held in living rooms, in bedrooms, and in the unmarked trailer. She meets prospective clients at coffee shops and truck stops. I don't want to over-dramatize; Linda isn't looking over her shoulder most of the time. She's not that careful. Although the black file box she carries with her at all times is equipped with a five-digit combination lock, she has never set it. She pays taxes and lists her occupation as "midwife." If she's pulled over while speeding off to a birth, she tells the cop she's rushing to deliver a baby and will even give out her client's name and phone number. If the officer doesn't look convinced, she opens her worn black leather bag and produces a bulb syringe.

Linda doesn't call her work civil disobedience. She's not political, but she clearly feels a sense of duty: "The way that births are going is horrible. It's an injustice to our women that we have a C-section rate that's so high, a death rate that's so high. I feel obligated to women and their babies," she told me over the phone before my visit.

Her clients feel entitled to their decision, and legally, they are. Midwifery may be illegal in places, but there's no law against giving birth at home. (There is, however, a chance that social services will get involved; in some cases, home birth has been regarded as neglect.) Neither Linda nor her clients seem all that bothered by her need for concealment. I point out the incongruity of a prenatal exam in an RV park to Nicole, a client who is due at the end of the month. She laughs. "I always wondered about that. Linda, do your neighbors ever wonder what you're doing in here?" Linda, also laughing, nods. "They know," she says. "The lady who runs the trailer park asked me and I told her. You know what? It's a lot worse if you lie." "I never lie to anyone either," says Nicole. "I just try to not give too much information."

THE "OFFICE" VISIT

Over the course of 2 weeks, Linda conducted roughly 30 prenatal, postnatal, and informational appointments, canceled five, attended three births, missed one birth, and drove approximately 1800 miles within a 150-mile radius. She missed three nights of sleep. Maybe she sat down to a handful of square meals during that time, but I can only remember four.

Prenatal and postpartum visits account for the bulk of Linda's life— her clients see her once a month until 38 weeks, then at 40 weeks, and at least once a week thereafter. After the birth, she visits the next day, then a week later, and more as needed. Her entire fee is $1500. For indigent families she charges less. Sometimes she never gets paid.

Linda checks blood pressure, pulse, and fetal heart tones. She tracks the woman's weight and belly growth. She does urinalysis at every visit, using a thin strip of reactive paper that picks up PH level, blood in the urine, albumin, ketones, glucose, and nitrates. The urine stick would reveal such problems as glucose intolerance, preeclampsia, a urinary tract infection, or a client's failure to get enough fluids. Early in their pregnancies she has her clients fill out a soup-to-nuts worksheet describing a full week of food intake. Linda devotes much of the visits to diet, mainly begging her clients to reduce sugar and simple carbs.

Linda gets a baseline hemoglobin in the first trimester and checks it again in the second. "At 20 to 22 weeks, I like to see a drop in iron. That means the liver and kidneys are functioning well," she says, explaining that dilution is a healthy response to the increase in blood volume during pregnancy. "If the iron is rising, then this lady is having a problem." Linda palpates the belly, noting the fetus's position, and listens to fetal heart tones with a handheld Doppler monitor, which amplifies the heartbeat as though on loudspeaker. She can discern the position of the placenta aurally as well: whereas the fetus has a faster heartbeat separate from that of the mother, the placenta's pulse beats with the mother's. If the placenta is lying low or near a cesarean scar, she will suggest an ultrasound; otherwise, many of her clients never get one.

Toward the end of the pregnancy, Linda makes sure the baby is positioned head-down and is descending into the pelvis. She determines this with her hands. At one prenatal, she called me over to feel a woman's 8-month-pregnant belly for the baby's head "engaging." She guided my hand down over the young woman's taut, almost conical abdomen just above her pubic bone and had me push gently with my thumb and fingers stretched wide, as though I were reaching for a softball. I could feel the solid contours of the head. Linda guided my hand from side to side gently. If the baby were still "high up," its head would bob freely. "Feel how it won't move? That means the head is engaged." Once the baby's head settles into the pelvic cavity, there's less chance of cord prolapse or a surprise breech.

Linda does not perform or recommend several screens that would be routine under physician care. The Group B Strep culture, for example, she believes is unnecessary, and she refers her clients to literature explaining why. The glucose challenge to test for gestational diabetes she finds redundant—if a client isn't tolerating sugar, she will know from the presence of glucose in the urine, and she'll adjust the client's diet accordingly or refer her to a physician for further testing. Other diagnostics simply require technology beyond Linda's scope, such as a complete blood workup, biophysical profile, genetic tests, amniocentesis, and ultrasound. She generally discusses these with her clients only if there is an indication or if they show an interest.

After the birth, Linda checks the baby for reflexes and anomalies and sends the state a blood sample called a PKU, which screens for some 50 diseases and abnormalities. She does not give antibiotic eye drops to newborns or administer vitamin K, unless the baby experienced trauma, and she recommends against circumcision. She gives her clients information on how to obtain a birth certificate, but she will no longer sign one.

One of the World Health Organization's guidelines for birth attendants is that they not only should be capable of attending healthy, uncomplicated pregnancies, but also should be able to diagnose abnormalities and refer high-risk cases. Linda doesn't have official physician collaboration as licensed midwives must. However, she has fostered relationships with two obstetricians who will offer second opinions, perform diagnostics, or repair perineal tears in a supportive atmosphere. One doctor, whom I'll call Dr. Smith, is the director of OB/GYN at a nearby hospital. When one client's fetus was diagnosed with an anomaly, Dr. Smith supervised the delivery in the hospital but allowed Linda to catch the baby. The other OB, let's call him Dr. Jones, is that rare breed of physicians still willing to attend vaginal breech deliveries. His wife, also a doctor, gave birth to their first child in the hospital and got an unwanted episiotomy. She gave birth to their subsequent children at home, including one who was breech.

Carolyn, a client of Linda's who is 7 months pregnant with twins when we meet, saw Dr. Jones for an ultrasound and consult. She asked him, "Can we do this at home?" He responded with two answers: the official line (no, you absolutely can't) and his personal opinion (of course you can). "It was really helpful," says Carolyn, "because with each question we asked, he was able to give us two answers so we could compare. He said most other doctors, even his own colleagues, would have just given one."

"If people ask me, 'I'm considering a home birth, what do you think?' I go over their risks and say these are the concerns, the choice is yours," the doctor told me, sipping an espresso at a bookstore. "As a physician I'll support you whatever your decision is. Isn't that my role? I'm just there to say hey, it's really your choice." Dr. Jones, who did separate fellowships in obstetrics and maternal–fetal medicine, tells me that what he knows about normal birth he learned from his wife. "In obstetrics, there are no forefathers. There are only foremothers. Guys didn't start this gig."

Home-birth midwives must also be equipped to stabilize a hemorrhage or resuscitate a baby—emergencies that don't wait for 911. Linda considers this her *raison d'être*. "An uncomplicated birth is straightforward;

anybody could do it. Policemen do it all the time," she tells me. "That's not why you're hiring a midwife. You're hiring a midwife because you want her there for complications." Some of Linda's clients are such believers in birth that they toy with the idea of going unassisted. To this, Linda is fond of telling the story of a birth she attended where the baby had its umbilical cord wrapped three times around its neck and needed resuscitation. "You never know when you're going to have a problem," she says. "It's like playing Russian roulette."

For the problems, Linda carries several medical supplies, including the drugs Pitocin and Cytotec, which she carries for their anti-hemorrhagic properties, although she's used them only once. She gets the Pitocin from a midwife in Montana, who procures the supply from a friendly doctor; Cytotec she gets from a nurse-midwife in state. She obtains her RhoGAM injections, for women with negative blood types whose babies are positive, from yet another midwife (the Rhogam prevents the formation of antibodies that would attack the next pregnancy). Other supplies—surgical scissors, cord clamps, latex gloves—are readily available online. "The hardest part is finding oxygen," says Linda.

An appointment with Linda can take hours. She can get the information she needs pretty quickly, but some families just need to talk. In addition, Linda is often recommending remedies for yeast infections, urinary tract infections, fatigue, constipation, heartburn, hemorrhoids, aching backs and feet, sagging bellies, colicky children, and so forth. She is extraordinarily patient. The most exasperated I saw her was over a woman who was eating only two bananas for breakfast. "You have got to get more protein," she scolded, raising her voice. "That's just not enough."

A typical day went like this:

Noon: Drive an hour and 15 minutes. Stop at a diner for a salad of iceberg lettuce and red French dressing.

2:00 p.m.: Prenatal visit with Kristy and John, a young, nervous Catholic couple planning their second VBAC, due in 4 weeks. Kristy planned to deliver with a supportive OB until a woman from her cesarean support group told her that the OB was performing abortions at Planned Parenthood, which Kristy couldn't abide. Barely showing, she called practice after practice but found none that were VBAC-friendly and willing to take such a "late transfer."

4:30 p.m.:   Drive toward city.

6:00 p.m.:   Postpartum visit with Sheila, a 37-year-old massage therapist, which begins with 30 minutes of chatting.

6:30 p.m.:   Check Sheila's baby girl's umbilicus and soft spot, then weigh her with a portable "fish" scale. Linda takes the baby, coos, then lays her on top of a sling across her lap. She hooks the sides of the sling to the brass cylinder gauge and raises it up over her head until the baby is lifted an inch off her knees, as though carried by a stork's beak. Arching her back and flexing her head to read the measurement, Linda records it as just a few ounces more than the baby's birth weight, which prompts a stern lecture on stimulating the baby during breastfeeding. "You need to make sure the baby isn't just content to be at the breast," Linda says, cradling the baby. "You need to tickle her toes or cheek to wake her up and make her suck. She's got to get that hind milk, which is full of all the nutrients."

7:00 p.m.:   Check Sheila's uterus. Linda palpates her abdomen, asks about bleeding, and feels for "muscle separation." She explains that these are the two abdominal muscles that drift apart to allow for belly expansion. More than cosmetic, she says, their reunification prevents a malpositioned fetus in the next pregnancy. Linda recommends crunch-like abdominal exercises.

7:30 p.m.:   Drive across town.

8:00 p.m.:   Stop at Jack in the Box for a chicken sandwich.

8:30 p.m.:   Postpartum visit with Sarah, now a mother of four, whose labor Linda missed only 2 days before. (Linda says Sarah called too late and pushed the baby out without her. Sarah birthed her second, a breech, unassisted as well.) Sarah is pleasant but taciturn, and I suspect that she was intentionally using Linda as backup rather than as a birth attendant. It's nearly

9 p.m., and she's in bed in her nightgown. Linda weighs the baby and checks for anomalies, gently counting fingers and toes, surveying color, checking fists for grab and feet for reflexes, spreading tiny legs and buttocks.

9:00 p.m.:   Make baby footprints on a certificate; Linda signs her name under "special friends at birth." Then she checks Sarah's perineum for tears and bleeding and asks about breastfeeding.

9:40 p.m.:   Answer cell phone. Although Linda never rushes an appointment, she also never ignores her phone, and here on Sarah's bed she takes a call, phone pressed between shoulder and ear, while snipping the cord clamp off the 2-day-old newborn.

10:00 p.m.:   Fill up at a gas station, purchase a bag of pretzels and a Pepsi.

Midnight: Arrive home.

Another day went like this:

7:00 a.m.:   Drive 2 hours to Amish village.

9:00 a.m.:   Prenatal with Leah, a mother of six, whose 32-week-old fetus is lying breech. "Yup, a nice, low breech. I feel the butt here, a leg here, a knee here," says Linda, kneading the woman's dough-like belly. "So what are we going to do for this baby?" Linda suggests a knees-to-chest position held 2 minutes, twice every day, which she explains "crowds baby's head at the fundus, encouraging it to get into a more comfortable position." Leah could also try a chiropractor familiar with the Webster technique, or Linda could try a version. "We do all we can to help babies turn first," says Linda, "but if baby decides to stay breech, we'll go ahead and have the baby come bottom first."

10:30 a.m.:   Prenatal with Beth, Leah's sister-in-law. Beth is 9 weeks along, having conceived soon after the birth of her last child, number three, a colicky baby who needs

to be held constantly during the visit. Discuss med-
dlesome mother-in-law.

11:00 a.m.: Recommend herbs that will stave off menstruation next
time and "give you a little more time between babies.
It's awfully nice to have a bit of time without," says
Linda.

Noon: Stop at a gas station. (Linda seems to avoid using her
clients' bathrooms.) Consume a hot dog while in line to
pay for it.

12:30 p.m.: Prenatal with first-timers Judith and her husband
Jacob. Discuss the concept of whole grains and fresh
vegetables.

2:00 p.m.: Prenatal with Deborah. Talk at length about preg-
nancy-induced depression and nutrition. Deborah is
trying to adhere to a raw-foods diet. She says a
neighbor cured his cancer with this regimen. Linda
straightens her spine and inhales deeply. "Raw food is
great if you're trying to stop cancer," she says. "But
you're not growing a tumor, you're growing a baby."

3:00 p.m.: Check Deborah's hemoglobin. Linda pricks her finger
and smears the blood droplet on a glass slide, which she
inserts into the hemoglobinometer. The contraption
looks like an elongated Polaroid camera and works opti-
cally. The viewer is divided into two chambers, and you
match the shade of the droplet on one side (which is
converted by infrared light to a grayish-green) by
scrolling to the correct shade on the other side.

4:30 p.m.: Prenatal with Sarah, mother of three, illuminated by a
kerosene lamp.

5:30 p.m.: Drive.

7:30 p.m.: Home.

TIME MANAGEMENT

The Midwives Model of Care™, written—and trademarked—in 1996 by
a coalition of organizations, emphasizes two things: that birth is normal

and that women need individualized care. The same principle that applies to birth—let it happen in its own time, on its own time, with few exceptions—applies to prenatal visits and phone calls as well. In other words, spend as much time with the woman as she needs. Pacing, therefore, doesn't often come naturally to midwives, and in a state where supply doesn't meet demand, a midwife's caseload can easily swell to unwieldy proportions.

Owing to the state's hostility toward midwifery, Linda is one of the few women in the region willing to attend home births, and she is by far the most liberal in terms of the clinical challenges she'll accept. So she's in demand and at capacity, and it seems to several people that she is exceeding capacity. She has a reputation for missing births, for taking too many clients due too close together, and for being a bit of a maverick. She regularly calls on another midwife, Valerie, who lives near the closest major city, for backup. And there were two or more times when two of Linda's clients went into labor simultaneously, and she moved (or tried to move) both families to the same location in order to care for them both.

One woman who apprenticed with Linda told me that the experience nearly gave her an ulcer. "At every birth my stomach was turning because I was waiting for the cell phone to ring and someone to say, 'Hey I'm in labor and I'm on the other side of the state,'" she said.

Linda told me several times that she needs to start containing her practice, turning down those women who live a little too far away or who call after the month they're due is booked solid. "I'm trying to reduce my load," she says one day while we're driving, although it's followed by a doubtful like-that's-possible chuckle. "Three or four births a month—that's workable. But five or six? In July I have six." Linda doesn't sleep much as it is, and she loses sleep worrying. "I'm not worrying about the birth and if it will go okay. Usually what I'm worrying about is that people are going to clash in calling me. If I've got two or three people that are coming up due anytime, then it's like 'Oh no, how am I going to make them all . . . ?'"

Beyond losing sleep, the demands of her schedule have secondary effects. For one, she can't leave home to, say, attend an educational seminar or a midwifery conference, let alone go on vacation. Along with being mobile, midwives must be accessible—tethered to a short radius of their homes, tethered to sobriety, and now practically conjoined to their cell phone. Aside from spontaneous trips, midwives must block out a full month to ensure a couple weeks of vacation, and that's something Linda feels she can't do.

One critic of Linda's got in touch with me after my visit to say she worried that I had observed a "bad example" of midwifery—that Linda is not only overtaxed but that she gives poor herbal advice, is stubborn, unwilling to hear criticism, doesn't keep her knowledge current, and appears threatened by competition. Another took issue with her nutritional advice (and habits) and her time management and agreed about the stubborn streak, but defended her skills. "She's a very competent midwife," she told me. "That's why people like her. But she misses births like crazy. I just think you can't realistically take that many people, that far away from each other, and think that you'll be able to give them all good care."

Valerie, who knows Linda's practice style and abilities best, would only distinguish herself as more conservative than Linda. "If they've got so much going on that I need to load them up with 15 different herbs, well then they don't need to be home, they need to be somewhere else," she told me. Linda excludes very few: VBACs, breeches, and twins are fair game. Over 35? "I don't consider age a risk factor by itself," she says. High blood pressure? "We'll try to get that down with diet and exercise before I will risk her out." Preeclampsia? Ditto. Triplets? "I would love to do triplets," she proclaimed to a roomful of clients and younger midwives gathered in her home for my benefit. She has so far delivered 9 sets of twins vaginally and 15 breech babies.

THE FAMILY ROOM

Stacy is a woman who no doubt lives too far away from Linda—130 miles—and that's just one mitigating factor. She is obese (300 pounds), she is thought to be 2 weeks past her due date, and her belly is measuring larger than average. No question, she would already have been induced under the care of a physician. Linda had tried to coordinate co-care with another midwife, but that midwife demurred. She felt it too risky because of Stacy's weight and because she is having her sixth child; and maybe also, it turns out, because of her discomfort with Linda's style. She wouldn't even be backup.

Linda and I drive toward Stacy in the afternoon, eating a bag of pecans, the flat horizon of the plains beginning to undulate into gentle hills, the low winter sun reaching through bare, silhouetted trees. Linda tells me that she's agreed to "help get labor going" with homeopathics and that Stacy will drink castor oil before we arrive. Linda says she hardly ever induces, but Stacy has been anxious all week, and her history leads Linda to believe that, for whatever reason, Stacy needs a little push.

We arrive at dusk. Stacy is warm and pretty, with a booming voice and an easy laugh, and she is large; her belly sags precariously. Upstairs in Stacy's bedroom, Linda moves her hands around Stacy's belly and then checks her cervix—about 8 centimeters dilated, she announces, but lopsided, with one side thinner than the other. Stacy offers us the living room on the mezzanine of their new split-level ranch. She and her husband Tom have set up the family room down on the first floor, next to a bathroom and the kitchen, with a portable birthing tub. Actually, it's a $20 kiddy pool. "They're cheaper and better than the $200 tubs," says Linda. Unlike the hard plastic things I remember splashing in as a kid, this is essentially an aquatic air mattress, decorated with delightful cartoon fish.

Stacy and Tom's living room is brightly lit and freshly painted. The news is murmuring on the wide-screen television, bouncing off the cathedral ceiling. Linda sits on the couch knitting a cap for the newborn-to-be—a tradition of hers. She gives Stacy homeopathic doses of blue cohosh and pulsitilla, alternating between the two every 15 minutes. Stacy is on a leather recliner with her hands inside her loose T-shirt, pinching and massaging her nipples, which is supposed to stimulate oxytocin production and summon contractions. For the next 40 minutes or so, we chat about her previous five births. As we talk, she reports contractions to Linda with about the same frequency and remove with which she might note a commercial break.

Stacy's first pregnancy was induced with Pitocin, which she endured without an epidural because she had refused to take a class mandated by the hospital. She describes herself as "terrified of needles" and categorically did not want one inserted into her lower back; therefore, she wasn't signed off for such pain relief.

She lay with a Pitocin drip in her arm, frozen with fear of the tube in her vein, from 8 o'clock on a Friday morning to 10 o'clock that evening, when the nurses turned it down and gave her a sedative. The next morning, they turned it up again. At 4 p.m. she had her first contraction. Four hours later, she says, the doctor came in and told her to start pushing. "Thank goodness I don't remember all this very vividly," Stacy says. "By the time it was time to push, I had been lying in bed for 2 days. I had the worst hemorrhoids ever. I mean, awful. I pushed for over 3 hours. I was in so much pain." Finally, the birth was assisted by a vacuum extraction and a liberal episiotomy, which tore further. Stacy doesn't recall how much, but she remembers a lengthy repair.

Stacy wasn't given the baby until the incision and tear were sutured. If the birth was "agony," the stitches were "torture," she says. The night was sleepless due to the pain from the hemorrhoids and stitches and the constant coming and going of nurses. "I couldn't lie on my back because my butt hurt so bad. I had to call a nurse every time I wanted to go to the bathroom because I couldn't move." The next day, the nurses drew a sitz bath across the hall, "But my hemorrhoids were so bad that—I can't even describe it," she says, swallowing. "They were touching the bottom of the tub before I had even sat down."

Back at home with her newborn, Stacy was in pain for weeks, unable to sit except on a donut-shaped cushion, and was feeling uncharacteristically down. "I had terrible postpartum depression," she says. "I was crying. There were times I felt I could have just thrown the baby into the wall. And I was just feeling guilty about not being able to take care of the baby, not being able to take care of my husband, not feeling happy that I had a baby, and not ever wanting to have another one."

"It was just bad," she goes on. "A very bad experience. When I found out I was pregnant with my second one, I just kept wanting to die. I did not want to have another baby. And now I think this is too funny, that we're having six babies. We've come a long way in 11 and a half years."

For the second baby, in a new city, she found a nurse–midwifery practice in a hospital. The supervising obstetrician assured her they didn't require IVs. "We can make this as invasive as you want or not," Stacy remembers her saying. When her due date came and went, Stacy was advised to take castor oil—with two scoops of vanilla ice cream, cola, and peanut butter cups, a "labor float" that would become her own birthing ritual—and the midwives broke her water. She wore a fetal monitor, and her perineum tore a bit along the episiotomy scar, requiring three stitches.

Other than that, the birth was normal and low-tech. At the suggestion of the midwife, Stacy gave birth lying on her side to minimize the hemorrhoids, which it did.

"Afterwards, I felt so good. I had the baby at 1:15 in the afternoon and went home late that evening, and then the next day I was up and down the stairs doing laundry. I fixed a big meal that night." Stacy never experienced the depression again, or the fear of getting pregnant, or hemorrhoids so big they impeded sitting. She had her third, fourth, and fifth babies on her side with nurse–midwives and labor floats at exactly 8 days post-due-date. "I would start out lying on my side but would always end up lying across the bed with my head hanging off one side and my butt hanging off the other," she says, laughing at the ceiling. "I don't know how that happens."

Stacy keeps talking like this through contractions, barely stopping for an extra breath. "There's a contraction," she says flatly, turning to Linda, and then continues the sentence. I ask how she ended up here, having a home birth, after having such good experiences in the hospital. Primarily it was the recent move; the nearest nurse–midwifery practice, an hour and 20 minutes away, told her to find care closer to home. "I did want to have the baby at the hospital. Because I know you've got the technology if you need it," she says. But the doctor she chose told her she was high-risk, which would mean she'd be "closely monitored." "Which meant I'd be hooked up to all sorts of machines," says Stacy. She called back the nurse–midwifery practice, and they recommended Linda.

Until it became a choice between a "high-risk" birth in the hospital and a home birth, Stacy had never considered the latter. "Having a baby at home never even entered my mind," she says. "Never. I'm not a home-birth kind of person, I don't think."

Still dutifully pinching her nipples, Stacy seems more distracted by the relative weakness of each contraction than by any discomfort—she is ready to have the baby. But gradually, they begin to demand more of her attention. In about 15 minutes, while she's descending the stairs carrying a cookie sheet—one of the several common household items Linda has her clients gather leading up to the due date—the contractions will demand her full attention. In one motion she is rid of the tray and down on her hands and knees, as though she were about to crawl back up the stairs. She rocks in this position, moaning, for several moments, then picks herself up, wipes her brow, and says, "Wow, that one got me."

Along with a cookie sheet, Linda asks the family to assemble several other supplies:

- Towels
- Toilet paper
- Heating pad
- Plastic tablecloths
- Meat thermometer (for water temperature)
- Olive oil (for perineum)
- Large mixing bowl (for placenta)
- Adult diapers
- Gatorade or Pedialyte

Objects that Linda carries and assembles on or near the cookie sheet:

- Flashlight
- "Chux" pads (large, flat, diaper-like absorbent pads)
- Latex gloves, sterile and nonsterile
- Distilled water
- Waterproof Doppler heart rate monitor
- Various tinctures and homeopathic preparations
- Surgical scissors, umbilical scissors, and clamp
- Plastic cord clamps
- Bulb syringe
- Syringe to extract cord blood and Eldoncard blood-typing kit
- RhoGAM injection (if needed)
- Oxygen tank and mask
- Fetal resuscitation bag and mask

With Stacy bowled over on all fours, kiddy pool preparation shifts into high gear. Linda and Tom drape the couch and floor with a green floral-print plastic tablecloth and old blankets, as if preparing to apply a new coat of paint. Tom pumps more air into the tub at Linda's request—she wants the sides firm enough for Stacy to throw her weight on them with confidence—and then attaches a hose to the sink. The hot water runs out before the tub is a quarter full, however, and we're reduced to boiling water on all four burners of the stove, which feels fittingly rustic.

Finally, the pool is ready. Stacy sits on her heels, submerges her belly, and drapes her arms over one side. Tom sits on the couch facing her. Linda is stationed at Stacy's rear, kneeling on the floor, rubbing her back during contractions, shining the flashlight on her bottom. Every few minutes, Linda reaches the Doppler around to Stacy's belly to check the baby's heart tones, and they broadcast through the room like a techno beat. The rest of the time is quiet. We're all resting, waiting.

"Oh Linda, I have to go the bathroom!" Stacy says, breaking the silence. She turns her head back, "I'm sorry." Linda is unfazed. "It's OK," she says quickly. "It's no problem." Linda grabs the plastic bowl meant for the placenta and begins scooping the water clean. In a flash, Tom appears from the kitchen with a far more efficient metal colander. Linda stretches her torso across the tub and draws the strainer through the water quietly, gracefully, almost meditatively.

It is at this point that I begin to fathom what supporting normal birth really entails. Linda is on her knees, sleeves pushed up, gloved hand in a soiled kiddy pool up to her bare elbow, gleaning diarrhea wisps with a spaghetti strainer by flashlight. I try to imagine a doctor doing this work and have great difficulty. This is not medicine. This is birth. It is messy, backbreaking, humble work.

Tom and I get more hot water in the tub, the steam giving off a new, organic odor. Stacy is glowing—flushed, perspiring, hair up in a ponytail. Tom is sitting on the couch holding Stacy's hands, periodically placing a cold washcloth on the back of her neck. Stacy hangs over the far side of the tub, and Linda hangs over the other side of the tub toward Stacy. The room is loud with sensory stimuli, and yet very quiet. Everyone is waiting.

Stacy asks to go to the toilet and has a few strong contractions while sitting on it. She grunts through them. "Stacy, do you feel like pushing?" says Linda softly, kneeling on the ceramic tile at Stacy's feet. "Babies come in all sorts of places and we can have this one right here if you'd like."

But Stacy declines, so we move back to the tub. Within minutes, she's moaning through monumental contractions. She's still present enough, however, to make a joke. "Jennifer, have you ever met any of those women who have 'orgasmic births'? Cause I'd really like to know how that's done!" Then there's another contraction, and more silence following it. With the next contraction Stacy's water bag breaks with a pop, and milky fluid diffuses throughout the tub. Again, the smell shifts, now hinting at vinegar and urine and something sweet. "Oooooh lord, please let this baby come," Stacy sings, and then "Ooohhh, it's burning. This is it, this is it." Linda hands me the flashlight and inserts two fingers in Stacy's vagina for a minute; I'm wondering why. Later, she tells me she was helping rotate the head, which was cockeye and was the reason why the dilation was lopsided. Linda tells Stacy the lip of her cervix is swelling a bit and has her place two pellets of arnica, an anti-inflammatory home-opathic, under her tongue.

Stacy turns onto her back for a few minutes, belly to the ceiling, clutching her husband's hand in one hand and grabbing the plastic of the tub with the other, head thrown back, as though bracing her body for impact.

Linda keeps Stacy apprised of baby's position—she can feel the head only an inch into the birth canal—and asks if she'd like to flip back onto hands and knees to have the baby. She does. "Is it almost time to push?" Stacy keeps asking. Linda reminds her that she'll know, that she won't be able to help but push when it's time to push. Finally the head appears. Stacy is grunting. Linda has a washcloth on the perineum, pro-viding counter pressure to prevent a tear. "Pah pah pah pah," Linda says, "Breathe through it, go ahead and ease the baby out."

At the point of crowning, an oval of wrinkly infant scalp expands and retracts at the vaginal opening like the window on a kaleidoscope. It's a one step forward, two steps back process: the woman pushes with a con-traction, the baby's head pokes out further and then slips back under a bit—Linda calls it "turtlenecking." It's easy to see how an attendant's rescue reflex could kick in here, as though the baby might sink back into primordial quicksand, back into oblivion.

Stacy is pushing the head out—I can see its wavy image under the water's surface—and Linda asks me to get the cord clamp and scissors ready. Then there's another big push and a baby floats up out of the water. Linda places it on Stacy's back, rubbing it with a towel. First silent, the baby now squirms and lets out a few cries. Linda later tells me she asked for the scissors because the cord was wrapped once around the baby's neck and she thought she might need to cut it right away, but she got slack and lifted it off with ease. It was a maneuver done so quickly I didn't even notice. One-third of all babies, she reminds me, are born with cord wraps.

The baby is pink and huge. Stacy catches her breath. "What's the sex?" she asks, still on her hands and knees. With Linda's guidance, Stacy flips onto her back and Linda passes the baby, cord still intact, under Stacy's leg and up to her breast. "Oh, it's a girl," she says, laughing with relief it seems. "Look at you, you are the most beautiful baby," she sings, letting the baby grasp her finger. Linda suctions the baby's mouth with the bulb syringe.

The newborn, already suckling at the breast, is so big that the cap Linda knitted looks doll-size by comparison (the baby later weighs in at 10 lb, 2 oz—delivered over an intact perineum). Even though everyone suspected that the baby was overdue, she's covered in vernex, the creamy, waxy substance present in the womb that also signals gestational age at birth—the less there is, the longer the gestation.

The respite after the birth seems short; against the blue plastic of the tub, the blood following birth has dyed the water a shade of Pinot Noir, speckled with vernex like curdled milk. Linda feels Stacy's uterus to make sure it has begun clamping down.

The normal amount of blood loss during birth, about a pint, is undoubtedly more than the uninitiated would be comfortable with. Judging by Stacy's pallor following delivery of the placenta and slight wooziness getting out of the tub, Linda suspects that Stacy lost slightly more than average. "It was something to watch, but not something that concerned me," Linda tells me later. Stacy's color returns on the couch, where she nurses the baby and cheerfully begins chatting again, comparing this birth to the others, repeatedly thanking Linda. The pool made the pain "so manageable," she tells her.

After resting on the couch, Stacy waddles to the bathroom with Linda, holding a chux pad between her legs. Meanwhile, her husband takes the dog out. I stay in the family room, holding the baby, and meditate on the scene. There are drops of blood on the couch, on the toilet, on the kitchen table. The placenta lies in an extra large stainless steel mixing bowl. The pool looks . . . promiscuous—a Bacchanalian vat of wine with morning-after bird shit floating about. This mess will be Tom's chore of the evening (of the year?), and he'll tackle it with the same aplomb with which he presented Linda the colander. "The placenta is for the family to deal with," Linda tells me later. "They can bury it in the backyard, throw it out with the trash, dump it in the lake. Whatever they decide." We don't see what they do with the placenta, but while we're cleaning and packing up, Tom creates suction with the hose and siphons the pool's contents onto the front lawn. As we drive off, the grass shimmers under a full moon.

MORE PHONE CALLS

It's midnight when we leave Stacy, but Linda and I won't make it home until 4 a.m. We stop at a gas station at half past midnight, where Linda gets a diet cola and sun chips—she hasn't eaten since the pecans. "I've been running on adrenaline," she tells me. We're 30 minutes from home when her cell phone rings: It's Isaac, husband of Mary, an Amish client, saying that he thinks his wife is in labor. She's been having strong contractions that seem regular. Linda hangs up and begins to think out loud which roads she should take, arguing with herself for a minute. Finally she whips the truck around and we're flying back down the dark country road. "Watch out for deer on that side," she says, accelerating. The roads get progressively smaller until we're crunching gravel, with the moon illumining the pastoral landscape for miles around. We're looking for a red handkerchief tied to the fence.

We arrive after 2 a.m., and it's a false alarm. Mary is not dilated, and the baby is still high up in the pelvis—she is days, perhaps more, from labor. As long as we're there, however, Linda wants to do a full prenatal check. She asks the husband for a lantern.

Two days later Linda makes the 4-hour round trip to Stacy for a postpartum check, and the day after that I meet her at the RV park, 90 minutes away from her home. I spend the 8 a.m. to 8 p.m. day observing mostly prenatal visits, with the exception of a postpartum visit from Sheila and her baby girl, who has gained some weight. We go to a restaurant afterward, where Linda orders the only full entrée I've seen her eat during my entire stay. At around 10 p.m. we say our goodbyes and drive separately back home. Or so I think.

Linda calls me at my motel the next morning. She didn't make it home. Jessica, a near-term first-time mother, whom we saw in the trailer, called to report regular contractions and "bloody show." So, again just half an hour from home, Linda turned her full load around and headed back toward the city so she could be nearby. She went back to the RV park and slept until 5 a.m., when Scott, Jessica's husband, called again. Before sunrise Linda was back to work.

Labor was going slowly, so Linda was able take a midday nap and then an afternoon break to meet Susan and Andy, a preppy city couple who are disillusioned with the obstetric practice they've been seeing. "They call me three words," 35-year-old Susan tells Linda over tea at a nearby Denny's. "I can't remember. . . ." She looks to her husband. "*Advanced maternal age*, that's it." "We just think there has to be a better way," says Andy. Linda tells them that she doesn't consider age alone a risk factor; that Susan can labor in any position she wants or even in a tub; that she'll try very hard to prevent a tear by giving perineal support; that she does not do episiotomies.

The couple are nodding in unison. Susan looks over her list of questions, seeming to dismiss several. "Do you often put moms on bed rest?" she asks. Linda begins to shake her head, "Or does that also not exist in midwifery?"

"So, if a woman is allowed to drink and eat, then is the likelihood of her having an accident higher?" asks Susan, off script. "An accident?" asks Linda, playing dumb. "Having bowel movements is a very normal part of having a baby. Because that head is right against your rectum; it's like a tube of toothpaste being squeezed out. When that's happening, we're like, 'Okay then! The baby's descending. This is good!'"

Susan hands Linda a birth plan and asks whether she recommends getting a doula. Linda gives the two pages a cursory glance and puts them down. Neither a birth plan nor a doula is really necessary at home, she tells the couple, "because I'm not going to do stuff that you don't want. In the hospital, you really don't have much say—your doula is a buffer between you and the hospital. Whereas at home, I view me and the couple as a team. We are cooperating to bring about a healthy birth."

Certain information Linda offers without much prompting, such as gruesome complications associated with circumcision. "Here, I brought some beautiful pictures for you to look at," she says, handing the couple printouts from an anti-circumcision website. Regarding her legal status and how it affects her practice, Linda is less forthcoming. In response to a question about caseload, she says that she cares for 20 to 30 women within a 100-mile radius, but the truth is that she will travel 150-plus miles from her home in opposite directions, which means she could conceivably be 4 hours away from a client. She says nothing about the law or the discretion required of families if interfacing with medical personnel. Later, I ask Linda whether she meant to discuss legality with them. She says it slipped her mind. "It's not the primary thing I think about."

Jessica's labor does not go as swimmingly as Stacy's. She is in far more pain, labor progresses much more slowly, and it is marked by Linda's biggest fear, the worry that keeps her up at night: another client, 150 miles in the opposite direction, calls at 11 p.m. to say that her contractions are 5 minutes apart. Linda calls Valerie, who is 3 miles away, detaches the trailer, and speeds off.

Valerie arrives with a jumbo rolly suitcase, leather bag, and wooden birthing stool. A little winded, she sits down on the couch, sighs, and confesses to me that she was just about to conclude a romantic evening with her husband. Then she turns to Jessica with all her energy.

Valerie tries her best to keep momentum going. She has Jessica shift positions, keeps her drinking, and encourages food. She holds a pot for her while she vomits, rinses the pot, and then returns with a glass of water and yogurt. "Midwives are just glorified waitresses," she says to me on a bustle through the kitchen, one of many playful asides of the night. (Another is "Someday I'm going to write a book called *The Clients Who Get Some and the Midwives Who Don't*.") Jessica moans rhythmically through the night, mid to high notes that float through the air like jumbled scales. We all sleep for a couple of hours, then, at 5:30 a.m., Linda calls. "You have a baby?" asks Valerie.

Valerie hangs up and paces around the living room, thinking out loud. "Is there any reason for me to do a vaginal check? Am I going to find out anything I don't already know? No, I'm not." She turns around to survey the couple's vast collection of board games and reminisces about playing "panic Scrabble" with Mennonite women in labor. It's played by combining the tiles from several different boards together.

When Linda returns at 9:20 a.m., she checks Jessica's cervix. She can now feel the baby's head, which she determines to be lying occiput posterior—facing front rather than facing the spine—which helps explain the lack of progress and Jessica's suffering. Posterior babies can't descend as easily into the birth canal and put tremendous pressure on the mother's lower back, called "back labor."

The two midwives sit at the kitchen table strategizing. Valerie turns to me, "At 24 hours, you start running the risk of things 'going south.' That either mom's going to give or baby's going to give." In this case, they're clearly also worried about the midwife going south. Linda tells Valerie that things have to move or she's going to crash. Bleary-eyed, she hasn't had a full night's sleep in 2 days, has driven 5 hours, and almost certainly hasn't eaten anything of substance since lunch, if she had any.

The next couple of hours play a bit like an athletic drill session. The midwives first coax Jessica to the shower, where they have her make figure eights with her hips, which successfully rotates the baby anterior. Back in bed a half-hour later, finally feeling some relief, Jessica wants to rest. The midwives give her 15 minutes and then propose walking and squatting— at least walking. Linda also gives Jessica homeopathic pellets of gessemium to help relax the cervix and gives her caulophyllum to intensify contractions. "We might want to talk about breaking your water next," Linda says to Jessica.

After a couple of reluctant laps from the kitchen to the bedroom, Linda has Jessica sit backwards on the toilet. When Jessica stands up, still facing the tank, Linda stands behind her, hands on Jessica's hips, and sways with her from side to side. "That's it Jessica, let your whole butt relax," says Valerie from the doorway. When Linda checks her cervix again, it is almost fully dilated, save for a "hair." Jessica rests another half-hour while the midwives have a snack and talk shop.

"I just wish I had taken better care of myself," says Valerie, explaining why she takes on only one or two births a month. I ask whether being a midwife led to unhealthy habits. "Oh, absolutely," she says. "Mostly eating fast food, being gone for days at a time, not sleeping, not having regular bathroom schedules. I mean, admit it," she turns to Linda. "Haven't you held your pee for so long that your eyes are darn near green?" Linda nods. "I try not to drink anything at a birth, especially if there's only one bathroom."

At around noon Jessica moves to the birthing stool, where Linda holds the remaining cervical "lip" back while Jessica pushes. The tableau is branded in my mind: Jessica is on the stool leaning on Scott, who squats behind; Linda is lying on the floor on her side, contorted underneath Jessica's bottom with her head resting on one outstretched arm and the other reaching up into Jessica's vagina. "This is called the side-lying midwife position," Valerie jokes out loud, but Linda barely cracks a smile. In between contractions she closes her eyes and looks as though she could fall asleep right there, frozen with her fingers inside Jessica.

Jessica's water breaks on its own, and the party moves again, this time to the living room, where Jessica can get on all fours and rest her head and chest on the couch. "Let yourself sink into the couch," Linda intones. "Relax your forehead, relax your jaw." Everyone is quiet between contractions, waiting. Then Jessica says she feels like squatting, so Linda gets the stool. "She's going to tear," Valerie whispers in my ear. Jessica pushes hard, but then Linda and Valerie both suggest hands and knees to avoid tearing. She flips back over.

Soon we're watching that anticipatory ebb and flow of the soggy, molded scalp, which lasts several minutes. Valerie whispers in my ear that the baby looks a little "dark," in a tone that's mildly concerning. Linda is on Jessica's bulging perineum with olive oil and a washcloth in one gloved hand and the other on her back, encouraging her to push with each contraction. "But it hurts!" screams Jessica. "I know it does, I know it does," says Linda. Jessica cries out and shudders with each push. "Just pa-pa-pa through the push, ease the baby out," guides Linda. "You're doing great, Jessica. That's it, pa-pa-pa-pa-pah. . . ." Valerie holds a wad of toilet paper at Jessica's anus and is taking heart tones with the Doppler, which crackles with static—the beats seem farther away than they have been.

Finally, the head emerges along with a burst of fluid and some blood that streams over the baby's face. With the next contraction, the baby slides out. Linda and Valerie lay the new baby boy on a towel and rub his chest and cheeks and head; Linda holds the cord with her thumb and forefinger, laying her ear on top of the baby's chest. "Hi little guy, come on, say hello." "Jessica, talk to your baby, reach down and touch the baby." "Come on little guy, come on." The incantations get progressively more forceful, the rubbing more insistent, until all of a sudden a full-blown neonatal resuscitation is in progress.

Linda is shouting for warm towels, for the heating pad, for the bulb syringe. She gives the baby a breath, then listens. Another breath, listens. Another. Then she begins two-fingered compressions, counting out loud.

Valerie is taking heart tones, which are hovering around 90 beats per minute (they should be well over 100); she sets up the oxygen tank and waves the tube in front of the baby's nose. The baby isn't moving and breathes only an occasional reverse sigh, then nothing. There's no crying or kicking. His color, which had been blueish at first with a few foreboding white spots on his face, is now rosier, but he seems uninterested in perking up. A peaceful, indifferent expression never budges from his mouth, as if he's unwilling to abandon a compelling dream.

After what seems like 10 or 15 minutes, Scott picks up the phone, presumably to call 911. "Dad? Hi. . . . We need you to start the prayer chain." He returns to the living room, kneels down, and begins repeating prayers. "Lord Jesus, breathe life into our son's body. . . . In the name of Jesus I command you to breathe." Jessica joins him. Later, Linda tells me she heard them speaking in tongues. Linda is doing chest compressions and continuing to command the little one to clutch life. Valerie holds the plastic fetal resuscitation bag, which she pumps twice for every five of Linda's compressions. Finally, Valerie looks up and says, "Why don't you call 911."

The giant suitcase Valerie had wheeled in, packed with everything from a blood pressure cuff to packets of instant coffee, lies open on the living room floor. Linda's leather bag is unzipped, her tray of glass bottle tinctures next to it. Blood and shit-stained pads, towels, and tissues are strewn about. A digital camera, with perhaps a dozen pictures of the baby's head crowning, sits atop the stereo. Linda looks up for the first time, her face flushed. "Cover up that bag," she barks. "Close that suitcase. We need to clean up this room." Valerie packs up the oxygen and moves it to the garage, and when sirens become audible, she packs up the resuscitation bag; Linda continues compressions and mouth-to-mouth.

Jessica is preternaturally calm. When the medics arrive, she is steadfast. While they work on the baby—they have only a child-size, not a neonatal, resuscitation bag; there's some arguing, and Valerie retrieves her bag and resumes pumping—they ask Jessica a battery of questions. Is this her first pregnancy? "Yes." Any problems during the pregnancy? "No." Any problems during the labor? "No." Had she received prenatal care? ". . . No. We did it ourselves."

The baby, now breathing some on his own, is airlifted to the hospital. Jessica stays behind with Valerie and Linda and births the placenta at Valerie's house (the midwives expect that the police are well on their way to Jessica's home and don't want to stay there). And Scott's parents drive him to the hospital. En route, Valerie calls to counsel the couple on their story: they should say they did in fact get prenatal care, from a midwife, but she didn't make it to the birth in time. "If they think you didn't get prenatal care, they might call in social services," Valerie tells them. Two hours later, Linda and Valerie drive Jessica to the hospital's Emergency Room entrance, where Scott and a nurse are waiting with a wheelchair. Neither midwife gets out of the van.

POSTPARTUM

Primary apnea and *secondary apnea* are technical terms recognized among home-birth midwives but rarely used by hospitals. This seems to be because in a hospital, there's no need to distinguish, since the neonatologist is called in to intubate at the first sign of a respiratory problem. Primary apnea, according to *Myles' Textbook for Midwives*, occurs when a baby doesn't initiate breathing on its own right away and often needs some sort of stimulation or even a breath. Shannon, a doula and client of Linda's, experienced this firsthand with the rapid birth of her fifth child, who arrived before Linda did. A friend who was there gave the baby a breath and was rewarded immediately with robust squawls. "I wouldn't call that a resuscitation," says the friend, who is also an L&D nurse. "She just needed a little kick in the pants."

Secondary apnea, the term Linda and Valerie used to describe Jessica's baby, occurs when there is no attempt to breathe after the first minute. Thus the distinction between primary and secondary apnea is a question of time. Exactly how many minutes transpired before Scott called 911 is hard to say, but it was many more than one.

Most midwives I talked to, licensed and unlicensed, in both states where midwifery is legal and states where it is illegal, said they would call 911 not in 10 minutes, not in 5 minutes, but 1 minute after birth if the baby weren't breathing. "Within that minute you should know if you need to start neonatal resuscitation, and that's when you should call 911. Because you can always call to cancel," says one of Linda's peers.

Why wasn't 911 called sooner? Was it ego? Hubris? Fear of the law? "I think she truly thought that the baby was coming around," says Valerie.

Linda recounted to me births in which resuscitation (ultimately successful) took as much as 20 minutes, and 911 was never called, although she says that in those cases she was getting much better response from the baby. In all, she can remember resuscitating five or six babies suffering from secondary apnea.

Valerie says she reacted differently. She tells me that once the baby came out and there was no pink color, no cord pulse, and no attempt at breathing—an Apgar score of zero—she and Linda "weren't on the same page." "If I were going to be in that situation again, I would insist that someone bring me the phone and I would call right then," says Valerie. "Even so, even so," she goes on, the baby, "hasn't suffered any brain injury. He's totally normal. So it's obvious that we picked up quickly enough so that there wasn't any damage done. And I think that we both learned a lot from the experience. We both agreed that if that situation ever happened again, our response would be a lot faster."

Valerie dismissed the notion that the delay was the result of fear of being caught, citing Linda's willingness to accompany women if they decide to transport to the hospital. But she admits that part of the reason they were so "weirded out" was the county's reputation for "arresting everybody in sight and asking questions later." It had looked to me, however, as though the specter of law enforcement had a measurable effect. I saw both midwives divert energy from providing care and toward self-preservation. A few days later, I ask Linda how the situation would have been different if she were licensed. She notes many things, among them that "we would have been able to identify ourselves as CPMs and work with the EMTs instead of having to hide," she says. "There would have been less risk to the baby."

Sitting in the hospital cafeteria with her husband the day after the birth, their baby boy in stable condition upstairs in the neonatal intensive care unit, Jessica took the analytical approach. "I said, 'Let's talk about what would have happened if I were in the hospital,'" she recalls. "I would have been on a Pitocin drip—they would never have let me labor that long—and could have ended up with a C-section. If they'd lost the heart rate at the same point, that's still too late to do a cesarean, so they would have got the baby out the same way. The only difference would be that he'd have been at the hospital sooner."

Linda is frank about this difference: "Knowing that you have a longer period of time before getting assistance—that's a risk of at home," she says. "But there are risks in the hospital. Life is full of risks, and you make the choice of which types of risk you want to take. A lot of the couples we see, they're saying, 'I don't want to take the risk that I'm going to have this and this happen to me in the hospital.' But then they should be seeing too that there are risks of being at home, and one of them is not having the immediate assistance of a NICU."

Labor felt more endless and unrelenting to Jessica than she had expected. The act was also less intuitive than she had expected. "I never felt the urge to push," she says. "It was hard for me to figure out how to push." Certainly the resuscitation is something she never envisioned happening. Still, she doesn't regret having a home birth and maintains she'd make the same decision again. "I told Scott if we weren't going to have home births, then I didn't want any more kids," she says. However, if there were a birthing center in the area, she might compromise.

Jessica's only qualm with hiring Linda again would be the distance between them. Otherwise, she feels both midwives were competent, helpful, and supportive. She never felt rushed, and, interestingly, she remembers 911 as having been called right away. Her only wish is that she'd been better prepared to deal with the hospital. Driving there in the van, she says Valerie and Linda gave her a crash course in neonatal intensive care and advised her on which interventions to accept and which to refuse. "They were kind of throwing stuff at me: 'You want to let him have the vitamin K shot, you don't want the eye drops, you don't want the Hep B vaccine," Jessica remembers. Initially, she says, both midwives were going to go into the hospital with her, but then they thought better of it. (Valerie says she knew the nurse who met the van to be simpatico and felt her presence was code for them to keep driving. "When they hear of a home-birth transport they try to jump on it," says Valerie of certain nurses. "I think that's one of the ways they help try to protect us.") "I probably would have been happier if they had come in," says Jessica of the midwives. "But I didn't want them to get in trouble either." Linda, however, did return to the hospital twice for postpartum checks; she examined Jessica in the breast pumping room.

What resentment Jessica does harbor is toward the first responders, who were carrying a resuscitation bag of the wrong size and put it on the baby backwards. She's also upset with the hospital, which she feels gave her a hard time about breastfeeding and stalled discharge even though the baby was passing all the required tests. (On day 10 a physician friend of Valerie's who was formerly a higher-up at the hospital called to complain, and on day 11 the baby was released). "We are considering suing the hospital over the Hep B shot," which was administered without parental consent, Jessica tells me 4 months after the birth. On the consent form where her or Scott's signature should be, the words "medically indicated" are handwritten in pen.

ADVANCING THE PROFESSION

Women often describe the final moments of childbirth as requiring surrender, a letting go of control, a plunge into the unknown. In order to support a physiological birth, the attendant must be willing to make that leap as well. "For me it's always been as much about my own courage as it has been about the courage of the mother," says Jane, a midwife in a neighboring state who has practiced without licensing for 25 years.

It is not surprising that in the risk-averse culture of the United States, normal birth is pushed outside the regulatory system. When I asked Dr. Jones, who now teaches OB residents the art of breech delivery, how he learned, he responded, "Well, the first breech I attended was my son's." His wife, seated next to him, asked the next question. "Didn't you do any in your training?" "No, except a twin," he said, smirking. His wife: "You never told me it was your first."

Without the training, Dr. Jones had to take a risk. He had to trust the labor process rather than labeling it pathologic in order to offer his wife another choice besides surgery, in order to advance his practice, and, as he sees it, in order to advance his profession. "If I have any influence on obstetrical care, it's what do the residents carry with them, what skills do they have to offer women? I'm just here right now. They're the next generation. Hopefully some of them will get a vision, that we're here to help women, not to choose for them."

Do illegal midwives take more risks than licensed midwives, and are those risks justifiable? Valerie Vickerman Runes, editor of *From Calling to Courtroom*, a legal handbook for unlicensed midwives, says that underground midwives are a select group. "Without licensure, the only people who are going to become midwives are women who are willing to deal with the legal hazards of doing so," she tells me. "There are a lot of women who want to become midwives but don't want to take the risk of going to jail."

Lisa Block-Wieser, the midwife in Tucson, Arizona, has practiced in all legal configurations. She began her career as an unlicensed midwife in California, where she narrowly missed a felony conviction when the law changed a week before her case was set to go to trial. Then she obtained licensing and practiced legally in New Mexico, and finally she became a certified nurse–midwife and moved to Arizona. To date, she has cared for more than 1200 expectant women and trained a dozen apprentices. In her opinion, the type of credential or license doesn't make the midwife, nor does it necessarily make birth safer. Illegal midwife, licensed midwife, nurse–midwife, "I still deliver babies the same," she told me. However, licensure does make birth safer because it creates accountability and increases the number of midwives, which means women don't have to go weeks without prenatal care while they search for a home-birth attendant. "If a woman can pick up a phone book and find a midwife, then that makes it safer," says Block-Wieser.

Furthermore, if a midwife can pick up the phone without fear, it makes birth safer. Jane, though she practices illegally, is able to practice much more openly than Linda; she has an office and serves on the board of the state's perinatal association. Her relationships with area physicians are so strong that she can confidently transport to the hospital and take part in her clients' care. "You know, after this many years and the great relationships I have with the doctors, I'm happy to be in the hospital when things aren't progressing at home," she told me. "Because I can take people to a hospital where they're going to get really well treated, where we're going to get to work as a team, and they're going to get a lot of what they're hoping for." She sees herself as part of a community of care providers, rather than as the lone outlaw midwife. "I don't need to be practicing out there on the edge," she says.

Linda rarely has good transport experiences. She cannot guarantee continuity of care, because when she walks into an emergency room, she must assume the identity of a caring friend, not a caregiver with important information about her client's condition. And she and her clients can face bitter hostility. She tells me that when she transported one woman after hours of not progressing, the doctor on call cut three epi-siotomies—"Snip, snip, snip. One, two, three," Linda says while miming a pair of scissors in her hand. "He did it to punish this woman for thinking she could have a home birth."

Transporting to the hospital is an essential component of maternity care in countries where midwives are primary birth attendants. The mid-wives handle the normal, and when events exceed normal, they transfer to the next level of care. Most transports are not urgent. Rather, they are precipitated by exhaustion or failure to progress or a request for pain relief, and many times a dose of Pitocin or an epidural will facilitate a vaginal birth. In the literature on out-of-hospital birth, about one-third of transports end in cesarean section. Still, in the United States, trans-ports for any reason are often regarded as failures or botched home births, and they tend to bias medical staff, who see only the minority of women who transport, not the 90% who give birth uneventfully in their living rooms.

"It's totally normal to transfer into hospital if the mother is not pro-gressing well and you need some help," says Betty-Anne Daviss, the midwife in Ottowa who coauthored the home-birth study with Kenneth Johnson. She is also a consultant to the International Federation of Gynecology and Obstetrics. "That's not a failure; it's just like any other part of medicine," she says, drawing a parallel between the general prac-titioner who refers her patient to a cardiologist when heart troubles arise. "That's the way medicine works. That is the way midwives and physicians work all around the world, and very well together," she says. The trouble, and the increased risk to mothers and babies, comes in states where medical and state authority don't recognize midwives' role in maternity care and react with hostility. "And that is a problem," says Daviss, "because what it means is that they're not willing to recognize the woman's choice in that community."

CHAPTER 7

_____

Criminalized

_____

THE UNITED STATES IS the only country to have made the modern home-birth midwife an outlaw. This status did not befall her until the early part of the twentieth century, when "the midwife problem" was a frequent topic in medical journals and at conferences. This was how physicians explained why so many women and babies were dying of complications in childbirth. Meanwhile, public health began investigating, and municipalities began collecting vital statistics. Programs to register and supervise midwives were launched in several cities and across the South, and reports of their conduct began emerging in the 1920s and 1930s. The problem, it turned out, was not the midwives.

An estimated 60,000 midwives were practicing in the United States in 1923[1]—nearly twice the number of practicing obstetricians today, caring for a population one-third of our present size. Epidemiological data were not collected in the United States until after 1900, but as the numbers came in, they tended to favor midwives over doctors, and home over hospital. Hospitals were rife with infection, and such simple antiseptic measures as hand washing still were not universal. Meanwhile, physicians were treating all manner of patients, moving from the birthing to the dying to the birthing.

One historian wrote that if he had to pick "one factor above all others as the detriment of high maternal mortality in the USA, I would unhesitatingly choose the standards of obstetric training in medical schools."[2] As the Flexner report of 1910 would reveal, physicians actually had little to no hands-on training in attending birth.[3] John Whitridge Williams, the prominent Johns Hopkins obstetrician, who himself referred to the "midwife problem," surveyed professors of obstetrics in 1912 and discovered that most were themselves untrained. Also, these professors had little faith in their pupils: 26 out of 43 surveyed felt that more women died "as the result of ignorance or of ill-judged and improperly performed operations in the hands of general practitioners as from puerperal infection in the hands of midwives."[4]

In New York City, some 1700 midwives delivered 40,000 babies in 1919, roughly one-third of the birthing population.[5] S. Josephine Baker, MD, was director of New York City's Bureau of Child Hygiene from 1908 to 1923 and spent her tenure overseeing the city's midwives (she was also credited with tracking down and quarantining "Typhoid Mary"). In a 1913 report, Baker found that half as many women died in childbirth under the care of midwives as died under the care of doctors.[6] The postpartum care given by midwives was "infinitely superior," she remarked to a colleague. The midwife washed the baby and mother, fixed meals, and visited frequently following the birth, doing "little homely duties" along with physical care, Baker noted, whereas "The average doctor for the same fee comes in a hurry, often uses his instruments too soon, often lacerates the perineum, and frequently leaves the house in a hurry, and generally makes not more than one or two calls on his patient afterward."[7]

Although birth steadily moved into the hospital between 1900 and 1950, infant and maternal mortality did not begin to decline until the 1930s; in fact, it rose during many of the years prior to World War II. "How many of you know that the death rate for women, in hospitals, is as great today as it was a hundred years ago—the decrease being so negligible that one hardly would know it?" challenged the obstetrician Rudolph Holmes to the physicians gathered at the 46th annual meeting of the American Gynecological Society in 1921.[8]

Holmes had brought with him the work of a New Jersey Department of Health epidemiologist, Julius Levy, MD, who had scrutinized maternal and infant deaths in four cities and across New Jersey counties, and concluded that midwives had lower infant and maternal mortality rates. In 1921 midwives attended 40% of the births in Newark but only 13% of the maternal deaths. Their maternal mortality rate was 2.2 per 1000; the rate among physicians in private or hospital practice was 8.7 per 1000. Levy found that between 1917 and 1921, the midwives' infant mortality rate—that is, infants that died within the first 30 days of life—was 26.9 per 1000 births, whereas private physicians' rate was 38.3, and in the hospital it was 45.7.[9]

"It is a reproach on the medical profession that a city like Newark may advertise the fact that it is safer to be delivered by a midwife than by a physician or in a hospital," Holmes railed, suggesting further that physicians were not only failing to support women's and infants' health but were perhaps making it worse with Pituitrin, with heroic "surgical manipulation," and with inductions for convenience's sake. He called for the development of an "obstetric conscience which will permit intervention only when intervention is imperatively needed."

Other reports suggested midwives' skill and safe practices, including an influential survey of 11 states issued by the White House Conference on Child Health and Protection, published in 1933.[10] *Maternal Mortality in New York City*, a landmark study of 2041 maternal deaths conducted by the New York Academy of Medicine from 1930 to 1932 and published in 1933, found that two-thirds were preventable. It also found, as Baker had, that fewer women died with midwives, even though the study design, like Levy's, favored physicians. That is, if a woman died in childbirth and had been in the care of a midwife at any time, the death was recorded to the midwife but not the physician; however, if the woman lived but had been cared for by both a physician and a midwife, the case was recorded to the physician, not the midwife.[11]

Still, the midwives were blamed. The New York Obstetrical Society released its own interpretation of the New York maternal mortality report in 1934, in which they exonerated obstetricians and blamed midwives and general practitioners for the deaths. In a public meeting that followed—held at the Waldorf Astoria—only nurses spoke out against the society's distortion; the obstetricians and physicians in attendance, including several female physicians, kept silent.[12]

Meanwhile, in medical journals, midwives suffered vicious attacks. They were called "dirty and unscrupulous,"[13] "gin-fingering," "filthy and ignorant and not far removed from the jungles of Africa," "pestiliferous," "often malicious," and "un-American." Even after Williams documented the ineptitude of medical education, he advocated the "gradual abolition of midwives in large cities."[14]

By 1930, all but ten states had begun to regulate midwives. The Massachusetts Supreme Court was the first to make midwifery illegal, in 1907. In the South, midwives were initially supervised rather than criminalized, although this policy had explicit segregationist motives. By the 1950s, midwifery survived only in pockets of the South and West. In 1957 there were just two midwives known in all of New York City.[15]

In Europe, midwives ran the maternity wards, but in the New World, midwives were maligned, forbidden to practice, pushed underground and nearly out of existence. How did this happen?

As medical science began to offer solutions to complicated births in the eighteenth and nineteenth centuries, men entered the previously all-female lying-in chamber. In Europe, midwives were not discarded but, rather, were educated in the new medical science and employed by state-run clinics—where they, in turn, educated medicine men in attending normal birth. Midwives handled the normal pregnancies, and problem cases were referred to the physicians, a system that is still in existence there.

Historians have several theories of what happened in the United States. For one thing, the Americans had no vital health statistics system until relatively late, whereas countries such as England, Sweden, and Prussia had epidemiological data on midwives' competence dating back to the 1700s and 1800s.[16] Even though the initial reports supported trained midwives, they came after decades in which the medical community had asserted the superiority of hospitals. Midwives were simply no match for organized medicine. They were isolated by language and geography, many were foreign-born, most were over age 50, and, of course, they were women. Furthermore, their clients' daughters were turning to hospitals for care—that was where one could access twilight sleep.

There was also the philosophical shift articulated by DeLee, the notion of childbirth as a procedure—an emergency rather than an emergence. If obstetricians were to be the legitimate providers of care in normal birth, birth could no longer be considered normal. A normal process was one that a specialist need not attend. "If the profession would realize that parturition viewed with modern eyes is no longer a normal function, but that it has imposing pathologic dignity, the midwife would be impossible even to mention," DeLee wrote in 1915.[17] To put it simply, childbirth was to be something that doctors did, not women. This approach was reflected in hospital advertising. A pamphlet from 1935 warned that "Every woman in childbirth is potentially a major surgical case."[18] Best to go to a surgeon, then.

Mothers and babies died in fewer numbers beginning in the 1930s; the rates then fell sharply in the 1940s with the advent of commercial antibiotics and bloodbanking. Organized medicine frequently makes a connection between hospitalized births and maternal and infant survival, but the conclusion drawn by several historians and epidemiologists is that the credit goes to better nutrition and living conditions, improved sanitation, effective antisepsis, antibiotics, and general advances in surgery that made the emergency cesarean a safe intervention. Marjorie Tew, a British health statistician goes even further, arguing that "if births in obstetric hospitals had not increased, perinatal mortality would have fallen by more than it actually did."[19]

Maternal and infant death remains very high in some parts of the globe. The reasons are complex: where malaria is prevalent, so are high rates of anemia, which increase the likelihood of a deadly postpartum hemorrhage. Ectopic pregnancies—often fatal—are more common in populations with high rates of HIV. Unsafe abortion can account for as much as one-third of "pregnancy-related" deaths. Poor living conditions, high fertility rates, child marriage, and conflict all contribute to infection and mortality, and women may die or suffer humiliating, debilitating injuries where emergency obstetric care is unavailable. Yet the solution proposed by international bodies such as UNICEF and the World Health Organization is not continuous electronic fetal monitoring and elective cesarean section but, rather, access to contraception and safe abortion, to trained birth attendants with midwifery skills, and to emergency obstetric care. Maternal deaths are consistently highest in countries with the fewest skilled birth attendants.[20,21]

"It is important to remember that it has never been scientifically proven that the hospital is a safer place than the home for a woman who has had an uncomplicated pregnancy to have her baby," a 1985 World Health Organization report called "Having a Baby in Europe" states.[22]

The WHO also maintains that "the midwife appears to be the most appropriate and cost effective type of health care provider to be assigned to the care of normal pregnancy and normal birth."[23] A woman having a baby in the United States has not been similarly encouraged. ACOG, the professional organization for American obstetricians, has actively opposed state legislation that would license non-nurse midwives and insists that the hospital is the safest environment for childbirth.[24] At its 2006 conference in Washington, DC, the group gave out an instructive bumper sticker to all attendees: "Home Deliveries Are for Pizza."

WITH WOMEN

The resurgence of midwifery in the 1970s was largely a product of counterculture-inspired women like Ina May Gaskin, who fell into the role of birth attendant in communities that were questioning authority, including medical authority. Gaskin was a college grad and mother. After a hospital birth with drugs, forceps, and an 18-hour separation from her baby, she turned hippie and in 1970 joined the "Caravan," a group that traveled the country spreading the gospel of intentional living. During the 5-month tour, Gaskin ended up attending several births in the back of a VW bus. The rest of the group would park their vehicles in a circle around the imminent bus, like a motorized herd of elephants, and wait for the baby's first cry. Gaskin and the other women learned by doing, picking up advice on managing complications from friendly obstetricians along the way. When the Caravan settled in Summertown, Tennessee, it called itself "The Farm" and continued to deliver its own babies.

The term *direct entry* is still used to describe non-nurse midwives. But the modern American midwifery movement is "direct entry" in the larger sense as well, in that it emerged an anachronism, disconnected from the lineage of midwives who had accumulated knowledge and skills and passed them on to one another for generations. With few exceptions, the women who resurrected midwifery in the United States had to start from scratch. They had to rediscover how to be "with woman" in labor, which is what the word *midwife* means.

Cynthia Caillagh was an exception. She trained with a traditional Cherokee midwife who had attended thousands of births in a Tennessee mountain community. Caillagh spent 2 years with her in the late 1960s.

"She learned her skills from another midwife, who learned her skills from a midwife," says Caillagh. "Knowledge was handed down, midwife to midwife." While many of her peers were essentially winging it—it wasn't until 1972 that there was even a contemporary text to go by[25]—Caillagh was learning methods of care that had survived for centuries.

Physicians had dismissed this empirical knowledge for centuries as well. But a handful of records of individual midwives practicing before even the invention of the stethoscope suggest that what know-how they had served women remarkably well for the time. Martha Ballard, a Maine midwife practicing in the late 1700s who kept a detailed diary, is the subject of the Pulitzer Prize–winning *A Midwife's Tale*, by Laurel Thatcher Ulrich. According to Ballard's records, she attended 998 births with 5 maternal deaths, even during several outbreaks of scarlet fever.[26]

Catharina Schrader, a Dutch midwife also practicing in the eighteenth century, is the subject of the book *Mother and Child Were Saved*, which reprints an excerpt of her diary along with an analysis of her records by the Dutch obstetrician G. J. Kloosterman. Schrader kept a log precise enough to note when a baby was born less than 9 months from wedding vows, labeling some babies "bastards" and some mothers "whores." Kloosterman attributed 14 maternal deaths out of over 3000 births to Schrader, a rate of 4.6 per 1000, similar to Ballard's. Of stillbirths and infant deaths, Kloosterman counted 140, which constituted a rate of 54 per 1000, "a figure that is only slightly higher than the figures found in Europe and the U.S.A. before 1945," he writes.[27]

Caillagh, pronounced (KAY-lee), has silver hair, an angular nose, high cheekbones, and a quick, loud laugh. It is an unusually windy winter day when we meet. We sit at the dining table in her new home, a modest house on gently sloping fields that are home to sheep, llamas, and dogs. Bags of fleece are piled up on shelves. Caillagh's voice is deep and firm. She smokes—a stubborn habit left over from her final days in Virginia, she tells me.

Caillagh is somewhat of an exile here in the Midwest—or a convicted criminal, depending on how you look at it. In 1999 she was charged with practicing medicine without a license, practicing midwifery without a license, and involuntary manslaughter in the death of Julia Peters, a Stafford, Virginia, woman whose birth she attended in 1997. The investigation and pretrial hearings stretched over nearly 3 years, during which time the case made headlines in local and regional newspapers and on the local TV news.

Halfway through our talk, she admits with pained laughter that she'd been dreading my visit. "This is the first place I've ever lived where I've never spoken of midwifery. You're the first person I've spoken to about it since the trial." She asked that I not reveal her present whereabouts.

The eldest of three siblings, Caillagh was expected to be a doctor, or a lawyer. Her mother was one of nine children who all earned college degrees. Caillagh excelled in school, skipping two grades, and by her sixteenth birthday was enrolled at the State University of New York at Buffalo, where she declared premed with intentions of becoming a family physician. "I wanted a small, rural family practice—it would have included all of it, birth to death. That's all I ever wanted to do."

But in college she had "what can only be described as an identity crisis." She recalls meditating on the origins of the word *diagnosis*. "It actually means to look at all possibilities and allow what you see most to begin to reveal solutions. So in and of itself, the art of medicine is the art of stepping back and asking questions. What med school was revealing itself to be was not an art, but a categorization of accepted standards," she says. "I withdrew and asked myself some really hard questions."

At the time, she recalls, feminism was just "getting its leg up out of the trenches." Caillagh joined that movement, as well as what she terms "hippie communities" in upstate New York, in which she shared what she knew about herbs and general healthcare, and "was attending one birth or another because we were all having births at home." Meanwhile, she also helped set up free women's clinics in Syracuse, Ithaca, and Buffalo. There, she did abortion and fertility counseling. She taught women how to use diaphragms and second-year med students how to do pelvic exams. She helped found a rape crisis center in Buffalo.

Caillagh's Cherokee grandfather had predicted that midwifery was what she was destined to do, and in the next few years she began to accept this. She trained with the Tennessee midwife, even living with her for periods of time, and adopted a sort of feminist-tribal ethic: "I realized that a midwife has traditionally always been a servant. She does not exist for herself. She exists for and through her community. This doesn't make her a slave; what it does is place her firmly in the center of the needs in the community." Caillagh speaks of community several times during our talk. It is the first and last thought she leaves with me. "I realized I was well suited to work with rural people, and with people who had a sense of their own identity and a sense that their bodies belonged to themselves, and who believed what they did with their bodies and with themselves contributed to the welfare of the community."

Caillagh's mentor was in her 90s and therefore had Caillagh do most of the physical work with clients. What is now done with electronic fetal monitors, ultrasounds, Doppler monitors, and even fetoscopes, Caillagh learned how to do with her hands. "In traditional midwifery, the process of really beginning to understand birth is understanding where a woman is by looking at her, by putting pressure on her back and feeling how the ligaments are letting go at the small of the spine; putting compresses on her hip and feeling the change in the hip motion," she tells me. "Front and back compresses will tell you exactly what her ligaments are doing. You can feel the descent of the baby with each contraction. Midwifery as hands-on support rather than a tool determiner is much more accurate." For the most part, she shunned internal vaginal exams. "Over the years I learned how to feel that the baby had finally done a rotation of its head, that it had finally done its arc into final position into the sacrum and was about to turn and come down. No internal was needed to know that."

She tells me that in some cases she could monitor a baby's heart tones during labor with her hands alone. "People were amazed. 'What do you mean you're not listening with the fetoscope during labor?'" she recalls, to which she would reply, "What do you think these fingers are feeling? I'm not annoying the woman to get the heart beat, I can feel it right here."

"Cynthia was by far the most experienced midwife in Virginia," Leslie Payne, another Virginia midwife who practiced illegally, told me. "She had a wealth of knowledge about herbs and techniques for aiding the body to do what you wanted it to do." Caillagh's practice melded traditional tactile methods with a self-acquired scientific and medical knowledge. Her library consisted of some 5000 books. "I had antique books from 1600s and 1700s. I had medical texts in endless quantities," says Caillagh. When the police raided her house, "they ran out of ways to transport all the books. It was almost funny if it weren't sad, the endless trips." What she got back of the collection she sold before moving out of state.

During prenatal visits, Caillagh used her hands, but also technology and diagnostics. A self-use, electronic blood pressure cuff always lay on her coffee table—she takes this out while we talk and fastens the Velcro around her bicep, pressing a button that makes it hum. Urinalysis dipsticks were always in the bathroom, and she used a series-10 Allen fetoscope to check a developing fetus's heartbeat. "I never used Dopplers. I'm not interested in them in the slightest," she tells me. "I don't think we're ever going to fully comprehend the dangers of ultrasonography in the forming fetus." Caillagh says her tools were merely modern incarnations of what midwives had been doing for centuries. "Urinalysis is ancient, it's not new," she says. "Midwives traditionally had women pee into buckets. They'd smell the urine; they'd drink the urine; they would pour it over a variety of herbs; they would add herbs to it. These are old skills. We've refined them, and we call them medical. But they're not new."

Caillagh rejected the "midwife" label for the first 20 years of her practice. "I never felt comfortable with the term, not as it's currently used. If we use the classic definition, to be with woman, to stand with woman—yes. But in terms of standing over, or to make decisions for— no." Her role, as she saw it, was to help women "find themselves in their process." She told me a woman "meets herself in childbirth." To this she added the *Our Bodies, Ourselves* model of "self-care." Her clients recorded as little or as much information as they wanted in a notebook that was ultimately theirs to keep once the birth was over; it was their responsibility to test their urine and blood pressure at prenatal appointments. She taught them how to do their own cervical checks.

"While all these tools were available, I was not making decisions about risk factors," says Caillagh. If she saw blood pressure rising, or protein in the urine (a warning sign of preeclampsia), she would lead her clients to information on "what these numbers might mean" and what options were available to restore normalcy. "In virtually all cases, women given enough information and the freedom of self-education and choice will make made good decisions," she says, slowing down for each word, tapping her mug on the table for emphasis. "And I think the significant detail was that at no time did I own their health or the information they were gathering. They felt compelled to act on that information because it was about their own bodies. And the choices were theirs."

This philosophy is perhaps what separated her not only from physicians but also from other midwives. That she refused to traffic in the currency of risk made her "other" among others. Limiting her scope of practice to "low-risk" women was incompatible with her definition of midwifery. "I did not use risking factors the same way that other midwives do. Twins were born at home all the time. There were two sets of triplets; breeches were nothing I even gave a second thought to." She tells me one of the last births she attended was a VBAC for a 48-year-old woman who had had *seven* previous cesarean sections. "There was no bleeding, beautiful labor, absolutely picture perfect," says Caillagh.

"You must understand that if you view the body as a self-healing, self-describing, self-navigating entity, if you trust it, then it will give you all the signposts it needs when it is failing in its own defense," she says. Traditional midwifery, she explains to me, is recognizing those signposts while promoting optimal health. Good nutrition, rest, and essentially taking care of oneself emotionally and physically, "these are as nourishing as almost anything else you can do," says Caillagh. "When you begin there, you see fewer problems."

Caillagh estimates that over the course of 33 years, she attended 2500 births. Women sought her out for her Socratic approach as much as for her skills and experience, and other midwives called her for advice. D'Anne Graham Remocaldo was pregnant with her fourth child when she found Caillagh. Each of her previous pregnancies had caused debilitating morning sickness; Caillagh helped her resolve it with diet. "I appreciated the way she did things," says Remocaldo. "I've grown tremendously from it."

Caillagh was known widely for successfully treating even serious prenatal conditions with diet and herbs, for stopping postpartum hemorrhages, and for resolving complications that would otherwise be dealt with surgically. She could turn babies who were entering the pelvis askew and could reconcile shoulder dystocia with position change; "prolonged labor" was language she never employed. Other midwives, sometimes hours away or out of state, would call her when they had exhausted their own reserves. "When they got to the one birth where they really believed the woman could do it but they were terrified themselves, they would call me in. Lots of breeches and twins; the births that had gone for three days where they were in over their heads. As long as my own clients were OK, I'd drive," says Caillagh.

At the same time, however, Caillagh tells me that some of these midwives politically resented her, especially as they began organizing for state licensure. A midwife like Caillagh, practicing "on the edge," was seen as a risk to all. A bad outcome could befall any midwife, but midwives who take on breeches and twins risk a poor outcome that is politically indefensible. Caillagh believed her responsibility was to the families in her community, not to the other midwives or to what she felt was an elusive grab at legitimacy. "I was at great odds with the ever-developing movement spearheaded by people like Ina May," she tells me. Although Caillagh was originally part of that movement, serving on early committees of the North American Registry of Midwives (which would develop the Certified Professional Midwife credential in 1994), she abandoned the effort because she felt that it would inevitably mean allowing midwifery to be defined by medicine.

Caillagh foresaw regulation selling out the breeches and twins and VBACs, leaving those women with no alternative but unassisted birth. "Would we end up with women staying at home with nothing, no help, no information whatsoever, having babies completely without support or access to information they critically needed?" she says. Where others saw protection from criminal prosecution, Caillagh saw a trap. "I was a midwife out of commitment to community and women," she tells me. "I felt that eventually, yes, I'd fall to Practice of Medicine Without a License. And I was willing to accept that."

INFORMED CHOICE

Julia Peters called Caillagh in the spring of 1997. She was about 4 months pregnant and was searching for a midwife to help her have a home birth—her previous three children had been born by cesarean, which, even in 1997, at the crest of the VBAC wave, made her an unlikely candidate. She was also a heavy smoker who continued smoking through pregnancy—another risk factor.

Peters's mother-in-law, Claire Peters, a registered nurse, made the introduction. She had met Caillagh through a friend who had given birth to twins at home. "I was so impressed with her," Peters told me. "When my Julie [she was known to those close to her as Julie] decided she wanted to have her baby at home, I was the one who contacted Cynthia, and I was the one who talked her into taking Julie as a client."

Caillagh remembers Julia Peters's phone call. "Before I would even see her, we spoke at length over the phone," says Caillagh. "I said, 'You need to understand that you're making a choice that is not only highly unpopular, but may be an enormous risk in your community. You live in an area where it's not unheard of for people to turn you in to social services.'" Caillagh then referred her to a number of books, from Nancy Wainer Cohen's impassioned *Silent Knife: Cesarean Prevention and Vaginal Birth after Cesarean* to what Caillagh calls "more middle-of-the-road books that discussed risking and factors that would lead a midwife to determine that a [VBAC] birth at home might not be safe." Caillagh told her the homework was mandatory. "I said it's very important that this is not just your heart. You have to be more informed than that."

A number of weeks passed before Peters called back and said she'd read the books and was still interested. Caillagh told her there was one more assignment. Since 1995 she had been giving each client an extensive intake package. It is a notebook-thick folder with hundreds of questions about diet, lifestyle, and medical history. "Absolutely every aspect of what they may or may not want to experience during the birth process was covered in all these documents," says Caillagh. "I said fill everything out and then we'll meet."

The packet also included an explanation of the "informed relationship" between midwife and family, making clear that it was illicit. This meant that Caillagh couldn't sign birth certificates or be known to any medical agency as "witness" to a birth. "In practical terms, this means that you face potential anger and outward displays of disgust or disapproval," she wrote.

Caillagh included her statistics: Among the 1000 births she attended in Virginia, she counted only 10 cesareans, 24 sets of twins, 218 VBACs (of those, just 2 transported to the hospital for repeat cesareans), and 112 breeches—all born at home.

Relatively new in the welcome packet when Peters called on Caillagh was a 17-page primer on the politics of home birth and Caillagh's philosophy on community. She required that any new client join a group called PenFam, the Peninsula Families for Natural Birth and Health. The leaders were "five moms wishing to create a support network for clients of our local direct-entry midwife as well as provide information for the general public about natural birth and health care."[28] Their unofficial purpose was to serve as gatekeeper to Caillagh.

When PenFam sprung up around Caillagh, it connected what can only be called a diverse group of people, as home birth tends to. Caillagh served fundamentalists and feminists, the unconventional and the disillusioned. Katherine Prown is a former women's studies professor who initially saw home birth as a "radical, fringe idea." But while finishing her PhD at the College of William and Mary, she became pregnant with her first child and devoted some library time to the medical literature. "I was just shocked," she told me. "The thing that made me batty was episiotomy. Especially in conservative Williamsburg, Virginia, you were not going to get out of that hospital without an episiotomy with a first-time baby." As Prown's belly grew, she argued about the procedure with her obstetrician, a woman she greatly respected for having provided abortions. But the arguments went nowhere. "She bought into episiotomy hook, line, and sinker." Prown, who would become one of Caillagh's most resourceful supporters, found Caillagh just shy of her eighth month.

Caillagh keeps invoking the word *community*, and finally I begin to understand the connection that is so clear and direct in her mind. The birth of a child is literally the making of community, the creation of the next generation, the transformation of a couple into a micro-community. Midwives help facilitate that process, and therefore midwifery is more than just ushering in new life, it is stewardship of culture. And Caillagh gives enormous weight to the childbirth process, as if what happens during those hours guides what happens in the years following and ripples out to the larger community. A woman meets herself in childbirth. This, she says, represents "our greatest potential for what we can be as a species, if we let it teach us." She has been called an essentialist and a romantic for making such statements, but she is unapologetic. Seen through this lens, the legal restrictions on midwifery take on elemental meaning. "What we've done is criminalized women's options," says Caillagh, "and more than that, we've criminalized the making of community."

Feminist and women's health groups, she adds, "have not taken birth seriously in any way, shape, or form." And in this way she feels abandoned by her own. She recalls sitting on a panel at a National Organization for Women conference on health in the 1990s with Esther Zorn, founder of the group Cesarean Prevention Movement, which would later become ICAN. "NOW was only interested in the abortion issue," she tells me. "And Esther and I could not imagine for the life of ourselves how the feminist movement could not understand that [the issue of] how women birth and where they might birth was equal in every conceivable way in its importance, and why NOW was not taking a position was beyond us."

When Julia Peters came to her, Caillagh says she was seeking to reclaim her body. Peters had her first child at age 19. On a September morning in 1986, she was induced with Pitocin. She never dilated more than 2 centimeters, and by 3 p.m. she was in surgery for "failure to progress" and "cephalopelvic disproportion," according to her medical records. In other words, she hadn't really labored at all when doctors decided the baby wasn't descending and was too big to fit anyway. The baby weighed 8 pounds, 12 ounces.

The next two cesareans were automatic. "She felt after three cesareans that she'd just given away her body and that she couldn't do it this time," says Caillagh. Claire Peters tells me that her daughter-in-law was adamant about not going back to the hospital. She called several midwives looking for care. But after she and her husband Daren met with Caillagh, they were taken. "I didn't even know about her illegal status at first," says Claire. "When I found out, I said, 'Julie, are you sure you want to do this?' She said, 'Oh, absolutely.' This is what she wanted to do. She even got some videos and said, 'If I have to, I'll do it myself.'"

AFTERPAINS

"Julie had a great birth," says Caillagh. She tells me a birth story without sanitizing it of wrinkles and stains. Labor began late on a Saturday night and simmered throughout, interrupting Peters's sleep but not intensifying. Early Sunday morning, Peters was up and about, excited, and the house began to fill with interested family members. Peters shooed them away to church.

Caillagh and her apprentice, Beth Haw, stayed with the Peters all day, but labor didn't pick up again until the evening. Caillagh never put arbitrary time limits on birth—a long labor was a problem only if the baby or mother had "had enough." Prown's labor, for instance, went on for 3 days. "I would have been sectioned so fast in a hospital," Prown told me. "I do feel very strongly that it was being at home with a skilled midwife that saved me from a cesarean." She had her next two children at home as well.

"This is what we see with first labors," Caillagh tells me. "A cranky first night, a miserable try-to-get-some-sleep day, and then it will cook again in the evening." And that was how it happened with Peters—even though it was her fourth baby, it was her first experience with normal labor. As the sun set, contractions rose. Caillagh says Peters smoked cigarettes throughout. "I have a rule with women, if you can make it to a different floor to get your cigarettes, you're welcome to them," says Caillagh. "It's your choice, I won't take that away from you, but I'm going to put them in places like the garage, where you don't want to be when a contraction is."

Later that night, Peters had found a routine of climbing the stairs, then lumbering back down to the kitchen, where she would stand in front of the open freezer and let the cool air flow over her brow. "A lot of that is just helping reposition the baby, get the head right where it belongs," says Caillagh. "About the third round of stairs seemed to work, because contractions petered out and she got tired." Julia lay down with Daren in their bedroom. "This is very typical," says Caillagh. "If you don't interfere with a woman at this point, she'll actually go to sleep. I've seen this so often, it's what's wrong with medicalized birth. Things keep gearing up and up and up, and she's getting more and more intense. And everyone around her says, 'She's at 9, she's at 10. Get everything ready!' If you leave a woman to her own devices, very often contractions will ease off, and she'll get anywhere from 15 minutes to an hour where *absolutely nothing occurs.*" Caillagh stretches these last words, tapping on the table.

The explanation is that as the baby's head enters the birth canal, the uterus needs time to shrink back down around the diminished contents in order for effective contractions to resume. Caillagh says this is exactly what happened with Peters. After a brief nap with her husband, "She bolted out of bed," says Caillagh. "I was sound asleep on the floor. And she said—absolutely classic Julia, incredibly strong, self-assured young woman—'That's it, it's time to get the baby out!'" Peters then swung her legs over the birthing stool, dropped into a supported squat, "and in two contractions that baby was down, and in one more contraction it was out," says Caillagh. It took less than ten pushes.

The baby girl, whom they named Alexis, was healthy and normal—and weighed 9 pounds, 2 ounces—as the hospital would later confirm. Peters was ecstatic. "She called me yelling, 'I did it! I did it!" recalls Claire. There was nothing untoward about the period following birth. "There was no unusual blood," says Caillagh. "Just the typical blood of birthing." The placenta came soon after. Peters stood up, birthed it onto some sheets, and then lay down in bed with Daren and began nursing the baby. It was then that the labor pains really kicked in, "afterpains." Caillagh says that this oft-ignored part of normal birth affects some women severely, even more so than the labor itself. The uterus is contracting back down to size, clamping down on blood vessels that developed to grow the baby, and the pains can be overwhelming. "She was contracting really, really well—and was really angry about it," says Caillagh.

She brought Peters some honey-lemon-salt tea and a banana—electrolyte balancers. She also offered to draw Peters an herbal bath and set about cooking a meal. Caillagh always did those two things following a birth—the bath was intended to relax and soothe the perineum and establish breastfeeding. Caillagh's meal was a signature mix of steamed sweet potatoes, beets, kale, onions, garlic, ginger—"any vegetable she loved," says Caillagh—over brown rice. The ingredients help tone the uterus, Caillagh tells me. "Nothing hard to digest, just something extremely nourishing that would get into her bloodstream very quickly. Even women who hated vegetables adored this dish."

While Caillagh was in the kitchen assembling ingredients, her beeper went off. Another client, a religious woman expecting her fifth child, was in active labor. Caillagh had attended her previous two births and knew she could progress very quickly. She returned upstairs. Peters didn't want to eat and was asking for a cigarette. "You have to understand that poor afterbirth care can lead to things like hemorrhage, all kinds of problems," Caillagh tells me. A hemorrhage occurs when the uterus is atonic—the muscle is flaccid. The woman must keep her blood sugar up, stay hydrated, and relieve her bladder to keep the uterus firm and contracting. Caillagh encouraged Peters. Peters said she felt like she had to pee but didn't want to get out of bed. "As I did with many women, I grabbed a bunch of towels and said, 'You know what? I'm going to throw these towels underneath you, and you can pee right onto the bed. You don't have to go anywhere you don't want to go.'"

Caillagh told Peters she would be 20 minutes down the road at another birth and that Haw would stay a while to make sure she ate and drank. She hugged her and Daren goodbye and took a load of laundry down to Haw—this was another facet of Caillagh's birth routine. "The house was always immaculate when we left," she tells me, although this detail, like many others, would later be held against her.

Caillagh had been at the other birth for an hour when Haw called. Peters was still refusing the food and drink, hadn't peed very much, and was arguing for a cigarette. "Beth was not finding a way to talk Julia into improving her self-care," says Caillagh. "Julia was becoming more and more angry about the afterpains, and she was becoming incredibly angry about Beth's insistence that 'you have to eat something, you must drink something.'" Caillagh's other client "hadn't started cranking yet—we were still in the talking, having fun phase," she says. Haw called back 20 minutes later. She told her mentor of 4 years that she was at a loss what to do and that Peters had passed a couple of blood clots—enough to prompt her to give a dose of Pitocin to prevent a bleed, because Peters still wasn't eating or drinking. Caillagh's client insisted she'd be fine and that Caillagh should check on Peters.

Caillagh drove back at dawn, stopping on the way at a convenience store for some ice cream and an energy drink, things she knew Peters liked and might be coaxed into consuming. Caillagh sat with Peters in her bedroom. "I asked her if she'd taken her blood pressure recently. She said yes, it was fine, but 'I cannot stand the afterpains, I cannot stand the cramping, I hate absolutely all of it,'" recalls Caillagh. "I got her to eat some ice cream and part of the banana while we simply sat there and talked. I said, 'Julia, you really do have to understand. These afterpains weren't something you were expecting. You were drugged for the other births, and you didn't breastfeed. And for some women it's very serious.' I said, 'If you cannot handle this pain'—and it was the first time I broached the issue with her—'there is no shame in going to the hospital. You go into the ER, you declare that you're having serious afterpains, stay for 5 hours, get the drugs to kill it, and get some sleep. You've lost nothing. You got the birth you wanted.'"

Caillagh then returned to her other client. I ask Caillagh whether Peters's afterpains concerned her, whether they could have been symptomatic of a larger problem. "No," she says. "Afterpains can keep going 3 days after a birth. For each woman it's very, very different." Having said that, severe afterpains are themselves a concern because they can precipitate problems. "I've seen women vomiting to the point that they're dehydrating. Suddenly, 4 hours after an otherwise gorgeous birth, they're in the hospital for postpartum hemorrhage because they've dehydrated so badly that there's not enough fluid in their system to keep them from bleeding. It's critical—they must eat and drink, they must," she says.

Caillagh's other client gave birth later that morning. Caillagh drew her a bath, cooked the ritual meal, cleaned up, and drove back toward the Peters's house. To her surprise, Haw's car was still there (normally the midwives would have stayed about two hours following birth). She went in—Claire Peters and a party of family and friends were eating take-out in the dining room. Upstairs, Peters had not slept at all. And she was complaining of muscle pain in her legs—they were wrapped in ace bandages. Caillagh found her sitting up in bed, holding her stomach. She suggested again that her client go to the hospital for fluids and pain medication. "I sat with her for a while. I said, 'Julia, you know, really, truly, this is too long. It is not in your best interest to keep doing this; you're only undoing yourself. Typically at this point after a birth, you've had enough hours to eat and sleep. You'd just be waking up now, refreshed, ready to really be with your baby. You've done none of those things.' I said, 'I'm going to go downstairs for a while. I want you and Daren to talk about this. Because then next time I come up, it's because it's time for me to go home. I've been gone a long time.'"

Caillagh says she sat down at the communal table and chatted with the family amid fast-food wrappers. Haw was doing a final load of laundry. Before she headed back upstairs, she pulled Claire Peters aside and encouraged her to take Peters to the hospital if things continued as they were. Caillagh used the word *spiraling*, which would also later be held against her.

Caillagh went back up to Peters and helped her take her blood pressure. "It was showing typical signs of dehydration—it was elevated, her pulse was up a bit. I said, 'Julie, do you need any more indicators that you need to make some choices here?'" Caillagh says Julia was kneeling on the bed, "beautiful color," and swiveled to make eye contact with Daren. She nodded and said she'd go to the hospital. "I said great, I think you're making a really wise choice." Daren asked whether he should drive or call an ambulance. Caillagh says she told him it was his choice. "There's no real emergency as far as I can see." Caillagh walked over to the bed, gave Peters a "great big hug, and said I love you and I'll see you tomorrow morning. I said, 'I think you're making a really good decision. Let them help you, you're going to feel so much better." Caillagh told them she'd be calling to check in, said her goodbyes to the family, and left with Haw in separate cars.

About 10 minutes after the midwives left, Claire Peters remembers her son calling down, "Mom, can you come up here?" She was standing in the kitchen holding Alexis and handed her off to Julia's mother. "I went upstairs, and when I walked in the room, Julie was on her knees," says Claire. "She was saying, 'I need air.'"

"Beth and I got past Fredericksburg, and we were about to stop for something to eat, and I figured I'd call the house to see what was going on," says Caillagh. They had been gone about an hour. Peters's friend Robyn picked up the phone. "She said, 'Cynthia, you don't know. She's dead.'"

"At this point I hadn't slept in three days," Caillagh tells me in a quiet monotone. "I called a good friend and said you need to come take absolutely everything out of my house—every record, every document, everything. I had a second car there, an old car that my 17-year-old had been using. He filled the entire car and took it and hid it on a reservation someplace. I took the other car and spent the night anonymously in a hotel that took cash."

INDICTMENTS

In 1918, the Virginia General Assembly passed legislation that required all practicing midwives to be registered with the state and supervised by the health department. A booklet enumerated several "Midwife Safety

Rules." Rule 3: "Never pass your fingers or any instrument into the birth canal of the woman for any purpose." Rule 5: "Never give drugs of any kind to hasten or increase labor pains." The pamphlet advised that the woman should be laid flat on her back with her knees up for delivery. "Do not let the patient bear down with her pains, this can cause tears," warned the pamphlet. "Never pull on the cord."[29]

In 1974, the Virginia Department of Health discontinued licensing midwives who weren't registered nurses, and by 1977, legislation prohibited practice by those who didn't already hold licenses.

In the summer of 1998, a special grand jury convened in Stafford to investigate what had gone wrong at the Peters home the year before. The jurors met in secret, as special grand juries do, and witnesses were questioned under oath by the commonwealth's attorney. No other attorneys were permitted. A recorder appointed by the court transcribed the testimony, which was sealed upon adjournment, as testimony under such circumstances usually is.

Special grand juries are essentially investigative arms of the state; they decide whether the evidence warrants a trial. And on September 8, 1998, exactly a year after Julia Peters died—hours before the statute of limitations on misdemeanors was to expire—the jurors delivered what's called a "true bill," or a decision to indict Callaigh and Haw on two counts: practice of medicine without a license and practice of midwifery without a license. The indictments were not made public.

The previous spring, Caillagh's supporters had retained the defense attorney Peter Greenspun for her representation. Stafford is a small town. Greenspun is a high-profile attorney—he represented sportscaster Marv Albert through his sex scandal and John Allen Muhammed in the 2002 DC sniper case. Greenspun knew an investigation of Peters's death had been in progress for months, and he began making phone calls and writing letters to Eric Olsen, the prosecuting attorney, requesting a meeting. Greenspun got no reply for weeks, and then finally, in late October, Olsen called to "invite" Caillagh to testify before a grand jury; Caillagh received a subpoena. Neither Caillagh nor her attorney was informed of the special grand jury that had convened in September or the indictments issued against her.

Greenspun continued his one-way correspondence with Olsen. "As you know, the statute of limitations on any misdemeanor charges has long since expired," he wrote on November 6, 2 days after Caillagh testified, 2 months after she had in fact been indicted for misdemeanor crimes. He asked whether the grand jury was investigating felony manslaughter allegations. Two weeks later, hearing no response, he wrote to Olsen again. Although he couldn't imagine that his client would have been charged with misdemeanors without his knowing, "if that has in fact occurred, please contact me immediately." This continued for weeks, with one phone call returned and still nothing said about the indictments.

On January 19, 1999, the commonwealth issued arrest and search warrants, and the charges against Caillagh and Haw were unsealed. The misdemeanors were lumped with new felony manslaughter charges. Also charged was Claire Peters for perjury in her testimony to the special grand jury—she paid her $5000 cash bail in the same county office where she had witnessed her son marry Julia in a civil ceremony years before. As Greenspun would later point out to the court, this charge eliminated the only witness with medical knowledge, aside from the emergency responders, who had seen Julia Peters's death: Claire Peters would not be able to testify on the midwives' behalf.

The commonwealth alleged that Julia Peters had hemorrhaged, a loss of blood that "would have been obvious to any trained or experienced person," according to court papers. Cited was the final autopsy report, issued more than 8 months after the death by state medical examiner Gina Fino, MD, and chief medical examiner Marcella Fierro, MD, which concluded that "Postpartum hemorrhage due to uterine atony" was the cause of death. The special jurors heard testimony that Peters's uterus had not contracted effectively, which led to sustained blood loss over the 11 hours following childbirth. Court papers called the death "entirely preventable," one that would never have happened if Peters had been in the hospital, with access to a blood transfusion.[30]

The pretrial hearings, which began in March 1999 and continued through January 2000, started out politely enough. "I've been doing this for 15 years and I want you all to understand what a joy it is, absolute joy for the court to have able, well prepared, obviously excellent lawyers arguing matters," the judge, James W. Haley, Jr., commented to Greenspun, who had now been joined by Jonathan Shapiro, Claire Peters's attorney, and David Bracken, Haw's attorney. "It is an absolute joy to have folks like you all in the courtroom."

Soon this decorum began to deteriorate. Shapiro kept filing motions for the release of his client's testimony to the special grand jury—the testimony in which she allegedly perjured herself—which was still under seal and to which he had no access. "I'm standing here before you as a defense lawyer," pleaded Shapiro. "I do not know how to begin to prepare a defense for Ms. Peters on a perjury charge when I don't know what it is." Greenspun kept filing motions for access to the special grand jury's report and testimony, also sealed, as well as for access to other relevant documents. "What—well, you have a copy, do you not, of what the autopsy report says? It says the woman bled to death," Haley told Greenspun before he granted the motion.

A month later, however, the defense still had no autopsy report, no pictures, no special grand jury report, no testimony. "To this moment, we have received not one page of information from the commonwealth about this case. We are now 4 months post indictment, 3 months post arraignment," Greenspun told Haley.

Soon after that, Greenspun and Shapiro were given access to Peters's testimony and the jury's report, but a larger matter arose: the 5 months between when the indictments were issued and when Caillagh was informed of the charges. At a hearing in July, Greenspun charged the court with violating Caillagh's right to a speedy trial. He wanted to know: who had ordered the indictments hidden? For what reason?

Greenspun had with him his paper trail of faxes and letters to Olsen, in which he repeatedly asked whether any charges were being brought and repeatedly got the brush off. "The commonwealth had an obligation" to make the charges known to the accused and her attorney, he said. "There is no excuse, there is no justification." He cited statute after statute, case precedent, federal law. Greenspun asked whether the judge had authorized a delay, for which he could find no court record. Haley didn't answer the question: "I have no idea, I mean, there may be and there may not be," he responded. Olsen finally spoke up and defended his evasive conversations with Greenspun. "Look where your conversations have led us," Haley shot back.

Judges and prosecutors are prohibited from discussing pending cases with each other—this is called ex parte communication—and Greenspun was suggesting that it had occurred. Haley was furious. He put Greenspun under oath. "You have accused the commonwealth attorney of lying. You have accused him of misconduct. You have presumed that there were ex parte contacts between this court and Mr. Olsen," the judge said. He called these allegations "reckless" and Greenspun's further motions "frivolous" and denied them all.

Greenspun would later offer to step down as Caillagh's attorney. "He felt that he would never get a fair trial," says Caillagh, though she would not let him resign. She recalls one particular hearing in which he again provoked Haley with a lengthy, meticulous legal argument, and derogatory remarks flew from the bench. Several people present that day remember Haley saying "We don't do things here the way you do them up in Fairfax." After another monologue in which Greenspun argued midwifery as custom, Haley responded that so too is the bygone Hindu practice of burning widows on their husbands' funeral pyres. "Custom," he declared, "can be changed by law."

CAUSE OF DEATH

Julia Peters was pronounced dead on arrival at Mary Washington Hospital in Fredericksburg, Virginia, at 2:15 in the afternoon on September 8, 1997. The emergency responders noted in their report that Peters was alive just before 1 p.m. when they arrived at her home. Peters was "extremely agitated," the responders wrote, "struggling, face down in bed, stating she couldn't breathe." They also noted that the bedding showed an "extreme amount of blood loss." The responders were able to insert an IV catheter, but Peters went into convulsions, then she went unconscious. By 1:15 they had initiated CPR.

The team moved Peters to the floor. Claire Peters held her daughter-in-law's head back, helping the team establish an airway. Peters's blood pressure started to drop, her heart rate slowed down. They applied the defibrillator to her chest and brought it back. By then there were three teams of emergency responders working on her. Finally, they asked Claire and Daren to leave the room.

The emergency room noted in its report that it was "unable to identify the source" of Peters's death. The diagnosis was acute cardiopulmonary arrest—heart and respiratory failure. An examination noted "a small amount of vaginal bleeding." Medical examiner Frederic A. Phillips, MD, wrote in the narrative description of his initial report on

Peters that "Examination of her body grossly gave no clue as to the cause of her demise. However, I should think that embolism and bleeding would be high on the list." By embolism Phillips was referring either to the formation of a blood clot traveling to the lungs and heart, or to an amniotic fluid embolism, wherein amniotic fluid and debris pass into the mother's bloodstream.

In January 1998, the *Fredericksburg Free-Lance Star* ran a feature on Peters's death called "Cradle and Grave: A five-part series about Julia Peters, a young Stafford County mother whose decision to give birth at home may have cost her life." Staff reporter Jim Hall reported that the cause of death was "puzzling" to the state medical examiner's office. "The lab has ruled out pulmonary embolism, heart attack, or hemorrhage," wrote Hall.[31] After the charges were unsealed, however, the case hit the *Richmond Times Dispatch* and the *Washington Post*, and blood loss became the focus. That Peters had "bled to death" was printed in articles and stated on local network news, occasionally without the qualifying "according to court papers" or "allegedly."[32]

The defense rejected this explanation, seizing on the 8 months between Peters's death and the state's determination of the cause. Greenspun told reporters that expert testimony would reveal that the midwives were not negligent and that the cause of death was in fact not blood loss.

Caillagh is frank with me about the normal blood of birth: it looks like a lot. And it *is* a lot for the inexperienced—about a pint, which can look like even more when it is diluted by amniotic fluid or urine or bath-water. "This is something that's difficult to bring into a courtroom," says Caillagh. "Think of all the men, think of the male judge. How do you discuss the way blood dilutes? This is like a woman urinating into a toilet at the height of her menstruation. If her bladder's full and she's not using a tampon, you're going to see a lot of blood in the toilet. If you're not used to it, it's a frightening thing to look at. But it's nothing, it's absolutely nothing."

Caillagh lists for me the items at Peters's home that had been soiled: the sheets under Peters as she birthed, the sheets and towels she had peed on, and another set of sheets that she'd peed and bled some more on. None of this was abnormal, says Caillagh. She examined Peters following the birth and noticed no tearing and no abnormal bleeding. She says the difference between normal postpartum blood and a hemorrhage is obvious to anyone with even minimal training. In an e-mail dated May 1998, Caillagh wrote to a midwife colleague about the birth: "When I left for the next birth at 1 hour post birth, Julie's uterus was firm and centered at 3 fingers below the navel, and in fact, her largest complaint was (and would remain) the very strong afterpains that she was experiencing: these afterpains were doing a fine job of keeping the uterus well contracted. . . . " An excessive loss of blood, felt Caillagh, could not possibly have been the cause of Peters's death.

The commonwealth, on the other hand, was building its case around blood loss, citing the loads of laundry, the "blood-soaked" sheets and towels, and the Pitocin.

"She was not bleeding," says Claire Peters. "Not any more than anybody bleeds after they have a baby." She says not one emergency responder commented on blood. "If she had been bleeding they would have started her on IV fluids right away. But they didn't." When Claire heard about the hemorrhage allegation, she signed out Julia's medical records from the hospital. "There were so many inconsistencies in the reports," she tells me. For example, the EMT report states that Julia had no blood pressure and that intubation was "unsuccessful." "That's not true," says Peters.

The state also alleged that Caillagh and Haw fled as the ambulance was arriving. Caillagh tells me she had no compunctions about taking a woman or baby to the hospital in an emergency. "I couldn't care less about the hostility," she says. But Claire Peters understood that Caillagh would leave before an ambulance arrived and that the family was to offer no information about any midwives. Caillagh had already been investigated by the Department of Health once, and PenFam had an unwritten rule that families had a responsibility to protect her. If it wasn't an emergency requiring her physical support, Caillagh was not going to the hospital. In this case, there was no obvious reason for her to go, and neither Julia nor Daren was asking her to.

Throughout the legal aftermath, Daren Peters stood by the midwives, and by his mother. "No one knows the horrible last few minutes of Julie's life better than me. . . . Julie's death was sudden and unpredictable. I do not, in my heart, believe that Cynthia Caillagh or Beth Haw did anything to cause it, or could have stopped it," he wrote in a letter to the judge and prosecutor, reminding them that he was planning to testify on the midwives' behalf. He told a reporter, in reference to the charges against his mother, that "this justice system is a travesty."[33] Until the end, he blamed nobody. "The delivery of Alexis was perfect and so is she. That is what we will focus on."[34]

BLOOD LOSS

Caillagh's trial, scheduled before Haw's, was shaping up to be an event the likes of which Stafford had never seen. She faced 10 years in prison. The court allocated 2 weeks for the trial, not the customary 1 week, and it would call three times the usual number of potential jurors.

A succession of letters to the editor and commentaries in the local papers spoke to Caillagh's widespread support in the community and beyond, even from unexpected places. Dr. Patrick Neustatter, a Stafford County obstetrician, wrote an editorial in the *Fredericksburg Free-Lance Star*. "The unfortunate death of Julia Peters," Neustatter wrote, "is liable to put people off home birth. To my reading of the facts, this is unjustified. I see it not as a death attributable to the negligence of her attendants, as the deputy commonwealth's attorney would have us believe . . . but [as] one of those unavoidable events."

A handwritten letter arrived from Patch Adams, MD, of the Gesundheit Institute. "I ache that our society is so far removed from life," he wrote to Caillagh's supporters. "Both my children were born at home with midwives. I salute your important efforts. . . . Women (families) who want a home birth should be encouraged to have them, ideally with a midwife of their choice."

Caillagh's supporters were able to collect $50,000 for her defense, and Greenspun would ask for no more than that. They printed up "Legalize Midwifery" bumper stickers and "Ignorance is no excuse for the law" T-shirts, with the image of a witch hanging, and they packed the courtroom at the pretrial hearings and camped out on the courthouse lawn. As the trial was set to begin in January 2000, they arrived wearing white ribbons, to represent innocence, and dressed their toddlers in shirts that said things like "I was born at home and all I got was this lousy T-shirt."

Then there was a delay. Greenspun got a call from Olsen the morning of a hearing: a supplemental autopsy report had turned up in his office. Later in court that day, Greenspun moved to postpone the trial in light of the lost and found evidence. D'Anne Remocaldo sat in the courtroom that day and says she saw the judge become conciliatory toward the defense for the first time. Haley called Greenspun's request "well-founded,"[35] and for the next several minutes, the only sound in the courtroom was that of the judge and attorneys flipping through the pages of their calendars, searching for a new trial date.

That was the day Remocaldo began her own shadow defense. Soon after the hearing adjourned, Remocaldo called the clerk's office for Caillagh's case file—she wanted to see the report. Greenspun was giving away nothing specific about his defense strategy, "probably for fear I'd go and blab to the press," she tells me. What she found was a blood analysis ordered by state medical examiner Gina Fino, dated October 9, 1997.

Remocaldo is a brassy Texan, an evangelical turned zodiac-dabbling, "eclectic Christian" massage therapist. Her home in Richmond is decorated with female nudes hung on purple walls. She had her fourth and fifth children with Caillagh and named the fifth Caleigh in her honor. Remocaldo was one of Caillagh's most committed, and bracingly vocal, supporters. "In hospitals, strange people come in and want to stick their fingers in you," she told the *Richmond Times-Dispatch*.

The blood report showed that Peters died with a hematocrit of 22%—this is the percent of blood composed of red blood cells—and a hemoglobin of 9.8 grams per deciliter, the measure of those cells' oxygen-bearing capacity. The numbers are unremarkable for a 30-year-old heavy smoker who had just given birth. After her first cesarean at age 19, Peters's numbers were 28.3% and 10.2, respectively. Remocaldo called Greenspun and said she was taking the report to the press.

The blood report raised several questions: Why had Peters's hemoglobin been omitted from the final autopsy report? Why hadn't the blood report been in the file given to Olsen by the medical examiner's office? Or, if it had been there, why wasn't it entered into evidence and passed on to Greenspun? "There's a chance he didn't realize what it meant," says Remocaldo. "But that's when it gets into who knew what, when."

It turned out Greenspun had the hematology report all along—someone on the inside had informed him of its existence months before. He had promptly driven down to the medical examiner's office in Richmond and asked for a copy of Peters's file. He discovered that it was an inch thicker than what Olsen had turned over and that it included the lab report.

Caillagh's supporters seized on the report and wrote a press release titled, *Stafford Case Against Midwives Unravels Amidst New Questions*. Over a pizza lunch in Richmond, Remocaldo shared the press release and blood report with Jim Hall, the reporter who had written the sensationalist "Cradle and Grave" series, which reported that the medical examiner had ruled out hemorrhage as a cause of death based on lab results. The release was sent to other reporters as well, stimulating articles citing new evidence that cast doubts on the prosecution's case. Days before the trial was to begin, Olsen called Greenspun and offered to drop the manslaughter charge in exchange for a plea agreement.

Postmortem blood analysis wouldn't have proved that a hemorrhage had or hadn't occurred, according to forensic pathologists. "You can't rely on the answers," says John Adams, MD, a pathologist based outside Baltimore with 40 years of experience, whom Greenspun was going to call to testify. The numbers are rarely solid when taken from a dead body, he explains, and regardless, they wouldn't support the diagnosis of a sudden hemorrhage because that happens too quickly for the blood's composition to change. Caillagh herself explains to me that even if Peters had bled slowly over many hours, the numbers might still have looked normal, because at a certain point the body compensates. "I had to explain to Peter [Greenspun] why the blood report in and of itself wasn't important," she says.

Jack Daniel, MD, a pathologist who worked in the Richamnd medical examiner's office at the time of Peters's death, explains to me that without solid labs, a hemorrhage diagnosis would have had to rely solely on circumstantial evidence. "So if there were half a dozen completely blood-soaked sheets, that would clearly support the idea that she bled to death," he says. "But I don't think that was the case. As I recall, the big question was if she had bled to death, where the hell did all that blood go?"

MISSING INFORMATION

Caillagh says her first thought about Peters's death was to suspect an embolism. "I thought that she had either thrown a blood clot to the brain itself, or that it was an amniotic fluid embolism. I could not imagine what else it could be." Caillagh asked several physicians and midwives to review the case, including Marsden Wagner and Ina May Gaskin—both were going to testify on her behalf. The consensus was that amniotic fluid and debris had somehow entered Peters's bloodstream, eventually causing a clotting reaction in the blood and blocking circulation to the lungs and heart.

Research on the pathology of amniotic fluid embolism, or AFE, is ongoing, but the literature suggests that a sudden collapse is often preceded by pain, nausea, and malaise (symptoms that are unremarkable to midwives, nurses, and physicians alike), which quickly progress to a rise in pulse, a drop in blood pressure, extreme agitation, shortness of breath, and finally convulsions. Resuscitation efforts are usually ineffective, and many victims die or are permanently brain damaged. Even in 2006, death due to AFE was considered unavoidable. "AFE is an unpredictable, unpreventable, and, for the most part, an untreatable obstetric emergency," concluded a 2006 review article.[36]

Before AFE was recognized, women who expired this way were often labeled as experiencing "obstetric shock," thought to be caused by hemorrhage. It wasn't until a Chicago pathologist noticed that many women seemed to go into shock before bleeding, or with no bleeding at all, that the condition was studied. The pathologist teamed up with a graduate student, and together they reopened obstetric shock cases from the Chicago Lying-In Hospital. In each of the deceased, they found that the arteries leading to the lungs were clogged with globules of white blood cells surrounding amniotic fluid debris. The pathologists published their landmark findings in the *Journal of the American Medical Association* in 1941, making the diagnosis of "obstetric shock" obsolete.[37]

Without using the term, the State of Virginia was essentially calling Peters's death obstetric shock. At the same time, proving that AFE was responsible would be impossible. The final autopsy report noted no "amniotic fluid constituents" found in Peter's pulmonary arteries, and no other AFE-related tests had been ordered on Peters's blood. Both Daniel and Adams tell me this is not uncommon: less than half of clinically diagnosed AFE cases are confirmed by autopsy, even when lung tissue is examined. "You can't just take one little piece of lung and see no embolism in it and say there was no embolism," says Daniel. "If I tell you that out of this room with 100 people there may be somebody who has HIV, I can't go in there, test one person, and come back out and say that nobody in the room has HIV. In pathology, that's called a sampling error."

Daniel says nearly all deaths are given a cause by the medical examiner. But in a case like Peters's, "in the end, you may just have to bite the bullet and put this case in the 1 to 2 percent category of 'We just don't know.' And it's going to hack everybody off that we don't know, but we don't know. It could have been AFE, it could have been bleeding to death, but we just don't have the beef on either one of them. And that's probably about as strong as Greenspun's case might have gotten."

Including Adams and Daniel, Greenspun had lined up ten expert witnesses to dispute the alleged cause of death, including the chief medical examiner for the State of Maryland at that time and the head of the Virginia Commonwealth University pathology department.

The case's political ramifications were indisputable, and they would be raised by the defense as well. The state's Joint Commission on Health Care resolved to study the issue of licensing midwives—one way to get a bill introduced—exactly the same week that Caillagh's case hit the papers, and the bill that emerged was subsequently killed during her pretrial hearings. Steve Cochran, a libertarian who became incensed by the legal restrictions on midwives after marrying one, had drafted the bill. "The two issues were fused together from the get-go," he says. A case in point was a session in which legislators read a letter from Eric Olsen suggesting that they vote against floating a bill. The letter, dated December 21, 1998—after the secret grand jury's indictments but before they were made public—states that "The investigation into the circumstances of Ms. Julia Peters's death is ongoing, but will be reaching a conclusion very soon. . . . I am unable to say more now, but it is my belief that your committee should consider refraining from making any recommendations on the issue of Direct Entry Midwifery until this investigation is complete."

Meanwhile, questions began to surface about the role of the state's chief medical examiner, Marcella Fierro, in the case. Why had she taken over Peters's autopsy report? Why had it taken 8 months to finalize the cause of death? And why was Peters's hemoglobin omitted? Suspicions about bias were raised by a lobbyist in the *Richmond Times Dispatch*—Fierro was married to a prominent obstetrician. Those suspicions would have a more solid foundation in January 2001, when Fierro testified before a House committee, which was again considering the bill that would license certified professional midwives. One of the delegates asked whether the medical examiner had seen "bad outcomes" arising from midwife-attended births. Fierro responded, "We do see, each year, a few deaths where there was no physician involved where the woman, generally it is due to postpartum hemorrhage, where this has not been recognized and the woman has been allowed to bleed for hours and hours and hours and then dies of shock. . . . The question in the deaths that we have seen has been a question of judgment and a failure to recognize serious complications." When another delegate asked Fierro how many such deaths were attributable to negligence of a midwife, she responded, "We don't have figures for that." The delegate pressed on: "So, you can't attest that there have been any?" Fierro: "I can only attest to what the medical examiner has seen."

"She should have lost her job over that," says Cochran, who founded the organization Virginia Birthing Freedom to support the bill. "There had never been any [midwife-attended] maternal deaths due to hemorrhage. If there had been, they would have made the papers, just like Cynthia's case did."

Jack Daniel, who worked under Fierro for 4 years and independently in Richmond thereafter, told me he could not recall any other cases like Peters's.

I reached Fierro by phone at her office in Richmond, where she has held the position of chief medical examiner since 1994. She could not recall any specific maternal deaths due to blood loss attended by a midwife. "I don't have any of the records," she said. But had she seen deaths, "each year, a few," as she had testified before the House committee? "Yes," she said. What years had she been referring to? "I don't know," she replied. I asked whether any of those deaths had made the papers. Had criminal charges been brought against the midwives? "To tell you the truth, I don't remember," she said.

I asked Fierro whether she remembered the charges against Caillagh and the circumstances surrounding the death of Julia Peters. She said she did. I asked her whether 8 months is usual for the state to release an autopsy report. "It's not usual; it depends on the investigation," Fierro said. "And they had to do an investigation. Cause of death wasn't a question, it was the manner of death. What were the circumstances under which this death occurred? That took a long time to investigate." She explained that the cause of death is the "disease, injury, or poison," whereas the manner refers to "Is this a natural death, an accident, a homicide, a suicide, or undetermined?" The manner of death, however, does not appear on the final autopsy report.

Fierro told me that to determine a hemorrhage, the examiner would first have to find the source of the bleeding; second, the body would show "extreme pallor;" and last "You find buckets of blood at the scene," she said. I asked her whether that is what had been found at the Peters home. "There was a lot of blood found at the scene, and in the washing machine," she told me.

I asked Fierro why the hemoglobin reading hadn't been included in the final autopsy report. "They may have confused the terms," she said. "I don't know. I don't remember."

INCAPACITATED

On May 5, 2000, Caillagh pleaded guilty to practice of midwifery without a license, to practice of medicine without a license, and to "abuse and neglect of an incapacitated adult." With this plea, Olsen dropped the felony charges against Peters and Haw. (Haw would plead guilty to practice of midwifery; Peters's charge would later be expunged.)

Caillagh says she and Greenspun hashed out the plea agreement over the phone the evening prior to her final court appearance. "He said, 'They're not gonna let you go,'" recalls Caillagh. The charge of practicing medicine was unavoidable—a drug had been administered—and Caillagh was ready to plead guilty to that. But Olsen wanted something else, something on the level of reckless endangerment, for which there is no statute in Virginia. "The closest thing they could come up with was neglect of an incapacitated adult—in essence, that a laboring woman is like a woman in a nursing home," she tells me. "I could not accept this. It was absolutely not going to happen."

Greenspun stayed on the phone with Caillagh until dawn and, by that time, had convinced her that it was the only way. "Peter said, 'Cynthia, I want you to understand something. I'm good, but the hate of you is worse. If this goes to trial, you will go to jail. I can't keep you from it, no matter what we bring in. The cards are stacked against you. I cannot guarantee that you will win on appeal."

For the midwife who believed in a woman "meeting herself" in childbirth, a guilty plea to neglecting an "incapacitated adult" was the ultimate capitulation. "Julie became a nonentity," says Remocaldo. "What Julie had wanted didn't matter to these people."

At the sentencing hearing, Greenspun brought with him a pile of four dozen letters of support for Caillagh, all pleading for the judge to spare her prison time. They were written by a psychologist, a probation officer, a Baptist minister, a family planning counselor, a football coach, a high school teacher, a museum curator. Women who birthed twins and breeches with Caillagh wrote letters; there was a letter from a woman who chose to give birth unassisted following the indictments. Like Remocaldo, she also named a daughter after Caillagh.

The letters were almost funereal: "We have never met another person who has given of herself so completely and unselfishly in helping others. We are all better people for having known her." "Because of her, I not only have two beautiful happy healthy children, I have the knowledge, wisdom and confidence to raise them. Cynthia didn't just bring my babies into this world. She midwifed me into motherhood and us into a family." "As a priest, many people call me a teacher and guide. In Cynthia's presence I have always felt like she was teacher and guide to me."

Haley did spare her prison time, suspending all 36 months of the sentence and all but $2500 of the fine. Before she was released from his courtroom, however, he addressed her directly. He asked whether she knew the song "Sometimes I Feel Like a Motherless Child." "His clear implication was that there was a child who didn't have a mother because of Cynthia," says Leslie Payne, who attended every hearing. "I wrote it down because I remember thinking that it was just so unbelievable." Caillagh pled out May 5, which also happened to be International Midwives' Day.

The next day, May 6, 2000, Virginia Governor James Gilmore declared Virginia's own Midwives' Day, to acknowledge "the positive impact that midwives . . . have had on improving infant mortality rates and decreasing the incidence of complications and unnecessary medical interventions in childbirth." One day a midwife is criminally convicted for her practice, the next day she's indirectly honored by the governor.

Caillagh was frequently caught between such contradictions. She was considered a "lay" midwife by the state, yet she was the most experienced midwife in the state, perhaps in the country. Caillagh was never actually put on trial, but everyone felt that she had been. In a sense, Caillagh's case marked the completion of a campaign the State of Virginia had launched in 1918. First, it mandated what position women should give birth in and limited what their midwives could do to assist them. In 1977, it pushed home birth and midwifery underground. And in May 2000, the state of Virginia made it clear that traditional midwifery was a crime.

In 2005, years after Caillagh had moved away, the Commonwealth of Virginia brought this history almost full circle. It passed a law licensing the Certified Professional Midwife, by overwhelming margins in both chambers. The law includes no practice restrictions, which means that as of early 2007, Virginia CPMs are not obligated to "risk out" women carrying twins or breech babies, or women desiring VBACs.

What that means for the midwives Caillagh left behind is that her case no longer hangs over their heads. Any practitioner who attends births will sooner or later encounter death, most likely of a fetus or newborn, especially in clients who decline testing for anomalies. Even in Sweden there are 2 to 3 infant deaths per 1000 births. "You cannot guarantee that a conception will result in a full-term pregnancy," Caillagh tells me, as she told her clients. "You cannot guarantee that a labor will result in a living child. And you cannot guarantee that the birth process itself will see a live mother. You cannot guarantee life. Yet we live in a society that wants those guarantees."

According to a state report, 64 women died of pregnancy-related causes in Virginia between 1999 and 2001, including four deaths due to amniotic fluid embolism and six due to hemorrhage.[38] Unlike Peters, none of those deaths made the front page or resulted in criminal charges against the birth attendant. If Julia Peters had died while in Caillagh's care in 2005—and Caillagh had been licensed—it might have made the news, but the fallout would have been an administrative hearing, not a criminal prosecution. If Peters had elected a fourth repeat cesarean and died in the hospital, it is very likely that nothing at all would have happened.

Even after what she went through, Caillagh still has a fierce libertarian streak; she is still wary of legislating midwifery, even while she is sympathetic to the impulse. True legitimacy and professional respect cannot be won by turning a bill into a law, she argues, not within a system that gives one group—doctors of medicine—the authority to define healthcare. Midwifery might survive this system, she says, but not traditional midwifery.

Caillagh tells me that long before Stafford, she felt traditional midwifery was "coming to its inevitable end," not only because of regulation but also because of fear. "To truly give birth you have to surrender to the process of birth, which is to suspend a conscious awareness. You must trust the instinctive internal self. And I think we've come upon a generation of women who don't know what that internal trust looks like," she says. Caillagh does retain a dim optimism—a farmer's knowing that the season will change. "I think there will come a time when we will remember or will rediscover—perhaps it will be so distant that we'll feel we have discovered—the intrinsic value of birth under one's own steam. Maybe we have to evolve back to a place where we realize all of this is folly. That we can't control health in the ways we think we can. And that in fact the most important and valuable thing we can give ourselves is a woman under her own steam, bringing her babies forth."

CHAPTER 8

Rights

IN 1999, LAURA PEMBERTON had a twin VBAC in hiding. She won't tell me where she went or who assisted her. Call her paranoid, but she had previously been "forced out of my home by armed men," as she tells it, while attempting a vaginal birth.

This happened in January 1996. Pemberton had been determined to give birth vaginally but could find no doctor or midwife willing to attend her because they feared that her uncommon cesarean scar, in the shape of an upside-down "T," would rupture. Her physician was initially supportive, but at 25 weeks he said he would not permit a VBAC. He estimated the risk of rupture to be between 3% and 6%. Pemberton scoured the medical literature and consulted far-flung experts. She weighed the risks of labor against the risks of repeat surgery and decided the former was safer and healthier for herself and her baby. With no other options, she and her husband decided to order supplies and go it alone.

Pemberton labored for 2 days in her home in Tallahassee, Florida, but began to have trouble keeping down food and drink. After hours without sustenance, feeling drained, and knowing she was dehydrated, she decided to go to Tallahassee Memorial Regional Medical Center for IV fluids; then she was going to return home. But when she got to the hospital, nobody would start an IV. They wanted her to sign a consent form for a cesarean instead. The attending physician came to her room, next a succession of obstetricians, and then the hospital administrator. Says Pemberton: "I was given an ultimatum: no signature, no IV."

Finally two nurses walked in, shut the door, and began to help her get dressed. "They told me there was chaos out in the hall like they'd never seen," she says. The nurses reassured her: her baby's heart tones were great, her cervix was dilating, her blood pressure was normal, the baby was descending, and, except for signs that she was dehydrated, everything was fine. Her uterus showed no signs of rupturing. The nurses directed Pemberton and her husband to a back door and down two flights of stairs that would lead to the parking lot. The couple was out the door before Pemberton had put her shoes on. "I was running down the stairs in labor, barefoot and pregnant," she says, allowing for a chuckle.

Pemberton is a tall, trim woman, with straight black hair neatly bobbed at her chin and a quick, wide smile that often comes with a wink. Her steady retelling of the story suggests she was capable of the same conviction and poise in the throes of labor, even with the obstetric police after her.

On the way home, her contractions grew stronger and, she says, she felt a renewed strength. The nurses had "put my mind at ease," she tells me. Giving birth at home without assistance, after all, had been an absolute last resort. "I was aware of the risk. That's why I wanted to do it in a hospital setting. Watch me, care for me, let me do this, and if there's a problem then I'll be there." But not one doctor would allow a trial of labor. "They put me in a position where nobody was there for me," she says.

At home, Pemberton felt the baby working its way lower in her pelvis. She told her family it was time. As her husband was making preparations, her 12-year-old daughter answered the phone. It was the sheriff. "This was my first contact with the law," says Pemberton, "and he spoke to my family as though we were criminals."

Now, the police were after her. The sheriff and the state attorney soon arrived at Pemberton's front door. She allowed them in. The sheriff's deputy soon joined them, and a squad of EMTs followed close behind. The attorney and officer stood over Pemberton, who was resting in her bedroom, barely dressed, and told her she had to go back to the hospital.

"He told me his hands were tied," says Pemberton of the attorney. "A judge had issued a court order, and he had no choice but to take me in."

Pemberton was allowed to get her bathrobe only. The paramedics strapped her onto a stretcher by her wrists and ankles, wheeled her into the ambulance parked outside, and sped away with the sirens on. Pemberton remembers neighbors watching.

At the hospital, a nurse led her to a room and gave her a hospital gown to put on. She and her husband went into the bathroom and locked the door. Pemberton remembers squatting there, bearing down as hard as she could, willing the baby to come. "I reached up and could feel the baby's head in my hand," she says. She pulled at the water bag, still intact. It slipped out of her grasp. There was knocking on the door, and finally she opened it.

Two doctors, the sheriff, two attorneys, and a judge crowded into the small exam room, with Pemberton in a hospital gown on the exam table, and conducted a hearing. "All these professional men in one corner, and me in the other, still dehydrated," she says. At no time was Pemberton offered an attorney.

In between contractions, Pemberton argued in her own defense. She said this was an informed decision based on months of research and preparation. The judge said the doctors felt she would rupture her uterus. She said that she'd been in labor for 2 days and that the hospital had found her and the baby in perfect health. The judge said Pemberton would do anything to avoid a cesarean. She rebutted that she'd gladly consented to a medically necessary cesarean with her last baby, for placenta previa. "The judge said that my unborn baby was in the control of the state and that it was the state's responsibility to bring that baby into this world safely," says Pemberton. "The judge looked at me and pointed his finger: 'We are going to do the C-section, and we are going to do it tonight.'"

Pemberton's obstetrician did one final exam before he began operating. She was 9 centimeters dilated, the baby was literally inches from being born, yet the surgeons went ahead with the surgery.

Pemberton's court-ordered cesarean is extreme, but she is not the only American woman to have had or to have been threatened with one. In 2001, Amber and John Marlowe arrived at Mercy Hospital in Wilkes-Barre, Pennsylvania, in labor, ready to have their seventh child.

A triage nurse did an ultrasound and shook her head; the baby had grown much too big for a vaginal birth, she told the couple. Amber assured the nurse that all six of her previous kids had been large—one 12 lb, 4 oz—yet she had birthed them vaginally with ease. The attending OB who examined her was unconvinced. He told the Marlowes a vaginal delivery would not be permitted: "If you don't like it, go somewhere else." So they did.

At Wilkes-Barre General Hospital it was the same scenario, except that the physicians told them not to leave. Marlowe spent 14 hours at this hospital, refusing a cesarean section. Meanwhile, unbeknownst to the couple, hospital attorneys were petitioning a local judge for custody of Marlowe's fetus so that the hospital could legally compel its surgical extraction—and they won.

Before anyone could execute the order, however, the Marlowes were in their car driving to yet another hospital, Moses Taylor Hospital in Scranton, where Amber swiftly pushed out a perfectly healthy 11 lb, 9 oz baby girl, with nary a tear.

Ashley Dees, the Texas woman who had trouble bonding with her first baby after an unplanned cesarean (see Chapter 4), found an OB supportive of VBAC for her next birth in September 2005, but that particular physician was unreachable when Dees went into labor. Dees labored at home as long as she could and then checked into the hospital, where things progressed quickly. "Nurses were yelling at me not to push," she recalls. "But I couldn't help it. Pushing was beyond my control." Her doctor still unavailable, nurses paged the OB on call. Dees says he walked into the room, said that VBAC babies die, and announced that he was going to do a cesarean. The doctor "walked across the room to my bed and injected something in my IV that stopped my contractions. Stopped them. Nurses unplugged monitors and threw the cords up on my legs and began to wheel me out of the room to the OR."

"I have a law degree, I know my rights," says Dees. "I just kept repeating, 'I do not consent to a C-section, I do not consent to a C-section.'" At this point her husband was physically barricading the door, everybody was shouting, and finally the attending OB appeared in the doorway. "I don't do VBACs," the doctor ordering the cesarean told him. "Well I do 'do' VBACs," said the attending, and told the nurses to hook the monitors back up.

The baby's head was crowning, but Dees could no longer feel the muscles to push. The attending asked if he could cut an episiotomy, to which Dees agreed, and her baby slipped out, "not peacefully, but vaginally," she says.

PREGNANT WOMEN'S RIGHTS

There is little way of knowing how many legal, physical, and psychological skirmishes go on in American labor and delivery wards. Thankfully, few are court-ordered. However, a 2003 survey of directors of maternal-fetal medicine programs found that 14% reported using the court system to compel women to have cesareans, and 21% believed that coercive tactics were "ethically justified."[1] According to the 2005 *Listening to Mothers* survey 57% of women who wanted a VBAC were denied the option, and most of the women surveyed who had episiotomies had no choice in the matter. Furthermore, a quarter of those who had cesareans felt pressured into it.[2] In my own research, I've spoken with many women whose membranes were "stripped" without their knowledge or consent, women whose membranes were being punctured before they could protest, women who were told they had no choice but to wear a fetal monitor and stay in bed, and women who were given only a choice between Pitocin and a cesarean.

Adults seeking medical care have both the right to receive treatment and the right to refuse treatment, and they have the right to know the risks and benefits of each treatment option, including the option of no treatment at all. The legal term is *informed consent*, which the American College of Obstetricians and Gynecologists calls a "fundamental ethical obligation of health care professionals."[3] The concept is predicated on autonomy, a patient's right to make decisions about her healthcare. Patients' rights are grounded in the Constitution—in the right to bodily integrity, to self-determination, to liberty, and to privacy. There are exceptions allowed: it is unnecessary to obtain informed consent from the unconscious, the incompetent, and the child. But unlawfully, pregnant women have been treated as an exception as well.

Lynn Paltrow is an attorney and executive director of the National Advocates for Pregnant Women (NAPW), an advocacy organization for women facing legal action related to their pregnancies. She has argued reproductive rights cases for 25 years, including one that was brought before the Supreme Court. I met with Paltrow over breakfast in New York City one morning, and naïvely asked, how, if ethics and law prohibit it, women like Laura Pemberton, Amber Marlowe, and Ashley Dees have been denied, or very nearly so, their constitutional rights. She took a sip of her coffee. "You're wondering how these things happen," she said. Then she introduced me to the Angela Carder story.

It is 1987, Washington, DC. Having fought off cancer since puberty, 28-year-old Angela Carder believes she is in remission and begins carrying a much-wanted pregnancy. At 25 weeks gestation, however, Carder checks into George Washington Hospital with severe symptoms. She learns the cancer is back in the form of an inoperable lung tumor, yet she is denied chemotherapy and radiation based on the premise that it would be a risk to her fetus.

While Carder and her family are waging a battle *for* medical treatment to save her life, Carder's health is deteriorating, and trouble brews on another front. "We have a woman who is critically ill, 26 weeks pregnant," says Paltrow. "She, her family, her doctors are all in agreement that they should do whatever they can to keep her alive. But a hospital neonatologist, who happens to be a woman, walks by and overhears a conversation about if she did die, should they perform an emergency C-section and try to rescue the fetus?"

Paltrow goes on: "The neonatologist not only doesn't bother to talk to Angela, but doesn't talk to her attending physician. She runs to the hospital lawyers and says, 'I can save 26-week-old fetuses, this fetus has a right to life, we need to rescue the fetus!' And the hospital attorneys, who clearly don't know this area of law and apparently didn't know basic concepts of bodily integrity and informed consent, call a judge in on an emergency hearing. And the question presented was 'What right does the fetus have?' And they appoint a lawyer for the fetus."

Carder is now breathing with the help of a respirator, and her family is now fighting *against* unwanted medical treatment, treatment that her own doctors say will hasten her death. Nearby in a room at the hospital, her fetus's attorney is joined by her attorney, an attorney for the District of Columbia, hospital attorneys, and a judge. Her fetus's lawyer argues that Carder should be ordered to have a cesarean because she's as good as dead already: "Sadly, the life of the mother is lost to us no matter what decision is made at this point."[4] The judge rules in favor of the fetus.

Carder is conscious for a conversation with her obstetrician, who tells her of the decision, but that he will do the operation only if she consents to it. She very clearly mouths to him, "I don't want it done." An appeal is set up on conference call—not once does a judge visit Carder to determine her wishes—and the decision is upheld. Carder's physician refuses to perform the cesarean, as do all the other OBs present. A staff surgeon is called in. Carder's baby dies in 2 hours; Angela Carder dies in 2 days.

Paltrow led the appeal as an attorney with the American Civil Liberties Union and won. The court ruled that "in virtually all cases the question of what is to be done is decided by the patient—the pregnant woman—on behalf of herself and the fetus."[5] ACOG reiterates this in its own ethics guidelines: "In the absence of extraordinary circumstances that, in fact, the Committee on Ethics cannot currently imagine, judicial authority should not be used to implement treatment regimens aimed at protecting the fetus, for such actions violate the pregnant woman's autonomy."[6]

"We got the court to say that this was wrong, and there have been a number of cases since then that have reaffirmed that in very strong and helpful language," says Paltrow, coming around to my initial question. "Now, the way the law usually works is that well-reasoned decisions, decisions based on full argument, tend to set precedent." Technically, the Carder case should protect pregnant women in all 50 states. There is never a situation where the court can compel an adult to undergo a medical procedure for the perceived benefit of another human being. Even if a father's kidney would save his own son's life, the state cannot compel that father to submit to surgery. The Carder appeal reaffirmed that women are not stripped of these constitutional rights when they become pregnant. "But none of that can counteract the enormous effect of 30 years of political advocacy claiming the rights of fetuses and denying the rights of women," says Paltrow.

To illustrate her point, Paltrow introduces me to another story, that of Theresa Hernandez. As of this writing, 30-year-old Hernandez sits in prison in Oklahoma City, awaiting trial on a first-degree murder charge for suffering a stillbirth and testing positive for methamphetamine. What is the connection between her case and Carder's? Fetal rights.

Hernandez is one of more than 300 women around the country who have been charged with abusing their children *before* they're born, on the basis of legislation and rhetoric that promote the fetus as a full person with constitutional rights. In South Carolina, the only state with a child abuse law covering "viable fetuses," Regina McKnight—22 years old and homeless when she suffered a stillbirth in 1999—is serving 12 years in prison for homicide. These women are being prosecuted for a crime that doesn't exist, argues Paltrow (she believes the South Carolina law will be found unconstitutional, even though the Supreme Court has so far declined to hear McKnight's case). "We have at least 30 or 40 appellate decisions now and 5 or 6 state supreme court decisions saying you can't do this; and we're seeing as many cases as we've ever seen," says Paltrow. "This notion that you can control and punish a woman in relationship to her pregnancy is so pervasive that legal precedent means very little."

As Paltrow is quick to point out, the campaign for fetal rights, led by those intent on re-criminalizing and stigmatizing abortion, has been a detriment to women who decide to carry their pregnancies to term. "You can't have a 'culture of life' if you don't value the women who *give* that life," she is fond of saying. The drug-addicted women Paltrow represents often identify as pro-life. But rarely do they have access to drug treatment—most programs won't take pregnant women for fear of liability. If incarcerated, many of these women will end up giving birth in shackles.[7] They may be denied custody of their children and forced to put them up for adoption. Ironically, the threat of such punitive action may drive these women to get abortions.

Drug screens, routinely ordered without a patient's express consent, similarly deter women from prenatal care. "We're getting lots of calls from women who say, 'I smoked a little marijuana while I was pregnant, it helped me with my morning sickness. They tested me during delivery, child welfare took my child and all of my other children. Can you help me?'" says Paltrow. "And you know, I just want to start crying. There's no question that that's an abuse of state authority. Child welfare laws are intended to protect children from people who can't parent, not from people who have done any number of things that may or may not be illegal."

Paltrow founded NAPW to focus on these prosecutions but tells me that in the past few years, her office has turned into a hotline for mothers who feel that the obstetric care they received violated their rights. An increasing number of calls, says Paltrow, are from women who were given episiotomies that they refused and therefore want to press assault charges. She's getting calls from women whose local hospitals have banned VBAC and want to bring a suit. And she gets calls from women who are being threatened with forced surgery. "We're getting more and more of these calls, and we don't have the staff to deal with it," she says.

Paltrow adds that an episiotomy that's not consented to *is* assault. "It is certainly a form of battery to cut somebody when they've told you not to." That's how the doctrine of informed consent was born—without consent, invading another person's body is a crime. But no lawyer would touch such a case, she says, first because there would be no money in it, and second because a medical procedure isn't considered "damage" in and of itself. What a woman may consider assault, the court considers standard of care. "But it does fit the definition of a crime," says Paltrow.

What women eat, drink, smoke, or inject during pregnancy, however, does not fit the definition of a crime. Paltrow argues that these prosecutions are purely punitive and that they disproportionately affect poor women and women of color. She also maintains that they must be seen in the context of a culture that celebrates the woman who conceives quadruplets after multiple fertility treatments—treatments that put the fetuses at risk for severe prematurity, neurological damage, and death— yet imprisons the woman who puts her fetus at far less risk with illegal drug use. "These issues are not just problems of fetal rights, they're not just problems relating to pregnancy. They're also profoundly about race and class and our legal system," says Paltrow.

And they are profoundly about how we treat women. Paltrow reframes the debate: "The question is not when do fetuses have rights, but at what point in pregnancy do women's civil rights end?"

IS VAGINAL BIRTH A PROCEDURE?

The question of pregnant women's rights lands on the doorstep of the hospital that bans vaginal birth after cesarean. Do women have the right to give birth vaginally?

Howard Minkoff, MD, vice chair of the ethics committee of the American College of Obstetricians and Gynecologists, answers by saying that you can't force a woman to have surgery. "Nobody can make her go to the operating room. If she shows up in labor, her right is to not be taken to the operating room against her will." Minkoff explains that patients' rights are both affirmative and negative. The former is a demand: Fix my broken arm. Give me a cesarean. Give me fluids. The affirmative right is limited. It has to be consistent with what the physician believes is good care. "You can't say, 'You know doctor, not only do I want a cesarean section, but while you're there, take out my gall bladder and my right kidney,'" offers Minkoff by way of example. On the flip side, a negative right is the right to refuse a treatment, and this, Minkoff says, is absolute. "Autonomy is an unlimited, unimpeded negative right. A pregnant woman, any woman, has the right to refuse *anything*."

Rarely does this come up, though. "Women are remarkably reliable shepherds of the well-being of their child," says Minkoff. "They almost always do what a physician would have wanted them to do." Those two things don't always jibe, however, and Minkoff says that when women refuse treatment, "the results are more demonstrative of physician fallibility than of patient errors in judgment. In other words, the patient ran away from the hospital because they said, 'You'll never be able to have this baby vaginally,' and she went somewhere else and delivered the baby vaginally." (Indeed, Wilkes-Barre General Hospital argued in its court petition that there existed an "imminent threat of irreparable harm" to the Marlowe fetus.) The concept of a pervasive "maternal–fetal conflict," says Minkoff, is misguided.

The maternal–medical conflict, however, is real. Physicians have a right to refuse to perform procedures that they don't deem safe. But "safety" is dictated increasingly by liability rather than medical evidence. "So the question becomes: Is there ever a circumstance for a physician to have the right to refuse a VBAC?" asks Minkoff.

Barbara Stratton is an activist in Baltimore, Maryland. When she found out that her local hospital, Frederick Memorial, instituted an official VBAC ban, she organized a grassroots campaign, drew a crowd of moms and babies to rally in the freezing cold, and, with the help of the International Cesarean Awareness Network, placed a front-page story in the *New York Times*, which was followed by stories in the *Washington Post* and *USA Today*. Two years later, hospital administrators reversed the ban.

But Stratton wants a legal solution for the hundreds of hospitals and legions of physicians nationwide who continue to tell women, "No VBAC." Stratton spoke with a state attorney general. She called up the state Medicaid office and the Joint Commission for Accreditation of Health Care Organizations, both of which require hospitals to have and honor a Patients' Bill of Rights. Her question is this: How can a VBAC refusal coexist with a patient's right to refuse treatment? "The answer we keep getting is 'We can't force any hospital that doesn't want to offer a certain procedure to offer one,'" Stratton tells me. "To which *we* say, VBAC is not a procedure, it's the end of pregnancy, it's the normal outcome, and if you take away VBAC, you are forcing people to *have* a procedure against their will."

Is vaginal birth a *procedure*, as Joseph DeLee famously made it out to be when he advocated "prophylactic forceps" in 1921?[8] No and yes. For a woman, vaginal birth is not a procedure. It is her body's way of con- cluding a pregnancy, that automatic sequence of hormones and muscle reflexes, the painful/ecstatic mother–baby dance we may never fully understand. And a woman has a constitutional right to refuse all proce- dures that would impede that process. For physicians, however, *attending* a vaginal birth is understood as a procedure, even if the woman's body does everything and all they do is catch the baby. They get paid for doing it, and they can be sued for doing it. Many hospitals share this point of view.

The choice between VBAC and repeat surgery "should be a personal decision," says Minkoff. At the same time, however, he says that a physician has a right to refuse to "participate" in a case that she feels is unsafe, and that a hospital that does not meet ACOG's standard of care— with 24-hour "immediate" surgical capabilities—is justified in having a "No VBAC" policy. "But then I think that the system owes something to the patient," says Minkoff. He compares the controversy over VBAC to the controversy over the morning-after pill, which some believe is equiv- alent to abortion. "If an individual pharmacist in a drug store will not give a woman emergency contraception, that's fine, but that drug store has to make sure it's provided."

Yet there are no simple remedies for a woman with a scar on her uterus who shows up to give birth vaginally at an unfriendly hospital, says Minkoff. The nearest hospital that meets ACOG's standard may be too far away, and there may not be a physician in the area who feels comfortable attending. On the other hand, you can't force a woman into surgery. So what is a small hospital to do? What is a physician whose insurance policy doesn't cover VBAC to do?

Do pregnant women lose their constitutional rights when their physician is not on call? Can hospitals ethically ban VBAC? Do insurance companies violate women's rights when they withhold coverage for vaginal birth?

It surprises me that these questions have not attracted more attention from bioethicists and reproductive rights organizations. There is extensive scholarship on court-ordered cesareans and other cases of explicitly forced medical treatment in pregnant women. On the subject of VBAC denials, however, almost nothing. Birgitta Sujdak-Mackiewicz, a PhD candidate at St. Louis University, wrote a paper on the subject and spoke at an American Society for Bioethics and Humanities meeting in 2006. "Most bioethicists haven't tackled this issue, which to me is bizarre," she told me. "Women are being forced into major abdominal surgery."

Although informed of this issue, women's rights groups have taken no action. Barbara Stratton called every women's health, reproductive rights, and feminist legal organization she could find to take on the issue: the National Organization for Women, the Center for Reproductive Rights, the National Women's Health Network, Planned Parenthood, NARAL, the list goes on. Not one group offered to platform the issue. Some had never heard of VBAC. "Groups say they're about reproductive rights, but it's really not about the full spectrum of reproductive rights; it's all just about abortion," says Stratton. Finally someone referred her to the National Advocates for Pregnant Women. Paltrow, who does see VBAC as a reproductive rights issue, is searching for a lawyer willing to try a test case, but thus far she has found none.

The National Organization for Women did pass a strongly worded resolution on VBAC in December 2005, after much lobbying by Stratton and other members of ICAN, but there has been no other sign of NOW's commitment to the issue.

I asked Paltrow whether vaginal birth is a procedure that can be denied. "I would argue it's not. It's not a procedure," she said. "And as is often the case with claims of fears of liability and institutional protection, those fears have very little foundation in reality." Susan Jenkins, the attorney formerly with the American College of Nurse–Midwives agrees, and argues that insurance companies settle cases that would have no legs in court, and that the climate amounts to hysteria. "None of this is evidence based, and it's certainly not based on law," she says. "I think the insurance companies are just out of control and are making bad judgments." In fact, forcing a woman into surgery can cost a hospital dearly. George Washington Hospital settled a civil suit brought by Angela Carder's family for an undisclosed sum and subsequently revised its policy to emphasize pregnant patients' rights and avoid future litigation.

From a legal standpoint, the moment a woman says, "I do not want a C-section" or "I do not want continuous electronic fetal monitoring," a hospital's or physician's fear of liability is irrelevant. The protocol is to document the patient's decision and move on. Caregivers' duty is to provide care and honor patients' rights.

But often that's not how it plays out in the delivery room. Like Pemberton, women are given ultimatums. Not only women seeking VBACs, but all obstetric patients, are told, in essence: you can give birth here *if* you don't go too far past your due date, *if* your water hasn't been broken more than a few hours, *if* your baby is head down, *if* your baby looks small enough, *if* your pelvis looks big enough, if your cervix is dilating fast enough, *if* you'll wear this monitor and stay in bed, *if* you'll have some Pitocin, *if* you'll let us break your water, *if* you'll lie on your back and push when we tell you to push.

The women with scars, with twins, and with breech babies are in the most extreme predicament. They are often forced to choose between a cesarean with a physician and a home birth with a midwife. In some cases, their only alternative is a home birth with no trained attendant at all. Those are not reasonable options for most women, so they accept surgery, no court order required.

But how different are these women from the women who are forced by lawyers or court orders? Is their consent fully informed? Is it given freely? A woman's right to refuse is naturally dependent on her willingness to confront entrenched medical and legal authority, which has the backing of the state. It's not unheard of for a woman who refuses treatment or chooses a home birth to be visited by social services.

Erica Lyon, who runs an independent childbirth education center in New York City called Realbirth, says she spends a lot of time in classes just "teaching women how to say 'No.'" She calls this "informed dissent." "We're teaching them to say no to the monitor, no to Pitocin, no to the Cytotec . . .," says Lyon.

There's a concept in law called "undue burden." The term, which is understood as an excessive difficulty or expense, applies to abortion: the Supreme Court has ruled that a state can't create so many obstacles to the procedure that the woman's right to it is rendered meaningless. Is it an undue burden for a woman seeking optimal maternity care in the United States to have to pay thousands of dollars out of pocket for a midwife that her insurance won't cover? to have to travel to another state to avoid a cesarean? to have to give birth in a motel? or labor in a parking lot? or spend her entire birth experience saying "No"?

Ashley Dees regrets going to the hospital for her VBAC and is planning to give birth at home next time. "There was no peace to it," she told me. "It wasn't like we birthed the baby, it was like we went and picked a fight. And I don't think it should be a fight to have a baby."

A SCATTERED MINORITY

Who owns birth? Women or doctors?

A perinatologist who experienced the births of his own children at home explains to me why the hospital is a strange place for normal birth. "If you're a first-time mom, you're strong, and you're scared to death. And when you're strong and scared to death, you can't relax and let the baby fall in your pelvis. You've never hurt like that before. So until you're completely tuckered out, you can hold that baby in there for a really long time—hours, a day. And nobody's helping you try to relax."

When you're not relaxed, you're not dilating. Medicine calls this "arrestive dilation" and treats it with synthetic oxytocin, which requires the use of an intrauterine catheter, then an epidural, "so intervention leads to intervention," he says. "Also, in the hospital you're typically monitored while sitting or lying, mostly lying, which is not a typical mammalian position during labor. Animals get up, move around, sit down, stand up, move around. They don't just lie there in labor."

There are reasons to be in the hospital, and advantages to modern technology, he acknowledges, "but does everybody need to be in the hospital? Whose choice is it? Is there a choice or is there not for delivering at home? Can you be supported at home? Is there somebody who can attend your birth?" he asks. "I would be on the choice side always; it's not my life. You choose, I support you."

Wisconsin state representative and obstetrician–gynecologist Sheldon Wasserman, MD, articulates a similar philosophy and voted in 2006 for a bill licensing certified professional midwives. "I believe very strongly that people have a right to decide. You have a right to decide on abortion, you have a right to decide on contraception. Don't you also have a right to decide where you have a baby, where you have your birth experience?"

The Wisconsin bill was signed into law by governor Jim Doyle in April 2006, in spite of strong opposition from the Wisconsin chapter of ACOG, which released a position paper asserting that the only legitimate midwives are nurse–midwives, who work in collaboration with physicians, and that the bill would create "less safety for childbirth in Wisconsin" and would "devalue the meaning of 'trained midwife.'" The group also noted that "other states are *coping* with this same issue and have asked to use this position paper in their *fight* against licensing professional midwives" (my emphasis).

Wasserman wishes his colleagues would relax, not only in the legislative arena but also in the delivery room. "Some women are seeking a different type of experience. I don't think we should be so threatened by that," he says.

Wasserman tells me about his mentor, an old-fashioned, unflappable man who taught him to respect the physiological process, catch the baby, put it on its mother's breast, and then "sit back and put your feet up." "Then I saw other doctors. As soon as the baby is out, it's clamp, clamp, cut the cord, suction the face, rush the baby over to the intensive care bed, call the neonatologists. Every single baby! I couldn't understand it. Where's the emergency? Just let the kid breathe!"

Wasserman is a committed "noninterventionist." He rarely induces, he refuses to do elective cesareans, he strongly encourages VBAC, he delivers twins vaginally, he encourages intermittent fetal monitoring so that his patients can walk around, and he gets up in the middle of the night. The day I meet with him, he's on call, and he had been back and forth to the hospital three times to attend three births, all vaginal, between 2:00 a.m. and 7:00 a.m. the night before. "Babies come when they want to come, not when I want them," he says, yawning.

As Wasserman talks, he almost sounds like a doula fending off the encroachments of the hospital's time clock and rituals. He tells me about the gratuitous interference he sees every day. "Just this morning," he tells me, a resident was delivering a baby and was about to clamp the cord. "I said, 'Slow down. No. No clamping. Put the baby—just put the baby on the mother.' 'But everyone else clamps,' she said. 'Well I don't.' 'Why don't you?' I said, 'Look at the baby, does it need to be clamped? Let the baby get its blood supply! Ten percent of all stem cells are in the cord. Stem cells are this big controversial thing, and you're cheating this baby out of its own stem cells!'"

Across the country, there are physicians who support midwives, practically and philosophically. I've never spoken with a midwife, illegal or otherwise, who didn't have some sort of collegial relationship with at least one obstetrician. This silent, scattered minority have also supported legislation to decriminalize midwives and home birth. But not without incurring the ire of their colleagues and in flagrant opposition to ACOG, which as an organization "does not support the provision of care by lay midwives or other midwives"[9] and "does not support programs or individuals that advocate for or who provide out-of-hospital births."[10]

Both of these statements, reiterated in 2006 by the executive board, come on the heels of the largest, most scientifically rigorous study of out-of-hospital birth in the United States to date, the study of 5000 planned home births attended by certified professional midwives in which 95% of the women gave birth vaginally and babies were born just as safely as those born in the hospital.[11] Without referencing that study or any others, the executive board's statement on out-of-hospital birth claims that the research to date has "not been scientifically rigorous. . . . Until the results of such studies are convincing, ACOG strongly opposes out-of-hospital births."

The statements also come on the heels of successful midwife licensure efforts in Wisconsin and Virginia, as well as formidable campaigns for midwives in Missouri and Indiana.

The legislative victories by midwives and other "allied health professionals" may have also prompted the American Medical Association to launch their 2006 "Scope of Practice Partnership," an initiative to quash efforts by nurse practitioners, midwives, chiropractors, and other providers. *Scope of practice* is the legislative term for the treatments a caregiver is authorized by law to provide. In the 1900s, physicians were the first group of providers to organize and obtain state sanction in the form of licensure, so in the beginning, their "scope" was all-inclusive.[12] In order for professions such as dentistry, podiatry, psychology, and nurse–midwifery to establish themselves, they had to wrest authority from physicians—a process that took decades, and one that seems to be facing a backlash. A senior director for the American Association of Nurse Anesthetists charged that the AMA is "essentially declaring war on providers who are not physicians."[13] And childbirth, with 4 million annual customers, is a market that U.S. physicians will be hard-pressed to give up.

"ACOG is a lobbying organization," says Andrew Garber, MD, the director of maternal–fetal medicine in New Jersey who works with licensed midwives. "It is also an educational organization, but lobbying is a big part of what they do. That's why they're in Washington." Acknowledging that giving birth out-of-hospital with midwives is safe is not in their best interest.

ACOG has several committees as well as an executive board, each of which meets about twice a year and releases statements, recommendations, and opinions. The obstetric practice bulletins come with a prominent caveat that "these guidelines should not be construed as dictating an exclusive course of treatment or procedure," but the reality is that what ACOG says becomes the legal "standard of care." For example, a recommendation that induction be offered after 41 weeks gestation may become Exhibit A in a malpractice suit against a physician for a stillbirth: the baby would have lived had the pregnancy not been allowed to continue beyond 41 weeks.

As influential as these statements are, however, the practice bulletins are difficult for the general public to access. Nor are they necessarily evidence-based. A 2006 analysis of ACOG obstetric recommendations found that only 23% were based on "good and consistent scientific evidence" and that nearly half were based primarily on consensus and expert opinion, the weakest level of evidence.[14]

And the various ACOG committee statements often contradict themselves. Nowhere is this contradiction more apparent than in ACOG's recommendations on VBAC.[15] Even though Minkoff and the ethics committee are clear—you cannot force a woman into the operating room—what else can be implied by a policy that restricts vaginal birth to certain facilities and to certain patients? Nowhere is the issue of women's autonomy addressed, nor has ACOG taken responsibility for the policy's effect, which has been that hundreds of hospitals across the country have officially banned vaginal birth for women with cesarean scars, leaving many, many women with no real choice whatsoever. "Right now there's no recourse for a woman being dragged into the OR," says Racquel Lazer-Paley, an attorney hoping to bring a large class-action lawsuit against hospitals that deny VBAC.

The committee responsible for the VBAC policy is the obstetric practice committee, chaired by Gary Hankins, MD. In my conversation with him, he did not address the issue of women's autonomy; only physicians' and hospitals' autonomy. In regard to the VBAC bans, Hankins said hospitals without 24-hour immediate surgical capabilities "shouldn't be in the business. I presume those hospitals cannot provide that service." But VBAC is unavailable and sometimes officially banned even at large teaching hospitals, as it was at Frederick Memorial in Maryland, and many physicians have taken the ACOG guidelines as reason enough to stop offering VBAC. ACOG has not come to terms with the probable and widespread ethics violations attendant on this policy, and to date has shown no intention of doing so. I asked Benson Harer, who was instrumental in revising the VBAC standard of care, what recourse a woman has if she can find no provider or facility in her region. "Well, she has to travel to where she can get it," he said. "We have the same thing with abortion. If it's not available in the State of Alaska, then you go to Washington."

A REPRODUCTIVE RIGHT

In 1990, the authors of *Our Bodies, Ourselves*, the National Black Women's Health Project, and the National Women's Health Network collaborated on a position paper titled *Childbearing Policy Within a National Health Program: An Evolving Consensus for New Directions*. They re-released it in 1994 during the Clinton administration, when there was great optimism for universal healthcare. The paper argues for a "Primary Maternity Care System," one in which midwives would serve as the primary caregivers and all women would have access to birthing centers:

> There is an urgent need to replace the present system of front-line, high-technology, acute and specialist care with a Primary Maternity Care System. . . . Our national health program should recognize the midwife as the appropriate caregiver for most childbearing women and should provide broad support for widespread implementation of a midwifery approach to care. . . . Similarly, the freestanding birth center is a small-scale, health-oriented, accessible and highly appropriate setting for Primary Maternity Care. Our national health program should encourage the development and use of such centers and support the choice of home birth. These forms of Primary Maternity Care are highly beneficial in that they are safe, enhance access, meet the needs of virtually all childbearing women, involve judicious use of technology, are associated with a highly favorable liability record, are well-received by childbearing women, and are highly cost-effective. . . . We are concerned that the data in support of Primary Maternity Care, which are extensive and readily available in medical and other professional journals, are widely ignored.[16]

"It was a cult favorite," says Carol Sakala, who worked on the document. But it fell to the wayside once the Clinton administration was over. "I like to say that reproductive rights is about everything but reproducing," says Sakala. Even the grant money available under the "reproductive rights" heading is for contraception, STD prevention, and abortion—"maternity care is just off the radar screen," she says.

What's interesting is that in the absence of an organized feminist response, there is a "birthing rights" movement emerging. Across the country there are "birth circles" and "birth meet-ups" in which women swap books and watch birth videos—Goorchenko's unassisted twin birth is a popular one—and "facilitators" talk to pregnant women about the realities of hospital labor management and the politics of home birth. Linda Bennett, the retired midwife who helps women connect with underground or traveling home-birth midwives, sees her work as parallel to the underground networks that led women to safe abortions before *Roe v. Wade*. "To me, reproductive rights should still be the focus," says Bennett. "I still trust women to be able to make the right choices for themselves, and that includes birth." Many of the illegal home-birth midwives, even those who are vehemently opposed to abortion, defend their criminal activity in terms of protecting women's *choices*.

One group, called the Trust Birth Initiative, has announced Labor Day as "Take Birth Back" day and is organizing women to hand out cards that say things like "Birth is safe, Interference is risky" at beaches and malls and parks. "The goal is to get women to question what is happening to them and encourage them to take charge of all the decisions about their own births," say the organizing materials.

Many leaders of this grassroots movement locate birthing rights within the larger framework of reproductive rights. "We absolutely believe that reproductive rights extend beyond the choice of whether to have a child, to where to have the child, with whom to have the child, and in what manner. And those choices are under attack," argues Elan McAllister, a New York doula who founded the consumer education group Choices in Childbirth.

Erica Lyon, the New York childbirth educator, puts it in some of the strongest language. Women are vulnerable in pregnancy, she argues. Even if they are highly educated, professionally successful, and in control of their lives in every way, they are relying on the external authority of healthcare providers and institutions during pregnancy and childbirth. "And if that external authority is not responsible for holding appropriate clinical boundaries, that woman is in an abusive situation," says Lyon. "If the information she's receiving does not give her power, she is in an abusive situation."

Childbirth Connection, the group that conducted the *Listening to Mothers* surveys, distributes a brochure called "Every Woman's Rights." There are 20 rights listed, including a woman's right to "choose her birth setting," to enjoy "freedom of movement during labor," to "give birth in a position of her choice," and to have "virtually uninterrupted contact with her newborn from the moment of birth."

Even Amber and John Marlowe, who narrowly escaped a court-ordered cesarean, see the right to a physiological birth in the context of their rights as citizens of a democracy. Their belief in this is so strong that the couple, who believe in the Bible and believe that abortion is murder, traveled to Washington, DC, in April 2003 to march in the pro-choice "March for Women's Lives." John Marlowe told me they marched because after Amber's ordeal, they realized that if the government can restrict a woman's right to abortion, then it can force a woman to have a cesarean. "We don't believe in abortion for any reason, period. But we marched pro-choice because this is America. Are we going to be a majority that gives up our choices to a doctor or a politician?"

So it surprised me to hear Wendy Chavkin, MD, chair of Physicians for Reproductive Choice and Health, a longtime advocate of abortion access and social justice, state that birth has no place under the umbrella of reproductive rights. I asked her, Do women have the right to choose where they give birth and with whom they give birth? "No," she said.

Chavkin penned an amicus curiae ("friend of the court") brief in support of Paltrow's appeal of the decision that forced Angela Carder to the operating room, yet she defends hospitals and physicians that have policies prohibiting vaginal birth after cesarean. Like many within the medical field, Chavkin has come to see physiological childbirth as an inherently dangerous procedure that can be withheld.

In the decades prior to *Roe v. Wade*, physicians decided whether women deserved "therapeutic" abortions. Feminists argued that the decision to have or not to have an abortion was one that women had a right to make because women were the ones who had to live with the consequences. Women's bodies, women's choice. Yet the argument for the right to abortion wasn't necessarily grounded in bodily integrity, but in equality: women could never achieve full social, economic, and political participation without control over their reproductive lives. Abortion was a proxy for equal rights.

This may explain why mainstream American feminist groups have been slow to recognize the right *to* reproduce along with the right to be free *from* reproducing. A focus of the second-wave women's movement was shaking off motherhood as what solely defined womanhood. So perhaps there has been a reluctance to watch over the process that makes women mothers. "I think this is the last leap for the feminist movement," says Erica Lyon. "This is the last issue for women in terms of actual ownership of our bodies."

In January 2007, Paltrow organized a "National Summit to Ensure the Health and Humanity of Pregnant and Birthing Women." One of her goals was to convince feminists that they need to pay attention to maternity care, and to convince pro-lifers that they need to let go of fetal rights. Women's autonomy means both the right to legal abortion and the right to a vaginal birth after cesarean—you can't have one without the other. Paltrow loves to tease out these unlikely connections. She points to the irony of there being hundreds of laws restricting abortion access but not one law prohibiting the shackling of incarcerated women in labor. The profusion of so-called "informed consent" laws mandating what information abortion providers can give their patients contrasts with there being only two states to mandate that hospitals disclose their cesarean rates. "There are not two kinds of women—women who have abortions and women who have babies," Paltrow told the crowd of 300 gathered in Atlanta over 3 days.

Chavkin, who declined an invitation to attend the summit, does not see childbirth as a reproductive right. To her, it is a medical issue, one that may need reform, but one that belongs under the purview of physicians. "To my mind, I'm all for people having a pleasant and wonderful birth experience," she says. "But my highest priority would be for them to have a safe birth experience."

But what's considered safe is political. What's safe changes. Thirty years ago obstetricians said VBAC was dangerous. Then they said it was safe. Now they've gone back to saying it's dangerous. ACOG says out-of-hospital birth isn't safe, but the research has consistently suggested that for women with normal, uncomplicated pregnancies it is not just safe, but *safer*, because those women are far more likely to have a normal, spontaneous vaginal birth and far less likely to experience harmful, unnecessary interventions.

When ACOG claims that home birth and midwives are unsafe, they imply that the women who choose it and the midwives who provide it are acting irresponsibly and selfishly. They stigmatize normal birth just as the political right has stigmatized abortion. And they stigmatize women.

"Our country has created a mythology of women who are irresponsible and don't care," says Paltrow. "We talk about welfare queens, crack moms, and murderous women who have abortions." A culture that allows such language to permeate our national subconscious inevitably dehumanizes all women, including mothers. Lyon argues that this thinking perpetuates a phrase often invoked in exam rooms and delivery rooms: *The goal is to have a healthy baby.* "This phrase is used over and over and over to shut down women's requests," she says. "The context needs to be that the goal is a healthy mom. Because mothers never make decisions without thinking about that healthy baby. And to suggest otherwise is insulting and degrading and disrespectful."

What's best for women is best for babies. And what's best for women and babies is minimally invasive births that are physically, emotionally, and socially supported. This is not the experience that most women have. In the age of evidence-based medicine, women need to know that standard American maternity care is not primarily driven by their health and well-being or by the health and well-being of their babies. Care is constrained and determined by liability and financial concerns, by a provider's licensing regulations and malpractice insurer. The evidence often has nothing to do with it.

Today women have unprecedented access to the information they need to make the best decisions for themselves—and therefore the best decisions for their babies. They are in fact in a far better position to make evidence-based decisions than their doctors. They have a right to make those decisions, and they *should* make those decisions.

The goal is to have a healthy family.

Effective Care

Each obstetric practice listed here was evaluated by the authors of *A Guide to Effective Care in Pregnancy and Childbirth*, based on a systematic review of the available medical evidence. The complete list, as well as the entire text of *A Guide*, are available at www.childbirthconnection.org.

Included among 40 "Beneficial forms of care":

- Physical, emotional, and psychological support during labor and birth
- Continuous support for women during labor and childbirth
- Active versus expectant management of the third stage of labor
- Unrestricted breastfeeding

Included among 125 "Forms of care likely to be beneficial":

- Adequate access to care for all childbearing women
- Social support for childbearing women
- Midwifery care for women with no serious risk factors
- Respecting women's choice of place of birth

- Freedom of movement and choice of position in labor
- Respecting women's choice of position for the second stage of labor and giving birth
- Maternal movement and position changes to relieve pain in labor
- Superficial heat or cold to relieve pain in labor
- Touch and massage to relieve pain in labor
- Trial of labor after previous lower-segment cesarean section
- Trial of labor after more than one previous lower-segment cesarean section
- Assessing the state of the cervix before induction of labor
- Encouraging early mother–infant contact

Included among 34 "Forms of care with a tradeoff between beneficial and adverse effects":

- Routine ultrasound in early pregnancy
- Routine elective cesarean for breech presentation
- Induction of labor for prelabor rupture of the membranes at term
- Induction instead of surveillance for pregnancy after 41 weeks
- Narcotics to relieve pain in labor
- Epidural analgesia to relieve pain in labor
- Early amniotomy in spontaneous labor
- Prophylactic antibiotic eye ointments to prevent eye infection in the newborn

Included among 96 "Forms of care of unknown effectiveness":

- Bed rest for
  - women with pre-eclampsia
  - impaired fetal growth
  - triplet and higher-order pregnancy
  - to prevent preterm birth
- Sweeping of the membranes to prevent post-term pregnancy
- Early versus late clamping of the umbilical cord at birth

- Early use of oxytocin to augment slow or prolonged labor
- Active management of labor

Included among more than 120 "Forms of care unlikely to be beneficial":

- Routinely involving obstetricians in the care of all women during pregnancy and childbirth
- Not involving obstetricians in the care of women with serious risk factors
- Advice to restrict sexual activity during pregnancy
- Prohibition of *all* alcohol intake during pregnancy
- Routine use of ultrasound for fetal measurement in late pregnancy
- Screening for "gestational diabetes"
- Routine glucose challenge test during pregnancy
- Routine use of Doppler ultrasound screening in all pregnancies
- Bed rest for threatened miscarriage
- Routine cesarean section for multiple pregnancy
- Elective delivery before term in women with otherwise uncomplicated diabetes
- Elective cesarean section for pregnant women with diabetes
- Cesarean section for macrosomia to prevent shoulder dystocia without a trial of labor
- Induction of labor to prevent cephalopelvic disproportion
- Withholding food and drink from women in labor
- Routine intravenous infusion in labor
- Routine measurement of intrauterine pressure during oxytocin administration
- Frequent scheduled vaginal examinations in labor
- Routine directed pushing during the second stage of labor
- Pushing by sustained bearing down during the second stage of labor
- Breath holding during the second stage of labor
- Early bearing down during the second stage of labor
- Arbitrary limitation of the duration of the second stage of labor
- Instrumental vaginal delivery to shorten the second stage of labor

- Routine exteriorization of the uterus for repair of the uterine incision at cesarean section
- Silver nitrate to prevent eye infection in newborn babies
- Routine suctioning of newborn babies
- Medicated bathing of babies to reduce infection
- Routine measurements of temperature, pulse, blood pressure, and fundal height postpartum

Included among 41 "Forms of care likely to be ineffective or harmful":

- Requiring a supine (flat on back) position in the second stage of labor
- Routine use of the lithotomy position for the second stage of labor
- Routine or liberal episiotomy for birth
- Routine restriction of mother–infant contact
- Routine nursery care for babies in the hospital
- Routine supplements of water or formula for breastfed babies
- Samples of formula for breastfeeding mothers

APPENDIX B

The Cesarean Trend

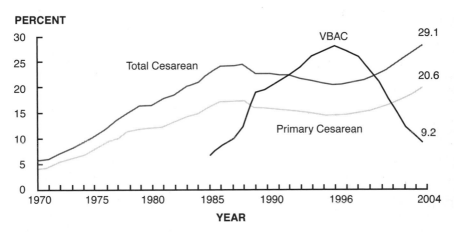

Figure B-1: Total and Primary Cesarean Rate 1970–2004 and VBAC Rate 1985–2004. *Source:* U.S. Centers for Disease Control and Prevention.

Notes

INTRODUCTION

1. George Blonksy and Charlotte Blonsky, 1965. Apparatus for Facilitating the Birth of a Child by Centrifugal Force. US Patent 3,216,423, filed Jan. 15, 1963, and issued Nov. 9, 1965.
2. Millie Sullivan Nelson, "Impact on the General Obstetrical Practitioner," (lecture, NIH State-of-the-Science Conference: Cesarean Delivery on Maternal Request, Bethesda, MD, March 27–29, 2006).
3. Eugene R. Declercq et al., *Listening to Mothers II: Report of the Second National U.S. Survey of Women's Childbearing Experiences* (New York: Childbirth Connection, 2006).
4. B. E. Hamilton et al., National Vital Statistics Report 35, *Births: Preliminary Data for 2005* (Atlanta, forthcoming).
5. Katherine Hartmann et al., "Outcomes of Routine Episiotomy: A Systematic Review," *Journal of the American Medical Association* 293, no. 17 (2005): 2141–48.
6. Declercq et al., *Listening to Mothers II.*
7. Hamilton et al., *Births: Preliminary Data for 2005.*
8. Steven L. Clark and Gary D.V. Hankins, "Temporal and Demographic Trends in Cerebral Palsy—Fact and Fiction," *American Journal of Obstetrics and Gynecology* 188, no. 3 (2003): 628–33.
9. K. D. Kochanek and B. L. Smith, National Vital Statistics Report 52, no. 13, *Deaths: Preliminary Data for 2002* (Atlanta, 2004).
10. World Health Organization, *The World Health Report 2005* (Geneva, 2005).

11. C. Abou Zahr, World Health Organization, *Maternal Mortality in 2000: Estimates Developed by WHO, UNICEF and UNFPA* (Geneva, 2004).

12. Nicholas D. Kristof, "Health Care? Ask Cuba," *New York Times*, January 12, 2005.

13. Stacie E. Geller et al., "Morbidity and Mortality in Pregnancy: Laying the Groundwork for Safe Motherhood," *Women's Health Issues* 16 (2006): 176–88.

14. World Health Organization, *World Health Statistics 2006* (Geneva, 2006).

15. T. A. Wiegers, J. van der Zee, and M. J. Keirse, "Maternity Care in the Netherlands: The Changing Home Birth Rate," *Birth* 25, no. 3 (1998): 190–97.

16. Gina Kolata, "New York Is First State to Try to Curb Caesareans," *New York Times*, January 27, 1989.

17. New York State Department of Health, *New York State Hospital Labor Intervention Statistics 2004* (Albany, 2006).

18. Florida Department of Health, Health Outcome Series, *Cesarean Deliveries in Florida Hospitals 1993–2004* (Tallahassee, 2006).

19. Washington State Department of Health, *Method of Delivery by County of Occurrence 2005* (Olympia, 2006).

20. Vermont Department of Health, Vital Statistics Report, *Type of Delivery by Place* (Burlington, 2003).

21. Tamara Henry, "Women Have Most Frequently Performed Surgery," United Press International, January 14, 1988; National Women's Health Information Center, U.S. Department of Health and Human Services, http//www.womenshealth.gov/faq/hysterectomy.htm (accessed January 2006).

22. Linda Lamb, "Making the Cut," *The (SC) State*, June 4, 2006.

23. G. B. Feldman and J. A. Freiman, "Prophylactic Cesarean Section at Term?" *New England Journal of Medicine* 312, no. 19 (1985): 1264–67; P. R. Overhulse, "The Cesarean Section Rate," *Journal of American Medical Association* 264 (1990): 971; R. W. Hale and W. B. Harer, "Elective Prophylactic Cesarean Delivery," *ACOG Clinical Review* 10, no. 2 (2005).

24. Childbirth Connection, *What Every Pregnant Woman Needs to Know about Cesarean Section* (New York: Childbirth Connection, 2004).

25. Kenneth C. Johnson and Betty-Anne Daviss, "Outcomes of Planned Home Births with Certified Professional Midwives: Large Prospective Study in North America," *British Medical Journal* 330 (2005): 1416.

26. World Health Organization, *Care in Normal Birth* (Geneva, 1997).

27. Marie Woolf and Sophie Goodchild, "Mummy State: Childbirth Revolution" *Independent on Sunday* (London), May 14, 2006.

28. Christiane Northrup (speaking at Birth On Labor Day (BOLD), Symphony Space, New York, NY, September 3, 2006).

29. Ian D. Graham, *Episiotomy: Challenging Obstetric Interventions* (London: Blackwell Science, 1997), 35–37.

30. National Institutes of Health, "Cesarean Childbirth," *NIH Consensus Development Conference Statement Online* 3, no. 6 (1980): 1–30, http://www.consensus.nih.gov/1980/1980Cesarean027html.htm (accessed February 2007).

31. World Health Organization, "Appropriate Technology for Birth," *Lancet* 2, no. 8452 (1985): 436–37.

32. Murray Enkin et al., *A Guide to Effective Care in Pregnancy and Childbirth* (Oxford: Oxford University Press, 2000), 362.
33. Robbie E. Davis-Floyd, *Normal Childbirth: Evidence and Debate*, ed. Soo Downe (Oxford: Churchill Livingstone, 2004), xii.

CHAPTER 1

1. "Roofs Fly, Trucks Move, Tourists Gape," *The Miami Herald*, August 14, 2004.
2. FL Dept. of Health, *Cesarean Deliveries in Florida Hospitals 1993–2004*.
3. Joyce A. Martin et al., National Vital Statistics Report 55, no. 1, *Births: Final Data for 2004* (Atlanta, 2006).
4. Joyce A. Martin et al., National Vital Statistics Report 54, no. 2, *Births: Final Data for 2003* (Atlanta, 2005).
5. Martin et al., *Births: Final Data for 2004*.
6. Steven L. Bloom et al., "Fetal Pulse Oximetry and Cesarean Delivery," *New England Journal of Medicine* 355, no. 21 (2006): 2195–202.
7. Eugene R. Declercq et al., *Listening to Mothers: Report of the First National U.S. Survey of Women's Childbearing Experiences* (New York: Childbirth Connection, 2002); Declercq et al., *Listening to Mothers II*.
8. Lauren Neergaard, "Test May Help Pick Time to Induce Labor," Associated Press, June 5, 2006.
9. Robbie Davis-Floyd, *Birth as an American Rite of Passage* (Berkeley: University of California Press, 1992), 299.
10. American College of Obstetricians and Gynecologists, Practice Bulletin no. 10, *Induction of Labor* (Washington, DC, 1999).
11. Mark A. Zamorski and Wendy S. Biggs, "Management of Suspected Fetal Macrosomia," *American Family Physician* 63, no. 2 (2001): 302–06.
12. Emily Oken et al., "A Nearly Continuous Measure of Birth Weight for Gestational Age Using a United States National Reference," *BMC Pediatrics* 3, no. 6 (2003).
13. Ibid.
14. R. J. Sokol et al., "Risks Preceding Increased Primary Cesarean Birth Rates," *Obstetrics & Gynecology* 59, no. 3 (1982): 340–46.
15. Oken et al., "A Nearly Continuous Measure of Birth Weight."
16. Centers for Disease Control and Prevention, "Diabetes and Women's Health Across the Life Stages: A Public Health Perspective, October 2001," http://www.cdc.gov/diabetes/pubs/women/#2.
17. Richard W. Wertz and Dorothy C. Wertz, *Lying-In: A History of Childbirth in America* (New Haven: Yale University Press, 1989), 264.
18. Zamorski and Biggs, "Management of Suspected Fetal Macrosomia."
19. A. M. Gulmezoglu, C. A. Crowther, and P. Middleton, "Induction of Labour for Improving Birth Outcomes for Women at or Beyond Term," *Cochrane Database of Systematic Reviews* 4 (2006).
20. Savas M. Menticoglou and Philip F. Hall, "Routine Induction of Labour at 41 Weeks Gestation: Nonsensus Consensus," *British Journal of Obstetrics and Gynaecology* 109 (2002): 485–91.

21. Mary E. Hannah et al., "Induction of Labor Compared with Expectant Management for Prelabor Rupture of the Membranes at Term: Term PROM Study Group," *New England Journal of Medicine* 334, no. 16 (1996): 1005–10.

22. Max Mongelli, Mark Wilcox, and Jason Gardosi, "Estimating the Date of Confinement: Ultrasonographic Biometry versus Certain Menstrual Dates," *American Journal of Obstetrics and Gynecology* 174, no. 1 (1996): 278–81.

23. Kathleen R. Simpson, "Perinatal Patient Safety: Management of Oxytocin for Labor Induction and Augmentation," *The American Journal of Maternal/Child Nursing* 29, no. 2 (2004): 136.

24. Kathleen R. Simpson and Kathleen E. Thorman, "Obstetric 'Conveniences' Elective Induction of Labor, Cesarean Birth on Demand, and Other Potentially Unnecessary Interventions," *Journal of Perinatal and Neonatal Nursing* 19, no. 2 (2005): 134–44.

25. Gail Hart, *Research Updates for Midwives: Some Thoughts on the Best of the Evidence,* self-published booklet (Portland, Oregon: 2005).

26. Simpson and Thorman, "Obstetric 'Conveniences.'"

27. Kathleen R. Simpson, Dotti C. James, and G. Eric Knox, "Nurse-Physician Communication during Labor and Birth: Effects on Clinical Outcomes and Patient Safety," *Journal of Obstetric, Gynecologic and Neonatal Nursing* 35, no. 4 (2006): 547–56.

28. Declercq et al., *Listening to Mothers II.*

29. John H. M. Pinkerton, *Advances in Oxytocin Research: Proceedings of a Symposium* (Oxford: Pergamon Press, 1965).

30. Kieran O'Driscoll, R. J. A. Jackson, and J. T. Gallagher, "Prevention of Prolonged Labour," *British Medical Journal* 2 (1969): 477–80.

31. Colm O'Herlihy, "Active Management: A Continuing Benefit in Nulliparous Labor," *Birth* 20, no. 2 (1993): 95–97.

32. James Thornton and Richard Lilford, "Active Management of Labour: Current Knowledge and Research Issues," *British Medical Journal* 309 (1994): 366–69.

33. Herlihy, "Active Management."

34. American Society of Anesthesiologists, "More Women Are Receiving More Pain Relief during Labor," news release, September 19, 2005.

35. Marsden Wagner, "Active Management of Labor," *Birth Gazette* 12, no. 2 (1996): 14–19.

36. D. Spelliscy-Gifford et al., "Lack of Progress in Labor as a Reason for Cesarean," *Obstetrics & Gynecology* 95, no. 4 (2000): 589–95.

37. Roger K. Freeman et al., American College of Obstetricians and Gynecologists, *Evaluation of Cesarean Delivery* (Washington, DC, 2000).

38. Ingrid VanTuinen and Sidney M. Wolfe, *Unnecessary Cesarean Sections: Halting a National Epidemic* (Washington, DC: Public Citizen's Health Research Group, 1992), 27–31.

39. Barbara Bridgman Perkins, *The Medical Delivery Business: Health Reform, Childbirth, and the Economic Order* (Piscataway, NJ: Rutgers University Press, 2004), 38.

40. Barbara Katz Rothman, "The Active Management of Physicians," *Birth* 20, no. 3 (1993): 158–59.

41. Joseph B. DeLee, "The Prophylactic Forceps Operation," *American Journal of Obstetrics and Gynecology* 1 (1920): 34.
42. Wertz and Wertz, *Lying-In*, 55.
43. Charles R. King, "The New York Maternal Mortality Study: A Conflict of Professionalization," *Bulletin of the History of Medicine* 65, no. 4 (1991): 476–502.
44. Brooke Anspach, "The Trend of Modern Obstetrics: What Is the Danger? How Can It Be Changed?" *Transactions of the American Gynecological Society* 48 (1923): 96–105
45. Joseph B. DeLee, "Symposium: To What Extent Should Delivery be Hastened or Assisted by Operative Interference," *American Journal of Obstetrics and Gynecology* 2 (1921): 299.
46. Anspach, "The Trend of Modern Obstetrics."
47. A. G. Diaz et al., "Vertical Position during the First Stage of the Course of Labor, and Neonatal Outcome," *European Journal of Obstetrics, Gynecology, and Reproductive Biology* 11 (1980): 1–7.
48. Amanda Carson Banks, *Birth Chairs, Midwives, and Medicine* (Jackson, MS: University of Mississippi Press, 1999).
49. Leigh Summers, *Bound to Please: A History of the Victorian Corset* (New York: Berg Publishers, 2001).
50. Constance L. Beynon, "The Normal Second Stage of Labor: A Plea for Reform in Its Conduct," *Journal of Obstetrics and Gynaecology of the British Empire* 64, no. 6 (1957): 815–20, reprinted in *Episiotomy and the Second Stage of Labor*, eds. Sheila Kitzinger and Penny Simkin (Seattle: Pennypress, 1984), 23–32.
51. Ibid.
52. WHO, *Care in Normal Birth*.
53. Q. De Marsh, H. Alt, and W. Windle, "The Effect of Depriving the Infant of Its Placental Blood," *Journal of the American Medical Association* 116 (1941): 2568–73, quoted in Doris Haire, *The Cultural Warping of Childbirth: A Special Report* (Seattle: International Childbirth Education Association, 1972).
54. G. C. Anderson et al., "Early Skin-to-Skin Contact for Mothers and Their Healthy Newborn Infants," *Cochrane Database of Systematic Reviews*, no. 2 (2003).
55. WHO, *Care in Normal Birth*.
56. "The Talk of the Town," *New Yorker*, February 1954.
57. U.S. Department of Health and Human Services, *The CDC Guide to Breastfeeding Interventions* (Atlanta, 2005).
58. Bloom et al., "Fetal Pulse Oximetry."
59. H. Phillip, H. Fletcher, and M. Reid, "The Impact of Induced Labour on Postpartum Blood Loss," *Journal of Obstetrics and Gynaecology* 24, no. 1 (2004): 12–15.
60. Judith Rooks, *Midwifery and Childbirth in America* (Philadelphia: Temple University Press, 1997), 55.
61. U.S. Dept. of Health, *CDC Guide to Breastfeeding Interventions*.
62. Heather J. Rowe-Murray and Jane R. W. Fisher, "Baby Friendly Hospital Practices: Cesarean Section Is a Persistent Barrier to Early Initiation of Breastfeeding," *Birth* 29, no. 2 (2002): 124–31.

63. Carson Banks, *Birth Chairs*, 10.
64. Jason Gardosi et al., "Alternative Positions in the Second Stage of Labour: A Randomized Controlled Trial," *British Journal of Obstetrics and Gynaecology* 96, no. 11 (1989): 1290–96.
65. Adrienne Rich, *Of Woman Born: Motherhood as Experience and Institution* (New York: Norton, 1986), 178.
66. Graham, *Episiotomy*, 18.
67. H. J. Garrigues, "The Obstetric Treatment of the Perineum," *American Journal of Obstetrics and Diseases of Women and Children* 13 (1880): 231–63.
68. William Dewees, "Relaxation and Management of the Perineum during Parturition," *Journal of the American Medical Association* 13 (1889): 804–808, 841–848.
69. Graham, *Episiotomy*, 27.
70. R. H. Pomeroy, "Shall We Cut and Reconstruct the Perineum for Every Primipara?" *American Journal of Obstetrics and Diseases of Women and Children* 78 (1918): 211–20.
71. R. A. D. Gillis, "Episiotomy as a Means of Preserving the Pelvic Floor during Labor with a Simple Method of Suture," *American Journal of Surgery* 9, no. 3 (1930): 520–26, quoted in Graham, *Episiotomy*, 50.
72. DeLee, "The Prophylactic Forceps Operation."
73. W. R. Cooke, "Management of Birth Injuries," *American Journal of Surgery* 35, no. 2 (1937): 409–16, quoted in Graham, *Episiotomy*, 33.
74. Perkins, *Medical Delivery Business*, 41.
75. Judith Walzer Leavitt, ed., *Women and Health in America: Historical Readings* (Madison: University of Wisconsin Press, 1984), 141.
76. Graham, *Episiotomy*, 34.
77. Ibid, 110.
78. Anonymous, "Episiotomy," *Lancet* 13 (1968): 75–76.
79. Anonymous, "Pain after Birth," *British Medical Journal* 8 (1973): 565, quoted in Graham, *Episiotomy*, 82.
80. J. R. Green and J. L. Soohoo, "Factors Associated with Rectal Injury in Spontaneous Deliveries," *Obstetrics & Gynecology* 73, no. 5 (1989): 732–38.
81. Hartmann et al., "Outcomes of Routine Episiotomy."
82. M. J. House, "Episiotomy—Indications, Technique and Results," *Midwife, Health Visitor and Community Nurse* 17, no. 1 (1981): 6–9, quoted in Graham, *Episiotomy*, 89.
83. Stephen B. Thacker and H. David Banta, "Benefits and Risks of Episiotomy," *Birth: Issues in Perinatal Care and Education* 9, no. 1 (1982): 25–30; Thacker and Banta, "Benefits and Risks of Episiotomy: An Interpretive Review of the English Language Literature, 1860–1980," *Obstetrical and Gynecological Survey* 38, no. 6 (1983): 322–338.
84. Beverley Chalmers, "WHO Appropriate Technology for Birth Revisited," *British Journal of Obstetrics and Gynaecology* 99, no. 9 (1992): 709–10.
85. J. A. Pritchard and P. C. MacDonald, *Williams Obstetrics*, 16th ed. (New York: Appleton-Century-Crofts, 1980), 430.
86. F. Gary Cunningham et al., eds., *Williams Obstetrics*, 19th ed. (Norwalk, CT: Appleton and Lange, 1993).

87. Hartmann et al., "Outcomes of Routine Episiotomy."
88. Heidi Merkoff, Arlene Eisenberg, and Sandee Hathaway, *What to Expect When You're Expecting*, 3rd ed. (New York: Workman Publishing Company, 2002), 352.
89. Bloom et al., "Fetal Pulse Oximetry."
90. Michael F. Greene, "Obstetricians Still Await a Deus ex Machina," *New England Journal of Medicine* 355, no. 21 (2006): 2247–48.
91. Judith R. Kunisch, "Electronic Fetal Monitors: Marketing Forces and the Resulting Controversy," in *Healing Technology: Feminist Perspectives*, ed. Katherine Ratcliff (Ann Arbor: University of Michigan Press, 1989).
92. Perkins, *Medical Delivery Business*, 133–135.
93. Madeleine H. Shearer, "Fetal Monitoring: For Better or Worse?" in *Compulsory Hospitalization: Freedom of Choice in Childbirth?* vol. 1, eds., Stewart and Stewart (Marble Hill, MO: National Association of Parents and Professionals for Safe Alternatives in Childbirth, 1979), 121–133.
94. Victoria P. Rostow and Roger J. Bulger, eds., *An Interdisciplinary Review*, vol. 2 of *Medical Professional Liability and the Delivery of Obstetrical Care* (Washington, DC: National Academy Press, 1989).
95. Albert D. Haverkamp, "Does Anyone Need Fetal Monitors? Comments Made April 17, 1978 before the U.S. Senate Sub-Committee on Health" in *Compulsory Hospitalization: Freedom Of Choice In Childbirth?*, vol. 1, eds., Stewart and Stewart (Marble Hill, MO: National Association of Parents and Professionals for Safe Alternatives in Childbirth, 1979), 135–139.
96. Kunisch, "Electronic Fetal Monitors."
97. H. David Banta and Stephen B. Thacker, National Center for Health Services Research, *Costs and Benefits of Electronic Fetal Monitoring: A Review of the Literature* (Washington, DC, 1979).
98. Kunisch, "Electronic Fetal Monitors."
99. Institute of Medicine, *Assessing Medical Technologies* (Washington, DC: National Academy Press, 1985).
100. William Booth, "When Medical High Tech Isn't Necessarily Better: Fetal Monitors Widely Used, Often Unneeded," *The Washington Post*, October 29, 1991.
101. Robert Resnik, "Can a 29% Cesarean Rate Possibly Be Justified?" *Obstetrics & Gynecology* 107 (2006): 752–54.
102. Greene, "Obstetricians Still Await."
103. WHO, *Care in Normal Birth*.
104. Soo Downe, ed., *Normal Childbirth: Evidence and Debate* (Oxford: Churchill Livingstone, 2004).
105. U.S. Preventive Services Task Force, *Guide to Clinical Preventive Services: An Assessment of the Effectiveness of 169 Interventions* (Baltimore: Williams & Wilkins, 1989).
106. Iain Chalmers and Martin Richards, "Intervention and Causal Interference in Obstetric Practice" in *Benefits and Hazards of the New Obstetrics*, eds. Tim Chard and Martin Richards (London: Heinemann Medical, 1977).
107. Iain Chalmers, Murray Enkin, and Marc Keirse, eds., *Effective Care in Pregnancy and Childbirth* (Oxford: Oxford University Press, 1989).

108. Enkin et al., *A Guide to Effective Care in Pregnancy and Childbirth.*
109. Marjorie Tew, *Safer Childbirth? A Critical History of Maternity Care* (London: Free Association Books, 1998).
110. Wagner, "Active Management of Labor."
111. Enkin et al., *A Guide to Effective Care*, 297.
112. Gina Kolata, "Less Prenatal Care Urged for Most Healthy Women," *New York Times*, October 4, 1989.
113. Judith P. Rooks et al., "Outcomes of Care in Birth Centers: The National Birth Center Study," *New England Journal of Medicine* 321, no. 26 (1989): 1804–11.
114. Harry Fields, John W. Greene, and Kaighn Smith, *Induction of Labor* (New York: Macmillan, 1965).
115. Charles B. Reed, "Induction of Labor at Term," *Transactions of the American Gynecological Society* 45 (1920): 40.
116. Perkins, *The Medical Delivery Business*, 38.
117. Fields et al., *Induction of Labor*, 45–62.
118. Reed, "Induction of Labor at Term."
119. Fields et al., *Induction of Labor*, 12.
120. J. Stearns, "Account of the Pulvis Parturiens: A Remedy for Quickening Childbirth," *Medical Repository of New York* 11 (1808): 308–309, quoted in Thomas F. Baskett, "The Development of Oxytocic Drugs in the Management of Postpartum Haemorrhage," *Ulsters Medical Journal* (2004).
121. K. O'Driscoll and D. Meagher, *Active Management of Labour*, 2nd ed. (London: Bailliere Tindall, 1986).
122. Fields et al., *Induction of Labor*, 80.
123. Ibid., 81.
124. ACOG, *Induction of Labor.*
125. MD Advantage, http://www.mdadvantageonline.com/about (accessed December 2006).

CHAPTER 2

1. New Jersey Department of Health and Senior Services, Center for Health Statistics, *Births by Method of Delivery and NJ Facility Occurrence 2004* (Trenton, 2006).
2. WHO, "Appropriate Technology for Birth"; Jose Villar et al., "Caesarean Delivery Rates and Pregnancy Outcomes: The 2005 WHO Global Survey on Maternal and Perinatal Health in Latin America," *Lancet* 367 (2006): 1819–29.
3. Marian F. MacDorman et al., "For Low-Risk Women, Risk of Death May Be Higher for Babies Delivered by Cesarean," *Birth* 33, no. 3 (2006): 175–82.
4. Martin et al., *Births: Final Data for 2004.*
5. Governor Jon Corzine of New Jersey, Executive Department Proclamation, March 24, 2006.
6. New Jersey Department of Health and Senior Services, Center for Health Statistics, *Births by Method of Delivery and NJ Facility Occurrence 1992* (Trenton, 2006).
7. HealthGrades Quality Study, 3rd Annual Report on Patient Choice, *Cesarean Rates in the United States* (Golden, CO, 2005).

8.   American College of Obstetricians and Gynecologists, "Gallup Survey Reveals Women Ob-Gyns Benefit from 'Insider Knowledge,'" news release, December 9, 2003.

9.   R. Al-Mufti, A. McCarthy, and N. M. Fisk, "Survey of Obstetricians' Personal Preference and Discretionary Practice," *European Journal of Obstetrics, Gynecology, and Reproductive Biology* 73 (1997): 1–4.

10. Kimberly D. Gregory et al., "Using Administrative Data to Identify Indications for Elective Primary Cesarean Delivery," *Health Services Research* 37, no. 5 (2002): 1387.

11. Joshua Press, Michael C. Klein, and Peter von Dadelszen, "Mode of Delivery and Pelvic Floor Dysfunction: A Systematic Review of the Literature on Urinary and Fecal Incontinence and Sexual Dysfunction by Mode of Delivery," *Medscape* (2006).

12. G. M. Buchsbaum et al., "Prevalence of Urinary Incontinence and Associated Risk Factors in a Cohort of Nuns," *Obstetrics & Gynecology* 100, no. 2 (2002): 226–29.

13. G. M. Buchsbaum et al., "Urinary Incontinence in Nulliparous Women and Their Parous Sisters," *Obstetrics & Gynecology* 106, no. 6 (2005): 1253–58.

14. Press, Klein, and von Dadelszen, "Mode of Delivery and Pelvic Floor Dysfunction."

15. Hartmann et al., "Outcomes of Routine Episiotomy."

16. George B. Feldman and Jennie A. Freiman, "Prophylactic Cesarean Section at Term?" *New England Journal of Medicine* 312, no. 19 (1985): 1264–67.

17. W. B. Harer, "Patient Choice Cesarean," *ACOG Clinical Review* 5, no. 2 (2000); W. B. Harer, "Quo Vadis Cesarean Delivery?" *Obstetrical and Gynecological Survey* 57 (2002): 61–64; R. W. Hale and W. B. Harer, "Elective Prophylactic Cesarean Delivery," *ACOG Clinical Review* 10, no. 2 (2005).

18. American College of Obstetricians and Gynecologists, Committee Opinion no. 289, *Surgery and Patient Choice: The Ethics of Decision Making*, printed in *Obstetrics & Gynecology* 102, no. 5 (2003): 1101–06.

19. National Institutes of Health, "State-of-the-Science Conference Statement: Cesarean Delivery on Maternal Request," *Obstetrics & Gynecology* 107 (2006): 1386–97.

20. Carolyn Susman, "More Women Are Demanding Caesareans," Cox News Service, July 12, 2006.

21. Declercq et al., *Listening to Mothers II.*

22. Marie McCullough, "C-Section Trend Reemerges," *Philadelphia Inquirer,* March 25, 2001.

23. Laura Berman, "Too Posh to Push?" *Chicago Sun-Times,* August 9, 2004.

24. D. J. Tuffnell, J. West, and S. A. Walkinshaw, "Treatments for Gestational Diabetes and Impaired Glucose Tolerance in Pregnancy," *The Cochrane Database of Systematic Reviews* 4 (2006).

25. P. Woodgate et al., "Intramuscular Penicillin for the Prevention of Early Onset Group B Streptococcal Infection in Newborn Infants," *The Cochrane Database of Systematic Reviews* 4 (2006).

26. Perkins, *Medical Delivery Business,* 104.

27. K. M. Hofberg and I. F. Brockington, "Tokophobia: An Unreasoning Dread of Childbirth," *British Journal of Psychiatry* 176 (2000): 83–85.
28. Mississippi Department of Health, *Percent of C-Section Deliveries Performed during 2005* (Jackson, 2006).
29. Ibid.
30. Declercq et al., *Listening to Mothers II.*
31. Fay Menacker, Eugene Declercq, and Marian F. MacDorman, "Cesarean Delivery: Background, Trends, and Epidemiology," *Seminars in Perinatology* 30, no. 5 (2006): 235–41.
32. Wisconsin Department of Health and Family Services, St. Mary's Hospital, *Births Occurring in Milwaukee Birthing Hospitals 1989–2004* (Madison, 2006); Massachusetts Department of Public Health, Newton-Wellesley Hospital, *Massachusetts Births 2005* (Boston, 2007).
33. Mississippi Department of Health, South Sunflower County Hospital, *Percent of C-Section Deliveries Performed During 2005* (Jackson, 2006); New Jersey Department of Health and Senior Services, Kimball Medical Center, *Births by Method of Delivery and NJ Facility Occurrence 2004.*
34. Katherine Baicker, Kasey S. Buckles, and Amitabh Chandra, "Geographic Variation in the Appropriate Use of Cesarean Delivery," *Health Affairs* 25, no. 5 (2006): w355–w367.
35. NJ Dept. of Health, *Births by Method of Delivery and NJ Facility Occurrence 2004.*
36. LMS Medical Systems, *LMS and McKesson Expand OB Risk Management Offering*, press release, April 18, 2006.
37. The Center for Responsive Politics, http://www.opensecrets.org (accessed February 5, 2007).
38. D. M. Studdert et al., "Claims, Errors, and Compensation Payments in Medical Malpractice Litigation," *New England Journal of Medicine* 354, no. 19 (2006): 2024–33.
39. U.S. General Accounting Office, *Medical Malpractice: Implications of Rising Premiums on Access to Health Care* (Washington, DC, 2003).
40. Freeman et al., *Evaluation of Cesarean Delivery*, 13.
41. Declercq et al., *Listening to Mothers II.*
42. Jessica Adler, "Nature's Way: New Jersey Has One of the Highest Rates of Caesarean Section in the Country," *Herald (NJ) News*, May 9, 2006.
43. Cheryl Welch, "Doctor Won't Make the Cut: Feeling Pressure from Hospital for More C-Sections, She Leaves," *Star (NC) News*, June 5, 2005.
44. Declercq et al., *Listening to Mothers II.*
45. Joseph P. Bruner et al., "The All-Fours Maneuver for Reducing Shoulder Dystocia during Labor," *Journal of Reproductive Medicine* 43, no. 5 (1998): 439–43.
46. Joseph B. DeLee, "Symposium: To What Extent Should Delivery Be Hastened or Assisted by Operative Interference?" *American Journal of Obstetrics and Gynecology* 2, no. 3 (1921): 299.

CHAPTER 3

1. Luis A. Cibils, "Breech Presentation," in *Cesarean Section: Guidelines for Appropriate Utilization*, eds. E. Quilligan and B. Flamm (New York: Springer, 1995).

2. Judy Packer-Tursman, "Alternative Therapy Struggles to Bridge East-West Divide," *The Washington Post*, November 11, 2002.
3. Denise Grady, "Trying to Avoid 2nd Caesarean, Many Find Choice Isn't Theirs," *New York Times*, November 29, 2004.
4. Declercq et al., *Listening to Mothers II*.
5. Albert A. Plentl and Raymond E. Stone, "The Bracht Maneuver," *Obstetrical & Gynecological Survey* 8 (1953): 313–25.
6. Ibid.
7. NIH, "Cesarean Childbirth."
8. NJ Dept. of Health, *Births by Method of Delivery and NJ Facility Occurrence 2004*.
9. M. Hannah et al., "Planned Cesarean Section versus Planned Vaginal Birth for Breech Presentation at Term: A Randomised Multicentre Trial," *Lancet* 356 (2000): 1375–83.
10. American College of Obstetricians and Gynecologists, Committee Opinion no. 265, *Mode of Term Singleton Breech Delivery* (Washington, DC, 2001).
11. K. L. Hogle et al., "Impact of the International Term Breech Trial on Clinical Practice and Concerns: A Survey of Centre Collaborators," *Journal of Obstetrics and Gynecology Canada* 25 (2003): 14–16.
12. C. C. Rietberg, P. M. Elferink-Stinkens, and G. H. Visser, "The Effect of the Term Breech Trial on Medical Intervention Behaviour and Neonatal Outcome in the Netherlands: An Analysis of 35,453 Term Breech Infants," *British Journal of Obstetrics and Gynaecology* 112 (2005): 205–09.
13. John C. Hauth and F. Gary Cunningham, "Vaginal Breech Delivery Is Still Justified," *Obstetrics & Gynecology* 99 (2002): 1115–16.
14. Peter Bernstein, "Who Will Deliver Breech Babies Vaginally?" *Medscape* 9, no. 2 (2004).
15. Hauth and Cunningham, "Vaginal Breech Delivery Is Still Justified."
16. Andrew Kotaska, "Inappropriate Use of Randomised Trials to Evaluate Complex Phenomena: Case Study of Vaginal Breech Delivery," *British Medical Journal* 329 (2004): 1039–42.
17. Marek Glezerman, "Five Years to the Term Breech Trial: The Rise and Fall of a Randomized Controlled Trial," *American Journal of Obstetrics & Gynecology* 194 (2006): 20–25.
18. H. Whyte et al., "Outcomes of Children at 2 Years after Planned Cesarean Birth versus Planned Vaginal Birth for Breech Presentation at Term: The International Randomized Term Breech Trial," *American Journal of Obstetrics and Gynecology* 191, no. 3 (2004): 864–71.
19. Glezerman, "Five Years to the Term Breech Trial."
20. American College of Obstetricians and Gynecologists, Committee Opinion no. 340, *Mode of Term Singleton Breech Delivery* (Washington, DC, 2006).
21. M. Alarab et al., "Singleton Vaginal Breech Delivery at Term: Still a Safe Option," *Obstetrics & Gynecology* 103 (2004): 407–12.
22. A. Giuliani et al., "Mode of Delivery and Outcome of 699 Singleton Breech Deliveries at a Single Center," *American Journal of Obstetrics and Gynecology* 187 (2002): 1694–98.
23. Kenneth C. Johnson, "Randomized Controlled Trials as Authoritative Knowledge," in *Childbirth and Authoritative Knowledge*, eds. Robbie Davis-Floyd and Carolyn Sargent (Berkeley: University of California Press, 1997).

24. Kenneth C. Johnson and Betty-Anne Daviss, "Outcomes of Planned Home Births with Certified Professional Midwives: Large Prospective Study in North America," *British Medical Journal* 330 (2005): 1416.
25. Rooks et al., "Outcomes of Care in Birth Centers."
26. American Public Health Association, "Increasing Access to Out-of-Hospital Maternity Care Services through State-Regulated and Nationally-Certified Direct-Entry Midwives (Policy Statement)," *American Journal of Public Health* 92, no. 3 (2002): 451–483.
27. M. F. Greene, "Vaginal Delivery after Cesarean Section—Is the Risk Acceptable?" *New England Journal of Medicine* 345 (2001): 54–55.
28. Mark B. Landon et al., "Risk of Uterine Rupture with a Trial of Labor in Women with Multiple and Single Prior Cesarean Delivery," *Obstetrics & Gynecology* 108, no. 1 (2006): 12–20.
29. Edwin B. Craigin "Conservatism in Obstetrics," *New York Medical Journal* 104 (1916): 1–3.
30. M. Lydon-Rochelle et al., "Risk of Uterine Rupture during Labor among Women with a Prior Cesarean Delivery," *New England Journal Medicine* 345, no. 1 (2001): 3–8.
31. NIH, "Cesarean Childbirth."
32. Landon et al., "Risk of Uterine Rupture with a Trial Labor."
33. American College of Obstetricians and Gynecologists, Committee Opinion no. 143, *Vaginal Delivery after a Previous Cesarean Birth*, printed in *International Journal of Gynaecology and Obstetrics* 48, no. 1 (1995): 127–29.
34. W. B. Harer, "Vaginal Birth after Cesarean Delivery: Current Status," *Journal of the American Medical Association* 287 (2002): 2627–30.
35. Martin et al., *Births: Final Data for 2004.*
36. M. J. McMahon et al., "Comparison of a Trial of Labor with an Elective Second Cesarean Section," *New England Journal of Medicine* 335 (1996): 689–95.
37. "Case Records of the Massachusetts General Hospital, Case 9–1998, Cardiovascular Collapse after Vaginal Delivery in a Patient with a History of Cesarean Section," *New England Journal of Medicine* 338, no. 12 (1998): 821–26.
38. American College of Obstetricians and Gynecologists, Practice Bulletin no. 2, *Vaginal Birth after Previous Cesarean Delivery*, printed in *International Journal of Gynaecology and Obstetrics* 64 (1999): 201–08.
39. American College of Obstetricians and Gynecologists, Practice Bulletin no. 54, *Vaginal Birth after Previous Cesarean*, printed in *Obstetrics & Gynecology* 104 (2004): 203–12.
40. Martin et al., *Births: Final Data for 2004.*
41. Lydon-Rochelle et al., "Risk of Uterine Rupture during Labor."
42. MacDorman et al., "Risk of Death May Be Higher."
43. Anne D. Lyerly et al., "Risks, Values and Decision Making Surrounding Pregnancy," *Obstetrics & Gynecology* (2007), in press.
44. Don Mecoy, "Limited Delivery: State's Largest Malpractice Insurer Limits Birthing Choices for Some," *Oklahoman*, March 13, 2005.
45. Landon et al., "Risk of Uterine Rupture with a Trial Labor."
46. J. Zweifler et al., "Vaginal Birth after Cesarean in California: Before and After a Change in Guidelines," *Annals of Family Medicine* 4, no. 3 (2006): 228–34.

47. Lydon-Rochelle et al., "Risk of Uterine Rupture during Labor."
48. Landon et al., "Risk of Uterine Rupture with a Trial Labor."
49. R. Gonen et al., "Results of a Well-Defined Protocol for a Trial of Labor after Prior Cesarean Delivery," *Obstetrics & Gynecology* 107 (2006): 240–45.
50. Lydon-Rochelle et al., "Risk of Uterine Rupture during Labor."
51. Carol Sakala, *Vaginal or Cesarean Birth? A Systematic Review to Determine What Is at Stake for Mothers and Babies* (New York: Childbirth Connection, 2006), http://www.childbirthconnection.org.
52. ACOG, *Vaginal Birth after Previous Cesarean.*
53. Rita Rubin, "Battle Lines Drawn over C-Sections: Legal vs. Medical Risks," *USA Today*, August 24, 2005.
54. Rob Stein, "Once a C-Section, Always a C-Section?: Women Who Want to Try Labor on Later Deliveries Are Increasingly Refused," *The Washington Post*, November 24, 2005.
55. American Academy of Family Physicians, *Trial of Labor after Cesarean (TOLAC), Formerly Trial of Labor Versus Elective Repeat Cesarean Section for the Woman with a Previous Cesarean Section* (Leawood, KS, 2005).
56. Society of Obstetricians and Gynaecologists of Canada, Clinical Practice Guideline no. 155, *Guidelines for Vaginal Birth after Previous Caesarean Birth,* (Ottawa, ON, 2005).
57. Bridget M. Kuchn, "Study Downgrades Amniocentesis Risk," *Journal of the American Medical Association* 296 (2006): 2663–64.
58. Johnson and Daviss, "Outcomes of Planned Home Births."
59. Rooks et al., "Outcomes of Care in Birth Centers."
60. R. E. Anderson and P. A. Murphy, "Outcomes of 11,788 Planned Home Births Attended by Certified Nurse–Midwives: A Retrospective Descriptive Study," *Journal of Nurse Midwifery* 40, no. 6 (1995): 483–92.
61. O. Olsen, "Meta-Analysis of the Safety of Home Birth," *Birth* 24, no. 1 (1997): 4–13.
62. L. Mehl-Madrona and M. M. Madrona, "Physician and Midwife Attended Home Births: Effects of Breech, Twin and Post-Dates Outcome Data on Mortality Rates," *Journal of Nurse Midwifery* 42, no. 2 (1997): 91–98.
63. E. Lieberman et al., "Results of the National Study of Vaginal Birth after Cesarean in Birth Centers," *Obstetrics & Gynecology* 104, no. 5 (2004): 933–42.
64. K. L. Hogle et al., "Cesarean Delivery for Twins: A Systematic Review and Meta-Analysis," *American Journal of Obstetrics and Gynecology* 188, no. 1 (2003): 220–27.
65. Laura Kaplan Shanley, *Unassisted Childbirth* (Westport, CT: Bergin & Garvey, 1994).
66. New Mexico Department of Health, *New Mexico Selected Health Statistics Annual Report 2004* (Santa Fe, 2006).
67. Karen Rosenberg and Wenda Trevathan, "Birth, Obstetrics, and Human Evolution," *British Journal of Obstetrics and Gynaecology* 109 (2002): 1199–1206.

CHAPTER 4

1. Matt Clark and Mary Lord, "Too Many Caesareans?" *Newsweek*, October 6, 1980.

2. Sandra S. Friedland, "Rise in Caesarean Births Stirs Dispute," *New York Times*, December 13, 1981.
3. Robert Steinbrook, "'Runaway' C-Section Rates Reflect 'Crisis,'" *Los Angeles Times*, August 21, 1988.
4. NIH, "Cesarean Childbirth."
5. Ibid.
6. Ibid.
7. U.S. Department of Health and Human Services, United States Public Health Service Expert Panel on the Content of Prenatal Care, *Caring For Our Future: The Content of Prenatal Care* (Washington, DC, 1989).
8. Mortimer Rosen and Lillian Thomas, *The Cesarean Myth: Choosing the Best Way to Have Your Baby* (New York: Penguin Books, 1989), xi.
9. Sandra G. Boodman, "Campaign to Cut C-Section Rate Assailed," *The Washington Post*, January 12, 1999.
10. Jane E. Brody, "Health: Personal Health," *New York Times*, July 27, 1989.
11. VanTuinen and Wolfe, *Halting a National Epidemic*.
12. Gina Kolata. "New York Is First State to Try to Curb Caesareans," *New York Times*, January 27, 1989.
13. U.S. Department of Health and Human Services, Public Health Service, *Healthy People 2000: National Health Promotion and Disease Prevention Objectives* (Washington DC, 1991).
14. World Health Organization, "Appropriate Technology for Birth."
15. Edward J. Quilligan, "Making Inroads Against the Cesarean Section Rate," *Contemporary Ob/Gyn* Anniversary Issue (1983): 221–25.
16. Mary Gabay and Sidney M. Wolfe, *Unnecessary Cesarean Sections: Curing a National Epidemic* (Washington, DC: Public Citizen's Health Research Group, 1994).
17. F. Menacker and S. C. Curtin, "Trends in Cesarean Birth and Vaginal Birth after Previous Cesarean, 1991–99," *National Vital Statistics Reports* 49, no. 13 (2001): 1–16.
18. Gabay and Wolfe, *Curing a National Epidemic*.
19. Menacker and Curtin, "Trends in Cesarean Birth."
20. Eugene Declercq et al., "Maternal Risk Profiles and the Primary Cesarean Rate in the United States, 1991–2002," *American Journal of Public Health* 96, no. 5 (2006): 867–72.
21. Press et al., "Mode of Delivery and Pelvic Floor Dysfunction."
22. W. B. Harer, Jr., "Patient Choice Cesarean."
23. Susan Gilbert, "Doctors Report Rise in Elective Caesareans," *New York Times*, September 22, 1998.
24. U.S. Department of Health and Human Services, Public Health Service, *Healthy People 2010*, 2nd ed. (Washington, DC, 2000).
25. Freeman et al., *Evaluation of Cesarean Delivery*, 2.
26. ACOG, *Surgery and Patient Choice*.
27. Benjamin Sachs et al., "The Risks of Lowering the Cesarean-Delivery Rate," *New England Journal of Medicine* 340 (1999): 54–57.
28. NIH, "Cesarean Delivery on Maternal Request."

29. Jose Villar et al., "Caesarean Delivery Rates and Pregnancy Outcomes: The 2005 WHO Global Survey on Maternal and Perinatal Health in Latin America," *Lancet* 367 (2006): 1819–29.
30. MacDorman et al., "Risk of Death May Be Higher."
31. Menticoglou and Hall, "Nonsensus Consensus."
32. G. Smith et al., "Cesarean Section and Risk of Unexplained Stillbirth in Subsequent Pregnancy," *Lancet* 362 (2003): 1779–84.
33. I. Danel et al., "The Magnitude of Maternal Morbidity during Labor and Delivery, United States, 1993–1997," *American Journal of Public Health* 93, no. 4 (2003): 631–34.
34. Declercq et al., *Listening to Mothers II.*
35. P. McGovern et al., "Postpartum Health of Employed Mothers 5 Weeks after Childbirth," *Annals of Family Medicine* 4 (2006): 159–67.
36. Freeman et al., *Evaluation of Cesarean Delivery*, 2.
37. Ibid.
38. Betsy McCaughey, "To Catch a Deadly Germ," *New York Times*, November 14, 2006.
39. Gabay and Wolfe, *Curing a National Epidemic.*
40. Martin et al., *Births: Final Data for 2004.*
41. Freeman et al., *Evaluation of Cesarean Delivery*, 2.
42. D. Getahun et al., "Previous Cesarean Delivery and Risks of Placenta Previa and Placental Abruption," *Obstetrics & Gynecology* 107 (2006): 771–78.
43. Resnik, "Can a 29% Cesarean Rate."
44. S. Wu et al., "Abnormal Placentation: 20-Year Analysis," *American Journal of Obstetrics and Gynecology* 192 (2005): 1458–61.
45. Resnik, "Can a 29% Cesarean Rate."
46. Ibid.
47. E. Bujold et al., "The Impact of a Single-Layer or Double-Layer Closure on Uterine Rupture," *American Journal of Obstetrics and Gynecology* 186, no. 6 (2002): 1326–30.
48. R. Silver et al., "Maternal Morbidity Associated with Multiple Repeat Cesarean Deliveries," *Obstetrics & Gynecology* 107, no. 6 (2006): 1226–32.
49. S. E. Sarsam, J. P. Elliot, and G. K. Lam, "Management of Wound Complications from Cesarean Delivery," *Obstetrical & Gynecological Survey* 60, no. 7 (2005): 462–73.
50. U.S. National Center for Health Statistics, *Health, United States, 2004* (Washington, DC, 2004).
51. Enkin et al., *A Guide to Effective Care*, 362.
52. C. Deneux-Tharaux et al., "Postpartum Maternal Mortality and Cesarean Delivery," *Obstetrics & Gynecology* 108 (2006): 541–48.
53. U.S. National Center for Health Statistics, *Health, United States, 2004.*
54. Khalid S. Khan et al., "WHO Analysis of Causes of Maternal Death: A Systematic Review," *Lancet* 367 (2006): 1066–74.
55. A.M. Miniño et al, National Vital Statistics Reports 55, no. 19, *Deaths: Final Data for 2004* (Hyattsville, MD: National Center for Health Statistics, 2007).
56. Centers for Disease Control and Prevention, "Maternal Mortality—United States, 1982–1996," *Morbidity and Mortality Weekly Report* 47, no. 34 (1998).

57. Cynthia J. Berg et al., "Preventability of Pregnancy-Related Deaths: Results of a State-Wide Review," *Obstetrics & Gynecology* 106 (2005): 1228–34.

58. New York State Department of Health, Bureau of Women's Health and ACOG District II/NY, *Safe Motherhood Triennial Report 2003–2005* (Albany, 2006).

59. Florida Department of Health, *Pregnancy Associated Mortality Review Report 1999–2002* (Tallahassee, 2005).

60. Mississippi Department of Health, *Selected Death Statistics, Residents of Jackson 2004* (Jackson, 2006).

61. Stacie E. Geller et al., "Morbidity and Mortality in Pregnancy."

62. M. Tucker et al., "The Black-White Disparity in Pregnancy-Related Mortality from 5 Conditions: Differences in Prevalence and Case-Fatality Rates," *American Journal of Public Health* 97, no. 2 (2006): 247–51.

63. Sachs et al., "The Risks of Lowering."

64. Mary Vadnais and Benjamin Sachs, "Maternal Mortality with Cesarean Delivery: A Literature Review," *Seminars in Perinatology* 30 (2006): 242–46.

65. Edward Reynolds, "Primary Operations for Obstetrical Debility," *Surgery, Gynecology & Obstetrics* 4 (1907): 306–18.

66. R. M. Cyr, "Myth of the Ideal Cesarean Section Rate: Commentary and Historic Perspective," *American Journal of Obstetrics and Gynecology* 194, no. 4 (2006): 932–36.

67. Menacker et al., "Cesarean Delivery: Background."

68. Declercq et al., *Listening to Mothers II.*

69. HealthGrades, *Cesarean Rates in the United States.*

70. H. L. Minkoff and R. H. Schwarz, "The Rising Cesarean Rate: Can It Safely Be Reversed?" *Obstetrics & Gynecology* 56 (1980): 135–43.

71. Sakala, *Vaginal or Cesarean Birth?*

72. Anthony G. Visco et al., "Cesarean Delivery on Maternal Request: Maternal and Neonatal Outcomes," *Obstetrics & Gynecology* 108, no. 6 (2006): 1517–29.

73. S. Liu et al., "Maternal Mortality and Severe Morbidity Associated with Low-Risk Planned Cesarean Delivery versus Planned Vaginal Delivery at Term," *Canadian Medical Association Journal* 176, no. 4 (2007): 455–60.

74. NIH, "Cesarean Delivery on Maternal Request."

75. International Federation of Gynecology & Obstetrics, Committee for the Ethical Aspects of Human Reproduction and Women's Health, *Recommendations in Ethical Issues in Obstetrics and Gynecology* (London: FIGO House, 2006).

76. R. Al-Mufti, A. McCarthy, and N. M. Fisk, "Survey of Obstetricians' Personal Preference and Discretionary Practice," *European Journal of Obstetrics, Gynaecology, and Reproductive Biology* 73 (1997): 1–4.

77. Earl Ubell, "When Is a Cesarean Really Necessary?" *Parade*, October 25, 1992.

78. Christine Dell'amore, "NIH Panel: No Final Word on Caesereans," United Press International, March 29, 2006.

79. New York State Department of Health, *New York City Hospitals Cesarean Section Rates 2000–2004* (Albany, 2006).

80. World Health Organization, *Preamble to the Constitution of the WHO as adopted by the International Health Conference* (Geneva, 1946), http://www.who.int/suggestions/faq/en/index.html (accessed February 2007).

81. WHO, *Care in Normal Birth*.
82. E. Hemminki et al., "Ambulation vs. Oxytocin in Protracted Labour: A Pilot Study," *European Journal of Obstetrics, Gynecology, and Reproductive Biology* 20 (1985): 199–208.
83. Nicky Leap and Tricia Anderson, "The Role of Pain in Normal Birth and the Empowerment of Women," in *Normal Childbirth: Evidence and Debate*, ed. Soo Downe (London: Elsevier, 2004), 33.
84. O'Herlihy, "Active Management."
85. VanTuinen and Wolfe, *Halting a National Epidemic*.
86. K. R. Simpson and J. Atterbury, "Labor Induction in the United States: Trends and Issues for Clinical Practice," *Journal of Obstetric, Gynecologic and Neonatal Nursing* 32, no. 6 (2003): 767–79.
87. I. M. Usta, B. M. Mercer, and B. M. Sibai, "Current Obstetrical Practice and Umbilical Cord Prolapse," *American Journal of Perinatology* 16, no. 9 (1999): 479–84.
88. K. R. Simpson and G. E. Knox, "Common Areas of Litigation Related to Care during Labor and Birth: Recommendations to Promote Patient Safety and Decrease Risk Exposure," *Journal of Perinatal and Neonatal Nursing* 17, no. 1 (2003): 110–25.
89. A. Herbst, P. Wolner-Hanssen, and I. Ingemarsson, "Risk Factors for Acidemia at Birth," *Obstetrics & Gynecology* 90, no. 1 (1999): 125–30.
90. Cunningham et al., *Williams Obstetrics*, 18th ed. (Norwalk, CT: Appleton & Lange, 1989), 345.
91. J. G. Thornton and R. J. Lilford, "Active Management of Labour: Current Knowledge and Research Issues," *British Medical Journal* 309 (1994): 366–69.
92. Simon Cooper, "'Quick Birth' Drug Can Kill Babies: An Efficiency Drive in Maternity Wards Is Causing Alarm," *The Observer*, April 19, 1998.
93. Wagner, "Active Management of Labour."
94. Sarah J. Buckley, "Ecstatic Birth: The Hormonal Blueprint of Labor," *Mothering*, March/April 2002.
95. Emma J. Glasson et al., "Perinatal Factors and the Development of Autism: A Population Study," *Archives of General Psychiatry* 61, no. 6 (2004): 618–27.
96. Tew, *Safer Childbirth?*, 33.
97. Lucky Jain, "Implications of Labor on Neonatal Outcome" (lecture, NIH State-of-the-Science Conference: Cesarean Delivery on Maternal Request, Bethesda, MD, March 27–29, 2006).
98. T. Kolas et al., "Planned Cesarean versus Planned Vaginal Delivery at Term: Comparison of Newborn Infant Outcomes," *American Journal of Obstetrics and Gynecology* 195, no. 6 (2006): 1538–43.
99. Jain, "Implications of Labor on Neonatal Outcome."
100. M. J. Davidoff et al., "Changes in Gestational Age Distribution among U.S. Singleton Births: Impact on Rates of Late Preterm Birth, 1992 to 2002," *Seminars in Perinatology* 30, no. 1 (2006): 8–15.
101. Save the Children, *State of the World's Mothers 2006 Report* (Westport, CT: Save the Children, 2006), 27.
102. Heather J. Rowe-Murray and Jane R. W. Fisher, "Baby Friendly Hospital Practices: Cesarean Section Is a Persistent Barrier to Early Initiation of Breastfeeding," *Birth* 29, no. 2 (2002): 124–31.

103. U.S. Dept. of Health and Human Services, *CDC Guide to Breastfeeding Interventions.*
104. http://www.cesarean-art.com
105. Cheryl T. Beck, "Post-Traumatic Stress Disorder Due to Childbirth," *Nursing Research* 53, no. 4 (2004): 216–24.
106. "Caesareans Decline, but Rate Is Called too High," *New York Times*, May 13, 1992.
107. Declercq et al., *Listening to Mothers II.*

CHAPTER 5

1. NJ Dept. of Health and Senior Services, *Births by Method of Delivery and NJ Facility Occurrence 2004.*
2. Declercq et al., *Listening to Mothers II.*
3. I. Danel et al., "Magnitude of Maternal Morbidity."
4. Lamaze Institute for Normal Birth, "Six Care Practices that Support Normal Birth," http://www.lamaze.org/AboutLamaze/LamazeInstituteforNormal Birth/tabid/171/Default.aspx (accessed February 2007).
5. Declercq et al., *Listening to Mothers II.*
6. Northrup, speaking at Birth on Labor Day (BOLD).
7. Declercq et al., *Listening to Mothers II.*
8. J. Kennell et al., "Medical Intervention: The Effect of Social Support during Labor," *Pediatric Research* 265, no. 17 (1988): 2197–201.
9. John Kennell, "The Psychological Effects of a Supportive Companion (Doula) during Labor," in *Birth: Interaction and Attachment*, eds. Marshall H. Klaus and Martha O. Robertson (New Brunswick, NJ: Johnson and Johnson Baby, 1982), quoted in Davis-Floyd, *Birth as an American Rite of Passage*, 328.
10. Bari Meltzer Norman and Barbara Katz Rothman, "The New Arrival: Labor Doulas and the Fragmentation of Midwifery and Caregiving," in *Laboring On: Birth in Transition in the United States*, eds. Wendy Simonds, Barbara Katz Rothman, and Bari Meltzer Norman (New York: Routledge, 2007), 262.
11. Deborah Springer, "Birth Plans: The Effect of Anxiety in Pregnant Women," *International Journal of Childbirth Education* 11, no. 3 (1996): 20–25.
12. E. D. Hodnett, "Pain and Women's Satisfaction with the Experience of Childbirth: A Systematic Review," *American Journal of Obstetrics and Gynecology* 186, no. 5 (2002): S160–72.
13. Sheila Kitzinger, *Giving Birth: The Parents' Emotions in Childbirth* (New York: Schocken Books, 1977), quoted in Christine Morton, "Doula Care: The (Re)-Emergence of Woman-Supported Childbirth in the United States" (Ph.D. diss., University of California, 2002).
14. Barbara Katz Rothman, *In Labor: Woman and Power in the Birthplace* (New York: Norton, 1982), 93, quoted in Morton, "Doula Care."
15. Barbara Katz Rothman, "Laboring Then: The Political History of Maternity Care in the United States," in *Laboring On: Birth in Transition in the United States*, eds. Wendy Simonds, Barbara Katz Rothman, and Bari Meltzer Norman (New York: Routledge, 2007), 25.

16. Leigh Summers, *Bound to Please: A History of the Victorian Corset* (New York: Berg, 2001).
17. Ibid.
18. Ibid, 59.
19. Joseph B. DeLee, *The Principles and Practice of Obstetrics* (Philadelphia: W. B. Saunders Co., 1913), 255.
20. Herbert Ratner, "The History of the Dehumanization of American Obstetrical Practice" in *21st Century Obstetrics Now!* eds. Stewart and Stewart (Chapel Hill, NC: National Association of Parents and Professionals for Safe Alternatives in Childbirth, 1977).
21. Alice B. Stockham, *Tokology: A Book for Every Woman* (Chicago: Alice B. Stockham & Co., 1897), 105–09.
22. Ibid, 89.
23. Judith Walzer Leavitt, "Birthing and Anesthesia: The Debate over Twilight Sleep" in *Women and Health in America: Historical Readings* (Madison: University of Wisconsin Press, 1984), 179.
24. Leavitt, *Women and Health in America*, 141.
25. Grantly Dick-Read, *Childbirth without Fear: The Principles and Practice of Natural Childbirth* (New York: Harper, 1944).
26. Tony Cappasso, "Haven't Got Time for the Pain: More Women Are Choosing to Avoid Hard Labor," *State (IL) Journal-Register*, December 5, 1999.
27. Hawkins and Beatty, "Update on Obstetric Practice."
28. Suzanne Arms, *Immaculate Deception: A New Look at Women and Childbirth in America* (Boston: Houghton Mifflin, 1975), quoted in Rich, *Of Woman Born*, 173.
29. Denis Walsh, Amina El-Nemer, and Soo Downe, "Risk, Safety and the Study of Physiological Birth," in *Normal Childbirth: Evidence and Debate,* ed. Soo Downe (London: Elsevier, 2004).
30. Michel Odent, "New Reasons and New Ways to Study Birth Physiology," *International Journal of Gynaecology and Obstetrics* 75 (2001): S39–45.
31. Buckley, "Ecstatic Birth."
32. Ibid.
33. S. Torvaldsen et al., "Intrapartum Epidural Analgesia and Breastfeeding: A Prospective Cohort Study," *International Breastfeeding Journal* 1 (2006): 24.
34. Leap and Anderson, "The Role of Pain."

CHAPTER 6

1. Johnson and Daviss, "Outcomes of Planned Home Births."
2. National Immunization Survey, Centers for Disease Control and Prevention (2005), http://www.cdc.gov/breastfeeding/data/NIS_data/data_2005.htm (accessed February 2007).
3. New Mexico Department of Health, *2004 Selected Health Statistics Annual Report* (Santa Fe, 2006), http://www.health.state.nm.us/hdata.html (accessed February 2007).
4. Martin et al., *Births: Final Data for 2004.*

5. Rooks, *Midwifery and Childbirth in America*, 76.
6. Martha Mendoza, "Prosecutions, Jailings Highlight Debate on Safety and Choice," Associated Press, November 18, 2002.
7. Chad Umble and Tom Murse, "300 at Rally to Support Lay Midwife," *Lancaster (PA) New Era*, January 26, 2007.

CHAPTER 7

1. Neal Devitt, "How Doctors Conspired to Eliminate the Midwife even though the Scientific Data Supports Midwifery," in *Compulsory Hospitalization: Freedom of Choice in Childbirth?* Vol. 2, eds. Stewart and Stewart (Marble Hill, MO: National Association of Parents and Professionals for Safe Alternatives in Childbirth, 1979), 345–70.
2. Irvine Loudon, *Death in Childbirth: An International Study of Maternal Care and Maternal Mortality, 1800–1950* (Oxford: Oxford University Press, 1993), 295.
3. Wertz and Wertz, *Lying-In*, 55.
4. J. Whitridge Williams, "Medical Education and the Midwife Problem in the United States," *Journal of the American Medical Association* 58 (1912): 1–7, quoted in Devitt, 353.
5. Francis E. Kobrin, "The American Midwife Controversy: A Crisis in Professionalization," *Bulletin of the History of Medicine* 40 (1966): 350–63.
6. S. Josephine Baker, "The Function of the Midwife," *Women's Medical Journal* 23 (1913): 196–97, quoted in Devitt, 355.
7. G. Kosmak, "Does the Average Midwife Meet the Requirements of a Patient in Confinement?" *The Transactions of the American Association for the Study and Prevention of Infant Mortality* 3 (1912): 238–260, quoted in Devitt, 362.
8. Rudolph W. Holmes, "Fads and Fancies: A Comment on the Pseudo-Scientific Trend of Modern Obstetrics," *American Journal of Obstetrics and Gynecology* 2, no. 3 (1921): 225–237.
9. Julius Levy, "Maternal Mortality in the First Month of Life in Relation to Attendant at Birth" *American Journal of Public Health* 13, no. 1 (1923): 88–95.
10. White House Conference on Child Health and Protection, *Medical Service* (New York: Appleton-Century, 1932), 169–209.
11. Charles R. King, "The New York Maternal Mortality Study: A Conflict of Professionalization," *Bulletin of the History of Medicine* 65, no. 4 (1991): 476–502.
12. Ibid.
13. Arthur Brewster Emmons and James Lincoln Huntington, "The Midwife: Her future in the United States," in *Medicalization of Obstetrics*, ed. Philip K. Wilson (New York: Garland, 1996).
14. Devitt, "How Doctors Conspired."
15. Raymond G. Devries, *Regulating Birth: Midwives, Medicine and the Law* (Philadelphia: Temple University Press, 1985).
16. Devitt, "How Doctors Conspired."
17. Rooks, *Midwifery and Childbirth in America*, 25.
18. Devries, *Regulating Birth*, 40.
19. Tew, *Safer Childbirth?*, 27.

20. World Health Organization, *Millennium Development Goals, Population Dynamics and Reducing Maternal Mortality* (Geneva, 2004).

21. C. Ronsmans et al., "Maternal Mortality: Who, When, Where, and Why," *Lancet* 368, no. 9542 (2006): 1189–200.

22. World Health Organization, *Having a Baby in Europe* (Geneva, 1985), quoted in Wagner, *Pursuing the Birth Machine*, 14.

23. WHO, *Care in Normal Birth*.

24. American College of Obstetrics and Gynecology, Statement of Policy, *Out-Of-Hospital Births in the United States* (Washington, DC, October 2006).

25. Raven Lang, *Birth Book* (Columbus, MS: Genesis Press, 1972).

26. Laurel Thatcher Ulrich, *A Midwife's Tale: The Life of Martha Ballard, Based on Her Diary 1785–1812* (New York: Vintage, 1991).

27. Catharina Schrader and Hilary Marland, *Mother and Child Were Saved: The Memoirs (1693–1740) of the Frisian Midwife Catharina Schrader* (Amsterdam: Rodopi, 2006).

28. Christa Craven, "Educated, Eliminated, Criminalized & Rediscovered: A History of Midwives in Virginia." Ph.D. diss., George Mason University, last updated 2004.

29. Virginia State Department of Health, *Midwife Book for Virginia Midwives* (Richmond, 1930).

30. Christine Neuberger, "Mom Needed Transfusion, Affidavits Say: Two Midwives Indicted in Death After Delivery," *Richmond Times-Dispatch*, January 22, 1999.

31. Jim Hall, "Cradle and Grave," *Fredericksburg (VA) Free-Lance Star*, January 1998.

32. Maria Glod and Josh White, "Midwives Charged in Death of Va. Woman," *Washington Post*, January 21, 1999.

33. "Lay Midwife, Assistant Charged with Manslaughter in Mother's Death," Associated Press State & Local Wire, January 21, 1999.

34. Kiran Krishnamurthy, "Unlicensed Midwives Get Suspended Jail Sentences," *Richmond (VA) Times-Dispatch* May 6, 2000.

35. Kiran Krishnamurthy, "Separate Trials Sought in Case of Midwives," *Richmond (VA) Times-Dispatch*, January 15, 2000.

36. G. Tramoni et al., "Amniotic Fluid Embolism: A Review," *Annales Françaises d'Anesthèsie et de Rèanimation* 25 (2006): 599–604.

37. P. E. Steiner and C. C. Lushbaugh, "Maternal Pulmonary Embolism by Amniotic Fluid as a Cause of Obstetric Shock and Unexpected Death in Obstetrics," reprinted in *Journal of the American Medical Association* 255, no. 16 (1986): 2187–203; see also Deanna Isaacs, "Code Blue Birth," *Chicago Reader*, May 15, 1998.

38. Virginia Department of Health, Maternal Mortality Review Team, *Preliminary Report 2006* (Richmond, forthcoming).

CHAPTER 8

1. Sarah F. Adams et al., "Refusal of Treatment during Pregnancy," *Clinical Perinatology* 30 (2003): 127–40.

2. Declercq et al., *Listening to Mothers II*.
3. American College of Obstetricians and Gynecologists, Committee Opinion no. 321, *Maternal Decision Making, Ethics, and the Law* (Washington, DC, 2005).
4. George J. Annas, "She's Going to Die: The Case of Angela C," *Hastings Center Report* 18 (1988): 23–25.
5. Terry E. Thornton and Lynn Paltrow, "The Rights of Pregnant Patients: Carder Case Brings Bold Policy Initiatives," *Healthspan* 8, no. 5 (1991): 10–16.
6. ACOG, *Maternal Decision Making*.
7. Adam Liptak, "Prisons often Shackle Pregnant Inmates in Labor," *New York Times*, March 2, 2006.
8. DeLee, "The Prophylactic Forceps Operation."
9. American College of Obstetrics and Gynecologists, Statement of Policy, *Lay Midwifery* (Washington, DC, 2006).
10. American College of Obstetrics and Gynecology, Statement of Policy, *Out-of-Hospital Births in the United States* (Washington, DC, 2006).
11. Johnson and Daviss, "Outcomes of Planned Home Births."
12. See Paul Starr, *The Social Transformation of American Medicine* (New York: Basic Books, 1984).
13. Kaiser Daily Health Policy Report, "American Medical Association Examines Retail Health Clinics, Other Issues at Annual Meeting," June 12, 2006, http://www.kaisernetwork.org/daily_reports/rep_index.cfm.
14. S. P. Chauhan et al., "American College of Obstetricians and Gynecologists Practice Bulletins: An Overview," *American Journal of Obstetrics and Gynecology* 194 (2006): 1564–75.
15. American College of Obstetricians and Gynecologists, Practice Bulletin no. 54, *Clinical Management Guidelines for Obstetrician-Gynecologists* (Washington, DC, 2004).
16. Women's Institute for Childbearing Policy, National Women's Health Network, National Black Women's Health Project, and Boston Women's Health Book Collective, *Childbearing Policy within a National Health Program: An Evolving Consensus for New Directions* (Boston, MA: Women's Institute for Childbearing Policy, 1994).

Index